Mutualism and health care

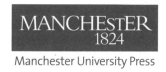

MANCHESTER
1824
Manchester University Press

Mutualism and health care

British hospital contributory schemes in the twentieth century

Martin Gorsky and John Mohan,
with Tim Willis

Manchester University Press

Manchester and New York

distributed exclusively in the USA by Palgrave

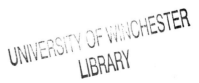

Copyright © Martin Gorsky and John Mohan 2006

The right of Martin Gorsky, John Mohan and Tim Willis to be identified as the authors of this work has been asserted by them in accordance with the Copyright, Designs and Patents Act 1988.

Published by Manchester University Press
Oxford Road, Manchester M13 9NR, UK
and Room 400, 175 Fifth Avenue, New York, NY 10010, USA
www.manchesteruniversitypress.co.uk

Distributed exclusively in the USA by
Palgrave, 175 Fifth Avenue, New York,
NY 10010, USA

Distributed exclusively in Canada by
UBC Press, University of British Columbia, 2029 West Mall,
Vancouver, BC, Canada V6T 1Z2

British Library Cataloguing-in-Publication Data
A catalogue record for this book is available from the British Library

Library of Congress Cataloging-in-Publication Data applied for

ISBN   0 7190 6578 X   hardback
EAN   978 0 7190 6578 1

First published 2006

15 14 13 12 11 10 09 08 07 06   10 9 8 7 6 5 4 3 2 1

Typeset in Jenson
by R. J. Footring Ltd, Derby
Printed in Great Britain
by CPI, Bath

Contents

Figures

Tables

Acknowledgements

The research on which this book is based was funded by grants from the Leverhulme Trust and the Economic and Social Research Council (ESRC) (grant no. RES-00-22-0044) and we are indebted to them for their support. John Mohan's work on this book was carried out while working at the Geography Department, University of Portsmouth, and he gratefully acknowledges institutional support and specifically assistance with typing and with production of illustrations. John Mohan would also like to acknowledge the support of an Erskine Fellowship at the University of Canterbury, New Zealand, during which parts of this book were drafted, and the hospitality of Ross Barnett and colleagues in the Geography Department during his stay there. Martin Gorsky began work on this book at the University of Wolverhampton, and completed it at the London School of Hygiene and Tropical Medicine, as a recipient of a Wellcome Trust University Award (2004–9). He is most grateful to colleagues at both institutions for their encouragement.

Our greatest debt is to officials of surviving contributory schemes (or 'health cash plans' as they are generally known today) who have facilitated access to the archival sources on which we have drawn. In particular, we thank: Graham Moore of the Westfield Health Scheme, Sheffield, who granted access to the records of Westfield's pre-National Health Service ancestor, the Sheffield and District Hospitals Council Fund; Liz Price, for access to records of the Patients' Aid Association, Wolverhampton; Carolyn Bell and Steve Fritz, for access to the records of the post-1948 British Hospitals Contributory Schemes Association; Bill Gaywood, of Medicash, Liverpool (formerly the Merseyside Hospitals Council); Des Benjamin, of HSA Healthcare (formerly the Hospital Saving Association); Peter Maskell, of Birmingham Hospitals Saturday Fund; Martin Wren, of Bristol Contributory Welfare Association; Richard Sear, of Healthsure; and Peter Green, of Bolton and District Hospital Saturday Council.

We are also grateful to the participants at a seminar we held to mark the end of this project, which brought together officials from several cash plans, academics, MPs, and representatives of think-tanks and the Department of Health. The seminar was hosted by the Institute for Historical Research, with some funding from the ESRC and the Society for the Social History of Medicine. We should particularly mention Rodney Lowe, Steven Cherry and

Calum Paton, who acted as discussants of the three papers presented, and whose comments were most helpful in revising them for publication.

Versions of papers based on this work have also been presented at: the Fifth International Conference on Urban History, Berlin, 2000; the Medicine and Society in the Midlands 1750–1950 Conference, University of Birmingham, 2003; the 6th Conference of the European Association for the History of Medicine and Health, Oslo, 2003; the 5th European Social Science History Conference, Berlin, 2004; the Stein Rokkan Centre workshop on the History of Medicine and Health, Bergen, 2005; and the 11th Medical Geography Symposium, Fort Worth, 2005. We are grateful to participants at those meetings for their comments. Our work on hospital contribution in Birmingham will appear as a chapter in J. Reinarz (ed.), *Medicine and Society in the Midlands 1750–1950*, to be published in 2007 as a supplement to *Midland History*, and we thank Jonathan Reinarz for his encouragement.

We owe a special debt to Bernard Harris, who commented in detail and with insight on the first draft of this book. Others who have commented on our work are David Gilbert, Nick Mays, John Benson, Virginia Berridge and Barry Doyle. We are most grateful to all of the above but take full responsibility for the final version of the book.

The primary research for, and the writing of, the book were divided in the following way: John Mohan extended an existing database on pre-war voluntary hospitals to include information on the schemes, and also conducted primary research at the Public Record Office (PRO), the British Library newspapers section and the British Library of Political and Economic Science (BLPES) at the London School of Economics; Martin Gorsky carried out archival work on the records of schemes in Glasgow, Edinburgh, Newcastle, Sunderland, Gloucestershire, Winchester, Bristol and Wolverhampton; Tim Willis was research fellow on the project and undertook archival work on schemes in Sheffield, Liverpool, Birmingham, Bolton and Leeds, on the records of the British Hospitals Contributory Schemes Association (BHCSA) in Leeds and London, and at the PRO. Gorsky was responsible for writing chapters 2, 5, 6, 7 and 8; chapters 1, 4, 10 and 11 were written by Mohan; and chapters 3 and 9 were co-authored by Gorsky and Mohan. We take joint responsibility for the whole of the final product.

For their courteous and efficient service we thank the staffs of Tyne and Wear Archives Services, Birmingham Central Library, Merseyside Record Office, University of Edinburgh Library Special Collections, Hampshire Record Office, the Mitchell Library, Glasgow (where Alastair Tough's advice was also invaluable), the National Archives of Scotland, the National Library of Medicine, Bethesda, Maryland, the Wolverhampton Archives and Local Studies Service, and the Bolton Archives and Local Studies Service.

Finally, we are grateful to several organisations for permission to reproduce copyright material, as follows. Parts of chapters 9 and 10 draw on a paper published in the *Journal of Social Policy*, 34, 3 (2005), pp. 447–67, and figures 9.1 and 9.2 appeared in the same article. We are grateful to the journal, and to Cambridge University Press, for permission to reproduce that material here.

The ideas advanced in chapters 7 and 8 first appeared in an article published in *Twentieth Century British History*, 16, 2 (2005), pp. 170–92, and we are grateful to the editors for permission to use the material here. Figure 5.1, 'Hospital Saturday' leaflets, and figure 5.3, *The Samaritan*, are reproduced by courtesy of Birmingham Library Services. Figure 5.2, 'The education of Mr Bowcher', appears by permission of HSA Healthcare and figure 5.4, 'League of Subscribers' annual report', by courtesy of Lothian Health Services Archive, Collections Division, University of Edinburgh Library.

And last, but by no means least, we would like to thank our families for their constant support during the period of writing this book.

Martin Gorsky
John Mohan

Abbreviations

AGM	annual general meeting
BHA	British Hospitals Association
BHCA	Birmingham Hospitals Contributory Association
BHCS	Birmingham Hospitals Contributors Scheme
BHCSA	British Hospitals Contributory Schemes Association
BHSF	Birmingham Hospital Saturday Fund
BMA	British Medical Association
BrHCA	British Health Care Association
BUPA	British United Provident Association
EHS	Emergency Hospital Service
HCP	health cash plan
HMC	hospital management committee
HSA	Hospital Saving Association
MHC	Merseyside Hospitals Council
MOH	medical officer of health
NALGO	National Association of Local Government Officers
NHI	national health insurance
NHS	National Health Service
NPHT	Nuffield Provincial Hospitals Trust
PEP	Political and Economic Planning
PMI	private medical insurance
RHB	regional hospital board
SHC	Sheffield Hospitals Council
SMA	Socialist Medical Association
VHC	Voluntary Hospitals Commission

Archives appearing in notes

BALSL	Bolton Archive and Local Studies Library
BCA	Birmingham City Archives
BLPES	British Library of Political and Economic Science (at London School of Economics)
BLSL	Birmingham Local Studies Library
BRO	Bristol Record Office

GRO	Gloucester Record Office
HRO	Hampshire Record Office
LHSA	Lothian Health Services Archive (at University of Edinburgh Library)
LMA	London Metropolitan Archives
ML	Mitchell Library, Glasgow
MMC	minutes of management committee
MRO	Merseyside Record Office
PAAA	Patients' Aid Association Archive
TNA: PRO	The National Archives: Public Record Office
TWAS	Tyne and Wear Archive Service
WALS	Wolverhampton Archives and Local Studies
WHSA	Westfield Health Scheme Archive

Chapter 1

Introduction

The British hospital contributory schemes movement was described in 1936 as 'one of the most outstanding examples of social organisation during the last two or three decades'.[1] Contributory schemes had flourished in response to the considerable financial challenges faced by the voluntary hospitals in the twentieth century, although their roots lay in the nineteenth-century Hospital Saturday and Sunday funds (described in chapter 2).[2] The aim was to elicit the support of working-class subscribers (people whose incomes were insufficient for them to be able to pay for treatment by a private medical practitioner) in the form of regular contributions to hospital finances. A small weekly contribution was levied, typically 2*d* or 3*d*, or a penny in the pound of wages, mostly through payroll deductions. The funds raised were either handed over directly to individual hospitals or pooled for distribution between groups of hospitals. The principal benefit of membership was free treatment in a voluntary hospital, without having to pass the means test set by the hospital almoner; at some hospitals, however, subscriptions were used to give free access to all the local population, regardless of membership. By the late 1930s over 400 schemes existed and the size of the movement was reflected in the formation in 1930–31 of a national representative body, the British Hospitals Contributory Schemes Association (BHCSA).[3]

At their peak, a widely accepted estimate is that there were at least 10 million contributors (the actual figure was probably nearer 11 million) and because benefits were extended to contributors' dependants[4] it is likely that over 20 million people were covered by the schemes. The largest scheme, the Hospital Saving Association (HSA), had approximately 2 million members organised through 14,000 local branches. The schemes generated substantial proportions of the income of many hospitals and they accounted for most of the growth in the resources of the voluntary hospitals in the inter-war period.

Recruitment and fundraising could involve substantial sections of the population in activities which ranged from door-to-door collections and the administration of workplace-based groups to major carnivals and fetes attended by thousands of people. Vigorous campaigns took place; the success of the Newcastle Royal Victoria Infirmary in pioneering contributory funds was attributed to its programme of 'education, education, and still more education' to inform local trades unionists about the Infirmary's functions.[5] The schemes were therefore significant vehicles for voluntarism and they also provided a new avenue of user participation in hospital governance, as contributors took seats on hospital management committees alongside the philanthropists and civic leaders who had hitherto dominated such bodies.[6]

For all these reasons the schemes were widely admired. William Beveridge described them as examples of 'self-help leading to the help of others'; their rapid expansion exemplified the 'driving force that emerges when local feeling can be combined with mutual aid'.[7] The movement was also said to epitomise voluntary initiative, to embody community enterprise, innovation and responsiveness: even in the individualistic voluntary hospital system, 'nothing quite so varied and variegated as the constitution and methods of the contributory schemes has emerged'.[8] The schemes were praised by overseas visitors, such as Douglas and Jean Orr, whose report on British insurance extolled their positive social benefits and the 'fraternal spirit' which they fostered.[9]

Given the scale and rapid expansion of the schemes, their absence from any of the major blueprints for the National Health Service (NHS) may be regarded as a puzzle: why was a movement of this size unable to exert any great leverage on the policy-making process? The possibility of funding a future NHS at least in part through the schemes was still under consideration by civil servants at the Ministry of Health late into 1943. They envisaged that the schemes might provide the finance for the maintenance of in-patients, as one element of a hospital income mix which would also include precepts from local rates and central government grants.[10] Ultimately, however, this option was rejected, with little public controversy. This decision reflected two sets of influences. First, it proved impossible to reconcile the existing schemes with the ideal of a national health service, because of variations in coverage and resources, and because of the difficulties of overcoming local loyalties and securing cooperation between schemes. Second, the schemes' representative organisation, the BHCSA, proved unable to articulate a collective interest and to exert influence on the negotiations concerning the form of the future health service. The possibility of developing the NHS along social insurance lines was therefore ruled off the agenda. Despite this the schemes did not disappear after the establishment of the NHS in 1948; support remained strong and many of them responded to such an extreme change in their external environment by searching for a niche which did not overlap with the public sector. They achieved this by offering low-cost insurance against various health-related contingencies; they also sought to retain the idealism that had motivated them in the pre-NHS era.

The starting point of this book is that a study of the growth and develop-ment of the contributory schemes is overdue and necessary in its own right. The book also seeks to contribute to a revised historiography of welfare, one that is no longer premised on a view of the ascent of state intervention as an unproblematic process of enlightenment and progress, and that is increasingly concerned with welfare outside the state.[11] In this regard, following Finlayson, this book also emphasises the 'moving frontier' between the state and the voluntary sector; it therefore explores in detail the strengths and limitations of this form of voluntarism and the response to the coming of the NHS.[12] In a wider context, it adds to knowledge of initiatives in civil society, which Walzer has described as the 'space of uncoerced human associations and the set of relational networks that fill this space'.[13] Academic and political commentators now attach considerable significance to strengthening civil society and promoting intermediate institutions to fill the space between impersonal, centralised states, and powerful, globalised markets on the one hand, and communities on the other. Contributory schemes were by any standards a major component of civil society in Britain, both before the establishment of the NHS and for several decades after it.

This study is also timely given the considerable current interest in organisational reform in the welfare state, exemplified in the possibility of a revived mutualism in health policy. Historical work such as this might appear to have little direct relevance today, but it is striking to observe the contemporary ring of some of the policy debates about the contributory schemes before 1948. These touch on such issues as how best to link hospital finances to demand, how to ensure that citizenship rights under the welfare state are balanced by an awareness of responsibilities, and how to guarantee democratic input and responsiveness in the hospital service. It is, of course, unlikely that there will be a departure from funding of the NHS from direct taxation. However, some proposals for health care reform have been advanced for other reasons, such as the enhancement of democracy and participation. These include, for example, proposals for a 'new mutualism' in public policy, as well as discussions of an 'associationalist' welfare state. An historical account of the contributory schemes can tell us much about the potential scope for such innovations.

Historiography

Despite the extent of the schemes, it is striking that there are relatively few references to them in accounts of the development of health care in Britain. Waddington traces the emergence of mass funding in the nineteenth century as a response to the funding pressures on London's hospitals, while Cherry's work on early Saturday funds argues that they manifested a new 'non-deferential' approach to hospital provision.[14] Abel-Smith's history of the British hospital system describes their growth, considers some of the problems of territorial demarcation which arose when schemes appeared to be competing for members, and discusses the implications for the medical profession of the shift away from philanthropy which was signalled by this new form of funding.[15] He did not discuss the contributory schemes' fate during the planning phase of the NHS, a neglect which his work shares with both broad-brush and fine-grained discussions of this episode.[16] Honigsbaum's account does refer to the schemes, albeit largely from the perspective of civil servants.[17] Abel-Smith merely observed that the schemes failed to press their case due to poor organisation and that they were therefore marginalised in policy discussions.[18] This verdict will be revisited, drawing on the records of the contributory schemes themselves and of their representative organisation, the BHCSA, to explore both the internal deliberations and the lobbying tactics of the BHCSA. Abel-Smith's explanation is augmented by detailed consideration of why policy-makers rejected the possibility of basing hospital finances on the schemes, and why the schemes themselves were unable to assert their position more forcefully.

What evaluations are there of the impact of the schemes? Webster argues that the schemes were a double-edged sword: they 'temporarily salvaged' the finances of the hospitals, but they also increased the demand for services.[19] For provincial hospitals (i.e. hospitals in England and Wales, excluding London) Cherry shows that, in aggregate terms, contributory schemes underpinned a significant expansion of hospital activity in the inter-war years. He points to the rapid growth in membership and income, especially in various locations not previously noted as major collecting centres. The schemes became, by 1936, the largest single source of income for provincial hospitals, and the second largest in Scotland. He also looks at the merits of different ways of evaluating the impact of the funds, such as the proportion of the cost of maintenance and treatment covered, compared with the proportion of hospital income derived from such sources. Overall, the picture presented by Cherry is a positive one, but he does note the problem of rising demand and also the evidence of diminishing returns – membership expanded but per capita income declined.[20]

Cherry also analysed the development of two individual contributory schemes, in Sheffield and East Anglia. He shows how both schemes developed efficient mechanisms for raising substantial sums, including contributions from employers in the Sheffield case, and he describes the important role played by the schemes in the integration of hospital services. These were places with 'very different economic infrastructures, social and political backgrounds', yet they had developed similar responses to the problem of hospital funding.[21] Work on the hospitals on Teesside by Doyle offers a more provocative evaluation: Doyle contends that mass contribution had enabled the voluntary hospitals to 'fund growth without resorting to paying patients or government grants'. Doyle demonstrates that the hospitals on Teesside were able to expand their activities greatly, but does not show whether this expansion was any more or less rapid than was the case elsewhere. He offers a positive verdict, contending that (at least in the case of the North Ormesby Hospital, Middlesbrough), mass contribution offered 'extensive patient access by right', and he therefore questions previous pessimistic accounts of voluntarism.[22] Cherry's view is more circumspect: he argues that 'contributory health insurance could not offer comprehensive health care at affordable rates for all the population'. This echoes an earlier assessment, by Mackenzie, that the two problems of the schemes were how to make them 'actuarially sound, and self-supporting'. The schemes pooled a limited range of risks – in that they were open only to those in a defined income bracket – and therefore had limited potential for cross-subsidy, while hardly any schemes covered the full costs to hospitals of treating their patients.[23] However, the latter may be an unfair criticism, in that the schemes never claimed that they would do so.

This study builds on the work of these authors in several ways. First, it uses case studies of individual hospitals, from the 1870s or earlier, to offer a new account of the coming of Saturday funds and workplace contributions (chapter 2). Second, it draws on a substantial database on pre-NHS hospital finances and provision, which has been extended to incorporate information on the finances and membership of contributory schemes. Conclusions about the growth and effect of the schemes are thus based on a much more extensive sample of hospitals than hitherto (chapter 3). It also investigates the 'free-rider' problem of imbalances between the distribution of contributors and users of hospitals, the attempts by schemes to develop reciprocal arrangements and joint planning structures (chapter 4) and whether the growth of contributory schemes was associated with rising demand for institutional treatment (chapter 3).

Turning from work on the financial aspects of the schemes to a consideration of motivations for subscribing to them reveals a more limited literature. The lofty promotional rhetoric of the schemes emphasised self-help, individual responsibility and commitment to the collective cause of the hospitals (chapter 5) but the existing literature has suggested that the appeal to subscribers lay primarily in the possibility of obtaining low-cost hospital insurance. Ross put this as follows:

> the principal purpose in the minds of their promoters was to strengthen the voluntary hospitals by giving them an assured income of a substantial amount ... the true ends which they promoted were, firstly, to serve their members by arranging for the provision of hospital service on very favourable terms and secondly to further the stability and efficiency of the hospitals in the general public interest.[24]

The schemes therefore had a quasi-insurance character. Walters similarly emphasises pragmatic necessity, arguing that the schemes were simply a response to the decline in the availability of free hospital care as more hospitals began to extract charges from patients.[25] This would imply that contributors would not invest membership with any great significance beyond the insurance aspect, a point echoed by Pickstone, who suggests a contrast between the attitudes of the rank and file, for whom membership was useful insurance, and those of scheme leaders, for whom the cause was a 'moral campaign and a source of civic pride'.[26] Johnson's study of working-class saving and spending habits includes the schemes in a discussion of insurance against the costs of sickness or hospitalisation. He argues that pragmatism and economic rationality alone are insufficient as explanations for the decision to subscribe to schemes; people took such decisions as part of 'a larger community or work group with its own customs, conventions and codes of conduct, and an important aspect of many financial decisions was the potential social integration or alienation that might result'. Drawing on testimony given to Mass-Observation,[27] he emphasises the importance of status preservation: members of contributory schemes would be excused from the embarrassment of means testing and would thereby preserve their self-respect.[28] In other words, he views the schemes in their wider social context, in which norms of respectability and workplace solidarity underpinned participation.

Johnson's assessment is broadly consistent with the rhetoric of the schemes. These issues are explored in several ways, using survey data to illuminate popular attitudes to contribution, along with publicity material and speeches from prominent figures in the movement. These show how ideas of citizenship were promulgated, through discourses which assumed particular gender norms and emphasised traditional British values, such as nationhood, voluntarism and self-reliance.

The question of democracy and governance has also exercised previous writers, who have offered mixed verdicts on the extent to which the contributory schemes were able to achieve representation on hospital governing bodies and to act as champions of consumer interests. Trainor notes that worker hospital governors in the late-Victorian Black Country largely acquiesced with the wishes of hospital trustees and played 'no more than a supporting role' in key decisions.[29] Waddington similarly observes that, despite the importance of sources of funds like Hospital Saturday funds – precursors of the contributory schemes – in late-nineteenth-century London, 'a separation existed between participation in a financial sense, and participation in an administrative sense'. Thus, the role of the working class in hospital governance was disproportionately small in relation to the funds they were providing.[30] In contrast, Cherry argues that, where contributory schemes were associated with individual hospitals, conflict over policy could arise and the influence of their representatives could be felt.[31] Thompson's work on voluntary hospitals in South Wales during the Edwardian era argues that in some cases the working class not only provided almost all the funds for the hospitals but were the only lay people represented on the governing body. This gave them a considerable degree of control over hospital policy.[32] Commenting on the Edwardian era, Doyle is convinced that the schemes represented a 'genuinely pan-class organisation in which middle- and working-class groups shared responsibility and management functions', and that this 'swam against the general trend of single-class organisations, spatial segregation and class politics ... there was a genuine communitarian element involved ... an exemplar of cross-class voluntarism.'[33] These contrasting verdicts are evaluated through original archival research into the records of several major schemes (chapter 6).

Moving into the post-war period, there is very little academic literature, which is surprising because, even after the principal reason for their existence disappeared in 1948, many schemes reinvented themselves, by offering a range of benefits such as convalescent home care, cash grants for in-patients and reimbursement of the costs of optical and dental treatment. By the early 1960s they had built membership back up to about 3.5 million (see chapter 9 for discussion of trends in membership). In Mossialos and Thomson's terminology the products offered would be regarded as supplementary insurance, since it covered services not generally offered by the state, whereas private health insurance would be regarded as complementary to the NHS.[34] Apart from Dawkins' brief history,[35] the place of the schemes in what Richard Titmuss referred to as the 'social division of welfare' is largely unexplored.[36] Most work on health care outside the NHS has concentrated on acute hospital provision and insurance[37] or on the purchase of alternative therapies.[38] The emphasis on acute in-patient care may be defensible in terms of turnover and political salience (the controversies surrounding the effect on the NHS of the private acute sector) but in terms of membership, or the number of treatment episodes, the reconstituted schemes are comparable in scale with the private acute hospital sector (see chapter 9). This book therefore investigates their development in relation to broader socioeconomic changes in Britain and in relation to changes in NHS policy. Parallels are also drawn with developments in the private hospital sector, where competition from commercial providers of hospital care and insurance has eroded the market share of not-for-profit providers.[39] We also discuss the ways in which these developments affected the schemes' ability to continue to adhere to their mutualist ethos. Finally, in the light of recent policy initiatives in the NHS, possible scenarios for the future development of the schemes are explored (chapter 10).

Contexts: voluntarism, civil society and economics

The wider academic context for this discussion is provided by three separate – though in fact related – sets of literature, pertaining to: the strengths and limitations of voluntarism; the role of voluntary associations in strengthening civil society and in creating social capital; and the economics of health insurance.

With respect to the first of these, the book draws on analyses of the existence and performance of voluntary institutions. Voluntary associations are appropriate in situations, as in health care, where consumers' imperfect knowledge may put them at risk; in these circumstances the absence of the profit motive promotes a bond of trust between producer and consumer. Voluntary responses also arise because of what is sometimes termed 'state failure', where there is a lack of popular consent for the provision of a particular social good.[40] Salamon has pointed to other positive qualities of voluntary institutions, such as innovation, responsiveness, flexibility and the ability to mobilise local feeling.[41] But there are also weaknesses of voluntarism, encapsulated in Salamon's term 'voluntary failure', such as the inability to provide a comprehensive and universal service. This might arise because of the absence of joint planning structures in the voluntary sector, and the consequent difficulties of collaboration, or it might be due to the patchiness of funding, perhaps arising from spatial variations in the wealth base or simply the unpredictability of philanthropic income.[42] Both the negative and the positive characteristics of voluntarism can be found in the contributory schemes (see chapter 4).

The virtues of voluntarism are extolled by critics of the centralised British welfare state. Thus, conservative commentators such as Seldon have argued that hospital nationalisation 'prevented the development of more spontaneous, organic, local, voluntary and sensitive services ... [that would have] better

reflected consumer preferences'.[43] Similarly, Green believes that, on the basis
of pre-1948 trends, hospital provision was expanding steadily and Seldon suggests, more dramatically, that the state simply 'mounted the already-galloping
horse' of voluntarism.[44] Contributors to recent discussions on the potential
for a revived mutualism in the NHS also point to the vibrancy of non-profit
institutions in the pre-NHS era.[45] These authors do not explicitly discuss
contributory schemes, although Green incorporates statistics on scheme
membership into estimates of the extent to which the population was covered
by various forms of insurance against the costs of health care before 1939. His
estimates have been ably criticised by Morris,[46] but perhaps comprehensiveness
and equity are less important to such commentators than the wider benefits to
society of a vigorous civic culture. Green does acknowledge this: he refers to
'taking the risk of under-government', which implies that reliance on the voluntary sector will leave some holes in the social safety net.[47] However, he advances
a strong moral argument for self-help. Participation in voluntary institutions is
a prerequisite for fostering civic virtues, rather than simply relying on 'socialist
materialism'.[48] Individual choice is the best way to secure welfare, and 'political
caring is a poor substitute for the mutual caring of civil society'.[49] In contrast,
state intervention is criticised by such writers because it involves a 'forcible
transfer of resources from the wealthy (and not-so-wealthy) to an ungrateful
population of dependants'.[50]

These comments raise the question of the link between rights and
responsibilities in the welfare state. Marshallian concepts of citizenship saw
the extension of social rights (including the right to state-provided welfare)
as a natural progression from the extension of civil rights and the gradual
widening of the franchise.[51] Over fifty years on, critics now accuse the welfare
state of having engendered a passive citizenship and a dependency culture,
which privileges rights over duties[52] rather than fostering the active engagement anticipated by its founders.[53] The welfare state is also charged with
an endemic bureaucratic rigidity and professional self-interest, which are
inimical to consumer interests.[54] Commentators have therefore restated the
case for active citizenship and voluntarism. Thus, Finlayson suggested that the
active, contributing citizen embodied characteristics of individual initiative,
self-reliance, freedom of choice and a genuine engagement in public affairs,
all virtues absent from the welfare state's 'citizenship of entitlement'.[55] With
their mass membership and procedures for popular participation in hospital
governance, the schemes offer a useful test of the existence of a broadly based
citizenship of contribution before the classic welfare state.

The second aspect of the literature examined concerns the value of voluntary organisations in strengthening civil society. Since Alexis de Tocqueville,
commentators have emphasised the significance of participation in voluntary
organisations in the shaping of public discourse and the articulation of collective values. Bellah *et al.* therefore argue that associations can play an important
mediating role between the individual and the centralised state, thus providing
a forum for the consensual shaping of public opinion and for educating the
public in the habits of taking initiative and accepting responsibility.[56] And, as

Fine and Harrington argue, theorists of civil society point to the 'crucial formative role' of activities organised on a small and local basis.[57] This is captured well by Deakin, when he talks of the 'rediscovery of the local' as a site for civil society.[58] Two questions about the schemes are prompted by Walzer's definition, quoted previously, of civil society as the 'space of uncoerced human associations and the set of relational networks'. Were the schemes genuinely 'uncoerced'? In other words, how spontaneous were their origins? And what was the nature of the 'relational networks' in which their members were engaged?

These broad arguments link to Putnam's influential work on the formation of social capital, which he defines as the networks, norms and trust that are generated through participation in non-hierarchical associational activities. Putnam conceptualises social capital as a replenishable stock of resources on which anyone in a community may draw, and which has beneficial collective and individual outcomes (e.g. improved health; economic development; more effective performance of governmental institutions).[59] There are criticisms of his work, especially some of its conceptual underpinnings and the causal efficacy which Putnam claims for social capital. Nevertheless, his ideas are valuable in the context of the schemes, for their rhetoric anticipated some of the arguments advanced in the literature on social capital. For example, did participation in the schemes galvanise whole communities in the manner implied by Putnam? Did the schemes cut across socioeconomic lines, and were they able to sustain commitment to the ideals which had inspired their foundation? And how do the surviving schemes relate to these desirable features of associational life? In its rhetoric, the contributory scheme movement strongly emphasised the importance of active citizenship, obligation to others and public participation. How far was this matched in reality, and to what extent was it sustained over time?

Third, the economics literature directs attention to the problems of incentive structures which confront health systems. In superseding traditional sources of funds, such as donations or legacies, did the schemes change the incentive structures facing hospitals? This question is explored with reference to reimbursement methods. It is also relevant to consider work on the effects of welfare systems on the behaviour of their beneficiaries. Le Grand argues that it can no longer be assumed that producers and consumers of welfare are public-spirited altruists (knights) or passive recipients (pawns). Instead, he contends, policy-makers now assume, to a greater or lesser degree, that people (whether producers or consumers of services) are all considered to be self-interested (in other words, they are knaves). In the most recent policy offerings from government it is implied that only if people are truly knavish will they exert the pressures on welfare institutions that are considered necessary to drive up standards.[60] Le Grand's work prompts consideration of the ethos and values of the schemes, which had an ambiguous character: while technically a gift, the act of contribution to a hospital was treated as conveying an entitlement to treatment. The problem of moral hazard, familiar to health economists, therefore arose, and was evident in a growth in demand for hospital treatment from scheme members. Several questions follow. Was it possible to restrain such demands? How far did contributors have consumer rights and how far could they exercise them? Were they permitted, for example, to obtain treatment from any hospital or, if not, how were their interests to be reconciled with those of the hospitals? It was clearly in the interests of the hospitals to promote the schemes, but it was also in their interests to limit their liabilities.

Contemporary debates about health care reform

Proposals for reforms of the NHS have been guided by two concerns. First, there are arguments that, despite its popularity, degree of equity and success in containing costs, weaknesses remain. These include, for example, the limited influence of consumer and community interests and the privileging of the hospital sector over community care.[61] The distinctive nature of NHS funding, which depends predominantly on direct taxation, has also come under scrutiny. Comparison with the facilities, health outcomes and public satisfaction in other Western countries has prompted the question of whether a social insurance model of funding might have delivered more resources.[62] The judgement of the 2002 Wanless report in favour of a tax-based system would appear to rule out any such alternatives, but if the current funding increases do not bear fruit the issue will certainly resurface in public discourse.[63] Consideration of alternative modes of funding would involve examination of a greater role for private insurance, as well as the idea of 'co-payments' for public services, such as charges for hospital amenities.[64] In these circumstances, the key issue would be whether an inclusive model of funding could be developed which would preserve the equity and comprehensiveness of the NHS. If this did not prove possible, the risk of fragmentation into an inequitable mix of private and public arrangements would have to be taken seriously.

A second reason why the NHS has been scrutinised relates to the more heterogeneous social and cultural landscape which presently confronts policy-makers. As a result, politicians are now prone to compare the NHS with the command economies of the former Eastern bloc, arguing that it was 'born in a world in which everyone was given the same rations' and that 'one-size-fits-all' models of welfare provision are not appropriate in today's more diverse and stratified society.[65] Regardless of the historical accuracy of these stereotypes,[66] the government's response has been to expand the scope for patient choice, to give patients – as individual consumers – greater voice (while simultaneously limiting other forms of representation and accountability) and to involve patients more actively in self-management of their conditions. This is an attempt to redress the imbalance between professional and consumer interests, but it raises expectations about what the NHS can deliver, thereby increasing the risk that the service will be perceived as having failed.

At the same time there is a perception that socioeconomic changes, especially insecurity in the labour market, are imposing new risks. Hence Taylor-Gooby refers to the paradox of 'timid prosperity': the coexistence of rising mass affluence with rising uncertainty about the future. When combined with socioeconomic polarisation, this has the potential to weaken support for the collective provision of welfare services.[67] Following Beck's influential analysis of 'risk society', it has been argued that citizens need to become more reflexive and proactive in taking responsibility for the assessment of the risks which confront them, and commentators foresee a welfare system in which 'collective welfare... is replaced by individualised risk management'.[68] However, this entails a shift in the character of the welfare state, away from anticipating and accepting collective responsibility for social problems, towards individual failings and individual responsibility. Rose has characterised this as a 'new prudentialism', in which insurance against future contingencies becomes a private obligation.[69] If risk is 'replacing need as the core principle of social policy formulation and welfare delivery', then the implication is that individuals will have to take more responsibility for assessing risk and protecting against it. The assumption is that state welfare must contract because proactive individuals will, to a growing extent, reject it or, at the very least, supplement a residual public welfare system by purchasing services privately.[70]

Reforms of the welfare state therefore need to satisfy some complex and contradictory objectives. In particular, can the desire for greater democracy and participation be reconciled with developing health services that are responsive to individual preferences and needs? What might this imply for the design of welfare institutions? If the burden of risk and choice is to be transferred from the state to individuals, what are the implications for equity, and what degree of inequality is perceived as tolerable?

Discussion of these issues was greatly stimulated by Hirst's vision of associative democracy as a potential alternative form of governance.[71] Hirst argued that the real problem with the welfare state was one of large-scale, inflexible, unresponsive organisation in both public and private sectors. He advocated a 'fusion ... between the voluntary and decentralised approach, which lost out to state welfare, and the conception of comprehensive, well-funded public services, which the national state appeared to provide and which localism and mutual aid could not'.[72] The argument for what he termed 'associationalist' welfare was that it would aid in the democratisation of civil society and the devolution of powers to voluntary organisations. Crucially, Hirst's proposals sought to empower individuals as consumers by giving them what are effectively vouchers, which they may use to choose, once a year, the voluntary associations they wish to be responsible for purchasing welfare services on their behalf. These would be democratic organisations, accountable to their members, but because the members would have the potential for exit, they would have to be responsive and innovative. The potential for inequity would be avoided because the system would be underpinned by a guaranteed citizen's income for all. Hirst believed that the role of the state in this system would be reduced to accreditation, regulation and gathering taxes.

Hirst was particularly concerned about the threat to social integration posed by growth in the use of private welfare services:[73] as an increasing proportion of the population were able to exit the public sector entirely, they were likely to become more reluctant to shoulder the tax burden necessary to pay for it.[74] Associationalist welfare might be one way of preventing this 'secession of the successful'.[75] In addition to a tax-financed basic package, individuals could purchase higher-quality or extra services but these would be provided by those same organisations delivering collective services. In this way the ability of welfare services to bridge social divides and promote social integration would be retained.

Various objections have been levelled at these proposals.[76] One is that individuals may not always be best placed to determine how to meet their welfare needs. The result may be under-consumption, leading (in the case of health care) to the postponement of treatment to the point at which it becomes excessively costly.[77] There is also the risk of inequality arising from the readiness of associationalists to accept a plurality of funding sources (donations, local taxation and the levying of charges).[78] Hirst's response to this was that inequalities already exist anyway, implying that welfare reform will have to accept that inequality, in some shape or form, will persist and the debate is therefore about what degree of inequality is tolerable.

Hirst did not refer to specific historical examples, although he did relate his proposals to pluralist traditions in British socialist thought which, as in the case of G. D. H. Cole, proposed similar reforms to the provision of welfare services. Hirst's goals of democratisation are shared by those advocating a new mutualism in public policy. Kellner, for example, argues that mutuality is a doctrine that 'individual and collective well-being is obtainable only by mutual dependence'.[79] These arguments prompt consideration of two issues. First, to what extent did the contributory schemes in the past match up to the desiderata identified by these commentators – equity, consumerism, accountability and participation? Second, to what extent might current or possible reforms to the NHS have implications for, or create new opportunities for, the surviving schemes?

At the time of writing no political party is openly suggesting radical changes in the funding of the NHS. However, the direction in which all parties (with some differences of emphasis) wish to move the delivery of health care is exemplified by the establishment of NHS Foundation Trusts, which have been liberated from a direct line of parliamentary accountability and given enhanced freedoms. Their governance structures are meant to involve increased scope for participation through the establishment of membership communities, whereby those with an interest in an institution are invited to sign up. In justification of this, a strong claim has been made for the importance of reviving earlier traditions of localism and mutualism. It is argued that representation through the membership community will enhance accountability and reduce health inequalities through the better articulation of local needs.[80] Historical precedent plays an important part in this argumentation, as in this depiction of pre-NHS hospitals from leading 'new mutualist' Hazel Blears, MP:

> local people had … provided the money and support to develop and maintain the hospital. The sense of affiliation felt for their local hospital was developed through a form of funding and governance that provided people with a real local relationship.[81]

Although Foundation Trusts do not directly replicate characteristics of the pre-war system, questions have been raised as to whether the aspiration to have more effective and participative structures of governance will be realised. If this is the likely trajectory of reform, it is relevant to explore whether concerns in the early twenty-first century about low levels of participation in elections to the boards of Foundation Trusts[82] have their antecedents in the governance of contributory schemes in the inter-war years. It is also worth considering whether the avenues for participation and involvement which characterised the early years of the schemes have survived in a rather different environment. And is there good evidence that local decision-making was really more responsive and accountable before the NHS?

Looking further ahead, another influence on the future development of the schemes is whether there will be scope for increased charges for NHS services. While the main political parties insist that this is not on the agenda, think-tanks have frequently suggested that only by extending charges can the NHS survive; there is now much common ground on this between think-tanks representing a broad swathe of political opinion.[83] Such proposals, if enacted as policy, might well open up new markets for health care products, but it is not clear what the attraction would be to individuals beyond the rather instrumentalist concerns of obtaining supplementary services. This might enable the remaining schemes to expand their activities as the boundaries between the public and private sectors become increasingly blurred, but it is not clear that it would be accompanied by increased involvement and participation. Some potential scenarios are reviewed in chapter 10.

Conclusion

This book has three main goals: to extend and develop work on the historical development of the contributory schemes; to relate this history to a range of debates about the advantages and disadvantages of ways of organising and delivering welfare services; and to place this history in the context of current and possible future developments in the welfare state. To achieve these goals the book is organised as follows. First, chapter 2 traces the emergence of mass contribution in the nineteenth century and describes the funds' early development, up to about 1920. Chapter 3 then analyses their growth and impact in the inter-war period and chapter 4 offers a geographical disaggregation of membership and finance, as well as a discussion of one of the key problems facing the schemes, namely the extent of cooperation and the demarcation of territory. Chapters 5 and 6 then discuss the schemes' procedures for ensuring participation, and evaluate the extent to which they were democratic and able to act as champions of consumer interests. Two chapters follow on the wartime and post-war discussions about the future of mass contribution. Chapter 7 concentrates on the perception of the schemes from the perspective of those responsible for translating general plans for an extension of health care into practical proposals, while chapter 8 examines the extent to which the schemes themselves were able to articulate a collective interest and press their case. Post-war developments are then explored in chapter 9, and in chapter 10 it is shown that some schemes found a new role as providers of health cash plans – low-cost insurance products dealing with services either not easily available on the NHS or with issues where NHS services were perceived to offer little consumer choice. In the process of this evolution, however, many of the democratic and participatory elements of the schemes were relinquished. Finally, the present position of the schemes and their response to current developments in the welfare state are considered in the concluding chapter.

Note on hospital names

The narrative is potentially complicated by name changes of the hospitals involved. For example, the Sunderland and Bishopswearmouth Infirmary and Dispensary later became the Sunderland Infirmary and subsequently the Royal Infirmary, Sunderland, while the Royal Hospital Wolverhampton began its existence as the South Staffordshire General Hospital and Wolverhampton Dispensary before becoming known as the Wolverhampton and Staffordshire General Hospital. For simplicity and economy, the general approach has been to use the name current at the end of the period in question, in both the text and the sources.

Notes

1 *The Hospital*, August 1936, p. 202.
2 S. Cherry, 'Hospital Saturday, workplace collections and issues in late nineteenth century hospital funding', *Medical History*, 44 (2000), pp. 461–88; K. Waddington, *Charity and the London hospitals, 1850–1898* (Bury St Edmunds, 2000), pp. 68–73.
3 A. T. Page, *Pennies for health: the story of the British Hospitals Contributory Schemes Association* (Birmingham, 1949).
4 J. Ross, *The National Health Service in Great Britain* (Oxford, 1952), p. 48.
5 The National Archive (TNA): Public Record Office (PRO), MH 58/204, Cave committee minutes, day 15.
6 S. Cherry, 'Accountability, entitlement and control issues and voluntary hospital funding c. 1860–1939', *Social History of Medicine*, 9 (1996), pp. 215–33.
7 W. Beveridge, *Voluntary action: a report on methods of social advance* (London, 1948), p. 292; British Library of Political and Economic Science (BLPES), British Hospitals Contributory Schemes Association (BHCSA) files, BHCSA 8/3, W. Beveridge, 'The role of the individual in the health service', speech by Lord Beveridge to the Bristol conference of the BHCSA, 1954.
8 W. Parkes, 'Contributory schemes and their relations with the hospital service', *The Hospital*, November 1934, pp. 290–2.
9 D. Orr and J. Orr, *Health insurance with medical care: the British experience* (New York, 1938), pp. 48–54.
10 TNA: PRO, MH 80/34, J. E. Pater, Contributory schemes, 28 June 1943; TNA: PRO, MH 80/34, NHS 27; BLPES, BHCSA files, BHCSA 14/2, Report of preliminary and informal conversation held at the Ministry of Health, Friday, 2 July 1943.

11   B. Harris, *The origins of the British welfare state* (London, 2004), pp. 5–8.
12   G. Finlayson, *Citizen, state and social welfare in Britain, 1830—1990* (Oxford, 1994).
13   M. Walzer, *Global civil society* (Providence, MA, 1995), p. 7, quoted in N. Deakin, *In search of civil society* (Basingstoke, 2001), p. 4.
14   Waddington, *Charity and the London hospitals*; Cherry, 'Hospital Saturday', p. 462.
15   B. Abel-Smith, *The hospitals 1800–1948: a study in social administration in England and Wales* (London, 1964), pp. 330–3, 387–8.
16   D. Porter, *Health, civilisation and the state: a history of public health from ancient to modern times* (London, 1999), pp. 215–16; A. Willcocks, *The creation of the National Health Service: a study of pressure groups and a major social policy decision* (London, 1967).
17   F. Honigsbaum, *Health, happiness and security* (London, 1989), pp. 158–63.
18   B. Abel-Smith, *The hospitals 1800–1948*, pp. 311–18, 323–37, 499.
19   C. Webster, *The health services since the war, vol. I* (London, 1988), p. 4.
20   S. Cherry, 'Before the NHS: financing the voluntary hospitals, 1900–1939', *Economic History Review*, 50 (1997), pp. 305–26, at pp. 317–21.
21   S. Cherry, 'Regional comparators in the funding and organisation of the voluntary hospital system, c. 1860–1939', in M. Gorsky and S. Sheard (eds), *Financing medicine: the British experience since 1750* (London, forthcoming, 2006); S. Cherry, 'Accountability, entitlement and control'; S. Cherry, 'Beyond national health insurance: the voluntary hospitals and hospital contributory schemes', *Social History of Medicine*, 5 (1992), pp. 455–82.
22   B. Doyle, 'The politics of voluntary health care in Middlesbrough, 1900–1948', in A. Borsay and P. Shapely (eds), *Medicine, charity and mutual aid: the consumption of health and welfare, c. 1550–1950* (Aldershot, 2006).
23   Cherry, 'Regional comparators'; M. Mackenzie, 'Recent tendencies in the development of general hospitals in England', *Quarterly Bulletin of the Health Organisation of the League of Nations*, 3 (1934), pp. 220–88, at p. 258.
24   Ross, *The National Health Service*, p. 48.
25   V. Walters, *Class inequality and health care* (Beckenham, 1980), pp. 33–4.
26   J. Pickstone, *Medicine and industrial society* (Manchester, 1985), p. 254.
27   The social research organisation Mass-Observation was founded in 1937; it recruited a team of observers and a panel of volunteer writers to study the everyday lives of ordinary people in Britain (for more details see www.massobs.org.uk/history.html, last accessed February 2006).
28   P. Johnson, *Saving and spending: the working-class economy in Britain between the wars* (Oxford, 1986), pp. 6, 73.
29   R. Trainor, *Black Country elites: the exercise of authority in an industrial area, 1830–1900* (Oxford, 1993), p. 329.
30   K. Waddington, 'Subscribing to a democracy? Management and the voluntary ideology of the London hospitals, 1850–1900', *English Historical Review*, 118 (2003), pp. 357–79, at p. 359.
31   Cherry, 'Accountability, entitlement and control', pp. 225–8.
32   S. Thompson, 'To relieve the sufferings of humanity, irrespective of party, politics or creed? Conflict, consensus and voluntary hospital provision in Edwardian South Wales', *Social History of Medicine*, 16 (2003), pp. 247–62, at p. 261.
33   Doyle, 'Voluntary health care in Middlesbrough'.
34   E. Mossialos and S. Thomson, 'Voluntary health insurance in the European Union: a critical assessment', *International Journal of Health Services*, 32 (2002), pp. 19–88.
35   V. Dawkins, *A study of the development of hospital contributory schemes in England and Wales* (Bristol, 1982).
36   R. Titmuss, 'The social division of welfare', in *Essays on the welfare state* (London, 1955).
37   B. Griffith, S. Iliffe and G. Rayner, *Banking on sickness: commercial medicine in Britain* (London, 1987); M. Calnan, S. Cant and J. Gabe, *Going private: why people pay for their health care* (Aldershot, 1993); J. Higgins, *The business of medicine* (London, 1988).

38 S. Fulder, 'Alternative therapists in Britain', in M. Saks (ed.), *Alternative medicine in Britain* (Oxford, 1992), pp. 166–82; U. Sharma, *Complementary medicine today* (London, 1995); M. Saks, *Professions and the public interest: medical power, altruism and alternative medicine* (London, 1995).
39 J. Mohan, *A national health service?* (London, 1995), pp. 161–7.
40 B. A. Weisbrod, 'Toward a theory of the voluntary non-profit sector in a three-sector economy', in E. S. Phelps (ed.), *Altruism, morality and economic theory* (New York, 1975), pp. 171–95; H. B. Hansmann, 'The role of nonprofit enterprise', *Yale Law Journal*, 89 (1980), pp. 835–901.
41 L. Salamon, *Partners in public service: government–nonprofit relations in the modern welfare state* (London, 1995).
42 *Ibid.*, pp. 45–7.
43 A. Seldon, *The litmus papers: a national health dis-service* (London, 1980), p. 5.
44 A. Seldon, *Capitalism* (Oxford, 1990), p. 250; D. Green, 'Medical care without the state', in A. Seldon (ed.), *Reprivatising welfare: after the lost century* (London, 1996), pp. 21–37, at p. 21.
45 For example, P. Hunt, 'Governance in public services', and H. Blears, 'Mutualism and the development of the NHS', both in S. Hogan (ed.), *Making healthcare mutual: a publicly funded, locally accountable NHS* (London, 2002), pp. 5 and 11.
46 S. Morris, *Defining the non-profit sector: some lessons from history*, London School of Economics Civil Society Working Paper No. 3 (London, 2000), p. 9.
47 D. Green, *Reinventing civil society: the rediscovery of welfare without politics* (London, 1993), p. 20; J. Wolpert, *What charity can and cannot do* (New York, 1996).
48 D. Green, *Community without politics* (London, 1996), p. 130.
49 *Ibid.*, pp. vii, 15.
50 C. Pierson, *Beyond the welfare state* (Cambridge, 1991), p. 201.
51 T. H. Marshall, *Citizenship and social class* (Cambridge, 1950).
52 D. Selbourne, *The principle of duty: an essay on the foundations of the civic order* (London, 1994); M. Ignatieff, 'Citizenship and moral narcissism', *Political Quarterly*, 60 (1989), pp. 63–74.
53 I. Culpitt, *Welfare and citizenship: beyond the crisis of the welfare state?* (London, 1992).
54 P. Hirst, *Associative democracy: new forms of economic and social governance* (Oxford, 1994); Green, *Reinventing civil society*.
55 G. Finlayson, *Citizen, state and social welfare in Britain, 1830–1990* (Oxford, 1994), pp. 8–9.
56 R. Wuthnow, 'The voluntary sector: legacy of the past, hope for the future?', in R. Wuthnow (ed.), *Between states and markets* (Princeton, NJ, 1991), pp. 3–29, at p. 22; R. N. Bellah, R. Madsen, W. M. Sullivan, A. Swiddler and S. M. Tipton, *Habits of the heart: individualism and commitment in American life* (New York, 1985), p. 38.
57 G. Fine and B. Harrington, 'Tiny publics: small groups and civil society', *Sociological Theory*, 22 (2004), pp. 241–56.
58 Deakin, *In search of civil society*, p. 17.
59 R. Putnam, *Making democracy work: civic traditions in modern Italy* (Princeton, NJ, 1993); R. Putnam, *Bowling alone: the collapse and revival of American community* (New York, 2000).
60 J. Le Grand, 'Knights, knaves or pawns? Human behaviour and social policy', *Journal of Social Policy*, 26 (1997), pp. 149–69.
61 J. Stewart, 'Ideology and process in the creation of the British National Health Service', *Journal of Policy History*, 14 (2002), pp. 113–34; P. Bridgen and J. Lewis, *Elderly people and the boundary between health and social care 1946–91: whose responsibility?* (London, 1999).
62 D. Green and B. Irvine, *Health care in France and Germany* (London, 2001), pp. 32–40, 80–2.
63 D. Wanless, *Securing our future health: taking a long-term view* (London, 2002), p. 4, para. 1.18; N. Timmins, 'A final chance for a return to health', *Financial Times* (18 April 2002).

64 E. Mayo and H. Moore, *The mutual state* (London, 2002).

65 A. Milburn, speech to Social Market Foundation, April 2003, and speech to Fabian Society, October 2001; J. Mohan, *Planning, markets and hospitals* (London, 2002), pp. 222–3.

66 J. Mohan, 'The past and future of the NHS: New Labour and the foundation hospitals debates', available online at www.historyandpolicy.org/archive/policy-paper-14.html (last accessed December 2005); J. Mohan, 'Milburn, Powell and Hayek: for and against planning in the NHS', *Journal of Health Services Research and Policy*, 9 (2004), pp. 54–6.

67 P. Taylor-Gooby, 'Introduction', in P. Taylor-Gooby (ed.), *Risk, trust and welfare* (London, 2000), p. 2.

68 U. Beck, *Risk society: towards a new modernity* (London, 1992); H. Kemshall, *Risk, social policy and welfare* (Buckingham, 2002), p. 121.

69 N. Rose, 'Governing advanced liberal democracies', in A. Barry, T. Osborne and N. Rose (eds), *Foucault and political reason* (London, 1996), pp. 37–64, at p. 58.

70 Kemshall, *Risk, social policy and welfare*, p. 1.

71 Hirst, *Associative democracy*; P. Hirst, 'Social welfare and associative democracy', in N. Ellison and C. Pierson (eds), *Developments in British social policy* (London, 1998), pp. 78–91; P. Hirst, 'Associationalist welfare: a reply to Marc Stears', *Economy and Society*, 28 (1999), pp. 590–7.

72 Hirst, *Associative democracy*, pp. 6–7.

73 T. Burchardt, J. Hills and C. Propper, *Private welfare and public policy* (York, 1998).

74 Hirst, 'Associationalist welfare'.

75 C. Lasch, *The revolt of the elites* (New York, 1995); R. Reich, *The work of nations* (New York, 1991).

76 M. Stears, 'Needs, welfare and the limits of associationalism', *Economy and Society*, 28 (1999), pp. 570–89.

77 *Ibid.*, pp. 577–8.

78 *Ibid.*, p. 586; Hirst, 'Associationalist welfare', pp. 594–5.

79 P. Kellner, *New mutualism: the third way* (London, 1998), quoted in J. Birchall, *The new mutualism and public policy* (London, 2001), p. 3.

80 Department of Health, 'The aims and purpose of NHS foundation trusts', www.dh.gov.uk/PolicyAndGuidance/OrganisationPolicy/SecondaryCare/NHSFoundationTrust/fs/en (last accessed December 2005).

81 Blears, 'Mutualism and the development of the National Health Service'.

82 R. Klein, 'Editorial: the first wave of NHS foundation trusts', *British Medical Journal*, 328 (2004), p. 1332; P. Day and R. Klein, *Governance of foundation trusts: dilemmas of diversity* (London, 2005), p. 14.

83 S. Ruane, 'The future of health care in the UK: think tanks and their policy prescriptions', in M. Powell, L. Bauld and K. Clarke (eds), *Social policy review 17* (Bristol, 2005), pp. 147–66.

Chapter 2

The emergence of hospital contributory schemes

The idea of a British hospital system funded by its users is one which began to emerge only in the late nineteenth century. Before this hospital organisation had taken three main forms. At the pinnacle of the institutional hierarchy were the voluntary hospitals. These were centres of acute medical care, funded by the philanthropy of the wealthy, managed voluntarily by local elites and staffed largely by consultants working on an honorary basis.[1] Public provision was the responsibility of the poor law, with the majority of beds located in workhouses and poor law infirmaries, and occupied predominantly by patients suffering from chronic diseases.[2] Local taxation, in the form of the poor rates, sustained these institutions, and although there had once been a 'broad identity' between ratepayers and recipients, the 1834 Poor Law Amendment Act had enshrined the principle of deterrence: this entailed the loss of civil rights for those whom it relieved and the stigmatisation of workhouse inmates, which lingered long into the twentieth century.[3] The application of the *general* rates to institutional care dates from the 1866 Sanitary Act, which empowered local authorities to spend revenues on isolation hospitals.[4] However, most taxpayers regarded access to these hospitals not as a universal right of citizenship but rather as a necessary evil to tackle infectious diseases.[5]

The origins of a funding system premised on payment by those who themselves expected to become patients lie not in the state sector, with its tradition of minimal provision for the necessitous, but in the voluntary hospitals. This chapter begins by tracing the history of medical charity and by identifying some of the earliest evidence for working people's subscriptions. It then discusses the two main channels for popular contribution which had developed by the end of the nineteenth century: local subscriptions taken in the workplace, firm and community, and organised collections of the Hospital Saturday and Hospital Sunday funds. Next it assesses the impact of these innovations up until 1914, with respect to hospital financing, admissions policies and the composition of management boards. Finally, it considers the funding crisis which followed the Great War, and the transformation of mass contribution from a generally marginal aspect of hospital income into a financial mainstay of the system. It argues that by the 1920s the traditional conception of hospital care as charitable dispensation was dead.

The early voluntary hospitals: charity and social class

The first major phase of voluntary hospital foundations occurred in the mid-eighteenth century, initially in London and provincial centres like Bristol and Cambridge. Their numbers multiplied through the Georgian and Victorian periods, so that by 1900 the large cities were typically home to several general and special hospitals, and many smaller towns had their own 'cottage hospital'. The movement was driven primarily by local philanthropic elites. Aristocrats might figure as donors or patrons, practitioners might be instrumental in identifying the need for an institution and the clergy might inspire hospital foundations,[6] but above all it was the urban middle class who funded and administered these hospitals. Motives for bourgeois charity, to the extent that they can be divined from the literature of exhortation, were many and varied. The new hospitals were identified with the eighteenth-century 'urban renaissance', in which open, transparent institutions were favourably contrasted with the closed, corporate bodies characteristic of 'old corruption'.[7] Sometimes hospitals represented consensual endeavour, when citizens set aside differences of sect and party, while at other times they reflected local political or religious tension, offering a visible rallying point for Tory/Anglican or Radical/Non-conformist factions.[8] Above all, voluntary action on the public stage was *de rigeur* for civic and business leaders seeking to proclaim their status in the pecking order of urban and national politics.[9]

Whatever the extraneous motives of philanthropists, the essence of the relationship between donors and recipients – the patients – was one of dependence. Before the twentieth century the benevolent middle classes did not expect to find themselves in hospital (they obtained their treatment elsewhere, from private practitioners): their subscriptions and donations entitled them to a fixed number of admission tickets (variously known as letters, notes, recommendations or 'lines') which they might give to people seeking access to the hospital. This allowed active philanthropists the opportunity to appraise the deservingness of putative patients before they gave them the means of admission.[10] The process of seeking entry to hospital therefore consolidated the ties of deference and paternalism – in workplace, parish, residential community or congregation – that characterised hierarchical social relations before the twentieth century.[11] Moreover, through supporting a healing institution in which abstemious behaviour, self-regulation and religiosity were inscribed in the rulebooks, donors could contribute to the public good.[12] For industrialists, the hospital meant the efficient preservation of human capital: the worker restored to productivity and recourse to the poor law averted.[13] Yet, alongside elements of social control, a genuine *caritas* inspired much philanthropy, and the manifest local popularity of voluntary hospitals demonstrates that they were never simply impersonal, disciplinary institutions.[14] Moreover, the subscriber admission system became progressively less important: accidents and emergencies had always been accepted without a ticket, and doctors assumed an increasingly significant role in admitting patients who met their clinical interests and teaching needs.[15]

The financial records of nineteenth-century voluntary hospitals illustrate the over-riding importance of the charitable middle class to their maintenance. At the outset, the bedrock of provision came from annual subscriptions. For example, in 1811 these furnished 75 per cent of income at the Royal Hampshire Hospital and 47 per cent at the Birmingham General Hospital.[16] Subscription was a pledged sum, which formally linked a hospital's utilisation capacity to its income through a system which awarded admissions privileges according to the size of the gift. Other principal sources of revenue were donations, fundraising events (such as the celebrated Birmingham Music Festival), legacies given at death and (as hospitals began to accumulate endowments and capital) the proceeds of investments in property or stocks. In the early nineteenth century such gifts came overwhelmingly from private individuals. Given the typical level of annual subscriptions, the absence of mass support is unsurprising; for Birmingham General Hospital, for example, the subscription around 1800 was either one or two guineas, when an unskilled labourer might earn 10s per week and a skilled worker 20–30s.[17] A small amount of 'corporate' giving also took place, such as parishes supplementing poor law provision, and businesses mixing paternalism with protection of their workforce.[18]

The financial dominance of wealthy private donors was mirrored in the administrative arrangements. Hospitals typically had a governing body (variously designated the 'court of governors', 'board of management', 'hospital committee', 'court of contributors', etc.) which met regularly to conduct their business. This included the oversight of financial affairs, the appointment of consultants and other staff, the upkeep of the fabric, the content of the rules and regulations and so on. Day-to-day running was in the hands of the matron and visiting doctors, although there was typically a house committee which met more frequently, and a group of 'visitors' appointed by the governing body to ensure the smooth functioning of the institution. Membership of these groups was open to all subscribers, the usual procedure being the annual nomination of a small number of individuals who would take the place of retiring governors. This would be ratified at an annual general meeting (AGM), again open to all subscribers, or, if contested, put to the popular vote. In practice it appears that seats on the board were not usually subject to election, and that interested volunteers were co-opted by existing members. Before the late nineteenth century, then, the patient was not directly represented in hospital government, which instead reflected the concerns of philanthropists and medical practitioners.

The precursors to mass contributory schemes

Workplace subscription

Intimations of change appeared in the early nineteenth century with the first references to 'sporadic' workplace collections within subscription lists, in 1820 in Dundee and 1822 in Bradford.[19] More generally, workers subscribed through guilds, friendly societies and firms. In Newcastle upon Tyne the coopers', bricklayers', tailors' and hoastmen's companies figure on subscription lists, along with various collieries, guilds and seamen's associations, and 'workmen' from the glass, iron, soap and merchant shipping industries.[20] Similarly, in 1827 Birmingham General Hospital's subscribers included collieries, iron founders, gas, canal, nail and gun companies, local friendly societies, including Odd Fellows' and Druids' branches, and trade clubs of miners and journeymen curriers.[21]

Early-nineteenth-century Glasgow provides an early example of organised subscription by manual workers. Here the Royal Infirmary had permitted 'Incorporations or Societies' subscribing three guineas annually to admit two patients a year. Thus in 1812 the subscription list included the Incorporations of Bakers, Barbers, Fleshers, Hammermen, Maltmen, Masons, Tailors, Weavers and Wrights, as well as the Dumbarton Glassworks Company, Lanark Cotton Mills Benevolent Society, Journeymen Bookbinders and Printers Society, Clyde Iron Works, 'trades of Lanark', weavers in Pollockshaw, Tobacco Spinners' Society and the Thread Makers' Society.[22] The 1830s saw the donations from guilds and journeymen's societies supplemented by more extensive contributions from 'Mechanics in the several public works'. The context for this was an ongoing tussle between the Infirmary and the city corporation and parishes over the cost of treating typhus patients. The Infirmary had admitted these without the usual 'subscriber's line', but had failed to persuade the city government to subscribe at a rate which would cover the cost.[23] A typhus epidemic in 1831 provoked a crisis, with the Infirmary opening a separate 'fever building' at its own expense.[24] Unable to offer support due to the simultaneous costs of the cholera epidemic, the city corporation backed the Infirmary in an extraordinary appeal through the Kirk Sessions: 'Personal safety is involved in the safety of the public; a Contribution is fairly due from every one, as a premium, for the protection and security afforded'.[25] Thus from 1833 subscriptions from Glasgow's 'Public Works' were listed separately in the Infirmary's annual reports, the term denoting businesses in the city's major industrial sectors: foundries, bottle-works, tobacco, weaving, spinning, distilling, shipbuilding, chemicals, cotton, flax, brewing, printing, building trades, and 'captains and crews of steam boats'.[26]

By the mid-century this separate tabulation was occurring elsewhere. In Bristol contributions from the 'working classes' were first described in 1846, and these began to be recorded in the published income statistics as the 'Workmen's contribution' from the 1850s.[27] At the outset these were not of much financial significance, but working-class generosity gave hospital governors a useful rhetorical device to embarrass 'those who have been blessed with the abundance of this world's goods' into giving more.[28] Similar rhetoric was deployed in Glasgow, where the governors liked to extol the 'example from the Operatives and Seamen' of 'good will' and 'independence of mind' to cajole the 'comparatively wealthy and comfortable' into giving more generously.[29]

Another forerunner was Sunderland Royal Infirmary, a hospital which rapidly came to depend to an unusual degree on workplace contribution. Its early subscription lists included small sums contributed by employees in shipbuilding, manufacturing and mining; in 1861 these amounted to £45 out of a subscription total of £698.[30] Small as they were, these sums persuaded the hospital's general committee to allow worker contributors admission tickets to the value of half the total subscription; the remainder supported an accident ward, which largely dealt with industrial injuries in the area's trades.[31] In 1864 the need for a new infirmary prompted governors to seek alternative sources of funding and they established an annual church-based 'Hospital Sunday' collection, conscious of the success of similar approaches in Leeds and Birmingham. Also, stressing the extent to which the hospital served the needs of the town's industries, they appealed to employers to establish workplace contribution schemes.[32] It rapidly became apparent that church collections, which by 1867 had raised only £266, would be insufficient to meet the capital costs of the new building.[33] Workplace collections were therefore prioritised and rapidly increased, both because the eligibility rights were attractive to labourers in heavy industries and because, from 1872, the Infirmary employed a collector who received a percentage commission.[34] By 1875 workers' funds were separately listed in annual reports and provided a large proportion of subscriptions (£933 out of £2,191); by 1881 they exceeded the amount raised by charitable subscription, with shipyards, collieries and railways the largest single contributors.[35]

Why did some towns innovate in this way? If Sunderland is typical, the answer lies in its socioeconomic characteristics. Following rapid population growth during the nineteenth century, with booming shipyards and collieries, Sunderland's middle class was relatively small and thus unable to sustain a philanthropic project like the Infirmary once demand for its services necessitated significant expansion.[36] The first employers' canvas for workplace subscriptions was undertaken in the early 1860s to support a paying accident ward and infectious diseases accommodation, in which employers could place workers or visiting seamen.[37] From the outset, then, the Infirmary catered to the peculiar needs of its town, and the early shift to mass contribution exemplified flexible adaptation. Indeed, the board of management publicly represented the institution as a unifying force in civic life, which was 'peculiarly free from the partiality, or tone of class, whether political, social or religious'.[38] The workers themselves did not regard the arrangement as entirely voluntary, given that it entailed a deduction from wages organised by the employer, and probably saw their subscription as a form of insurance for themselves and their dependants.[39] From the employers' perspective it bore some relationship to the existing welfare arrangements in colliery districts, where pit clubs and permanent relief funds were predominantly funded by deductions from wages.[40]

Hospital collecting funds

While some large urban hospitals were developing workplace subscriptions, two new forms of mass contribution appeared: the Hospital Sunday and Hospital Saturday funds. Saturday funds were distinguished from the existing workers' subscriptions in two respects: first, they were levied annually on a single day; and second, in the larger cities they were affiliated not to a single hospital but supported a range of local medical institutions.

Hospital Sunday had eighteenth-century antecedents. The practice of churches and chapels setting aside one Sunday each year for a sermon on hospital charity, followed by a collection, dates back, for example, in Edinburgh to 'Infirmary Sunday' in the mid-1700s, while in Aberdeen the custom began in 1784.[41] The later Hospital Sunday funds typically distributed not to a single hospital but to all medical charities within a given town.[42] A standing committee systematised and publicised the collections, and was able to exert a certain amount of influence on hospital policy through its allocative power. The first Sunday fund was established in Birmingham in 1859, having developed from an organised collection scheme begun around 1850.[43] Following publicity in the medical press it was adopted elsewhere; the largest, based in London, was founded in 1873.[44] Collections in London averaged 2*d* per head in the late nineteenth century, bringing contribution within reach of the small donor, though this was still essentially middle-class charity, with congregations in the wealthier areas raising the largest amounts and being rewarded with admission letters.[45]

Collecting funds which were avowedly directed at the working class date from the late 1860s. Some were connected to particular institutions, such as the People's Subscription Fund (1868) and the People's Contribution Fund (1877), which aided the London and University College Hospitals, respectively.[46] Other funds were associated with particular towns, such as Llanelly (1867) and Preston (1871). 'Saturday funds' followed the Sunday funds in taking an annual collection on a predetermined day (wages being customarily paid on Saturdays).[47] Early examples include those in Walsall (1863), Derby (1869), Coventry (1870), Manchester (1872), Birmingham (1873), Kidderminster (1873), Bradford (1873), London (1874), Wolverhampton (1874), Bolton (1877), Carlisle (1880) and Macclesfield (1885).[48] An indication of the rapidity with which they spread was given in 1889 by Henry Burdett in the first of his annual collations of statistics on the income of voluntary hospitals. Of 150 hospitals, 82 recorded receipts from Hospital Saturday, with the largest single sum, £2,680, going to the Birmingham General Hospital (15 per cent of its total income).[49]

What were the circumstances which led to the foundation of a Saturday fund? In Nottingham in 1872 the Sunday fund committee initially proposed that employers should organise workplace collections for the Nottingham General Hospital; the bosses' poor response prompted the establishment of a Hospital Saturday fund committee, consisting of nineteen 'works delegates', predominantly from the lace and hosiery industries, and managed by the existing chair and secretary of the hospital's weekly board.[50] Birmingham's fund originated in the efforts of Samson Gamgee, a surgeon at the Queen's Hospital, to raise finance for building works through a 'Working Men's Fund' in 1869. Pleased with its success, and buoyed by the advice of the Reverend Henn of Manchester's Hospital Saturday committee, in 1873 Gamgee proposed developing it into a permanent Saturday fund for 'the various medical charities' of the town.[51] A meeting of 'Gentlemen' and 'Artisans' was held, with the mayor in attendance, and a committee appointed, with Gamgee as secretary; it raised £4,700 from its first appeal.[52] County hospitals with rural catchments followed the lead of the industrial cities, as at the Royal Hampshire in Winchester, where a Saturday fund was initiated in 1883, in imitation of the 'plan found to work well in other towns'; it operated through the placing of collecting boxes by 'employers and tradesmen … on their counters'.[53] The sums collected remained small, only £86 in 1895–96, when total income was £6,065.[54]

Wolverhampton's Royal Hospital provides a useful case study of a Saturday fund, as here mass contribution became the mainstay of the hospital's finance: by 1938 its income was £60,340, of which £40,746 (68 per cent) came from what was by then the hospital's contributory association.[55] In 1845 (the earliest example) the annual report of the hospital noted 'the noble and generous aid rendered by the Working Classes, in the erection and furnishing of this Building'.[56] Small but regular sums in the 1850s came from 'Tradesmen's and Manufacturers' Boxes', which appear to have been kept in the workplace by employers to elicit contributions from their staff.[57] Workers' subscriptions were first listed separately in 1869, although they amounted to only £372, just 7.5 per cent of total income, notably from railway and iron companies.[58] Expansion followed a fundraising drive by hospital governors for a new wing, an isolation block, a laundry and wash-house and out-patient accommodation.[59] These threatened to push up annual costs, so governors appealed, noting the 'example set them by the workmen of Birmingham, who are doing their best for the Queens Hospital there'. This elicited a 'Christmas Box' of £500 in 1872, which, though insufficient, inspired the collecting fund.

The Wolverhampton Hospital Saturday fund was duly inaugurated in 1874, at a public meeting organised by hospital governors at the Agricultural Hall.[60] The mayor presided, alongside local MP Stavely Hill, chair of the hospital governors, Mr Briscoe, and four clerics, among whom was the hospital chaplain. Their audience, though it included 'representative men from nearly every works and manufactory in the town', was 'not as large as might have been expected': it was a Saturday evening, when most workers were enjoying their 'stroll out' or 'their drops of beer'. The speeches set out the rationale for the fund. The mayor appealed to urban patriotism, urging that 'free-will offerings' be made to the hospital, which 'would be the glory of the town'. Hill stressed the providential value of workers supporting an institution which they themselves might need in the future, while Briscoe detailed the financial case, warning that without an income boost 'the operations of the Hospital and its work of usefulness must be curtailed'. A Mr Fowler appealed both to Christian charity – that peculiarly English capacity for 'strong sympathy' – and to self-interest – the need to support scientific advance, to guard against occupational health risk, and to gain the right 'to enter a hospital without … any taint of pauperism, or in any way impugning that feeling of independence which ought to be cherished by every man'. Conversely, Rupert Kettle deployed a discourse of duty: better-paid workers such as they were the beneficiaries of 'the principle of free competition' and now had an obligation to support 'those persons whom they had run over in the race of competition ... bustling along for their own wealth, profit and gain'. Following brief addresses by two workmen, the meeting concluded with the establishment of the fund. Local foremen were to found workplace committees to organise the annual collection, while a tradesmen's association would oversee the placing of collecting boxes in shops. On the appointed day the money would be brought to the Agricultural Hall to be received by the mayor and representatives of the Staffordshire Bank.

Workers' contributions: an explanatory framework

With these examples in mind, what conclusions can be drawn about the emergence of workers' contributions? First, the different funds and schemes were initiated by local elites, and it is therefore strictly incorrect to suppose, as did the great hospital publicist Henry Burdett, that it was the 'spirit' of the friendly societies which 'gave birth' to them.[61] Though well supported, workers' contributions did not emanate from the labour movement, nor were they spontaneous manifestations of self-help. Instead, hospital governors and municipal politicians typically acted in response to the growing population pressure on hospital facilities which marked the mid-nineteenth century and which traditional forms of charity proved incapable of addressing.[62] Some hospitals arrived at this through their own trajectories, while for others an immediate impetus was the success of the Sunday funds elsewhere; competitive urban boosterism and emulation of pioneer cities such as Liverpool, Manchester and Birmingham therefore had some effect. Second, as the Wolverhampton case illustrates, a new language of appeals marked a reconfiguration of the triangular relationship between institution, donors and recipients. Henceforth, the hospital's claim to support was founded increasingly on the service it provided to users, thus undermining the patient's dependency upon the subscriber. Third, and related to this, the rhetoric which held Saturday fund contributions to be 'free-will offerings' (and hence a form of philanthropy) disguised a shift in entitlement. This did not yet amount to a direct insurance arrangement, although a *quid pro quo* was implicit in the allocation of subscribers' notes to the works committees.

Above all, it was hospital managers and local employers who encouraged workers' contributions. Employers' interests were also evident in another trend in hospital subscription, the gradual supersedence in the later nineteenth century of the individual subscriber by firms.[63] By 1861 in Birmingham, for example, the General Hospital received subscriptions from eighty-one of the region's firms, notably from the glass, metal, gun and toy trades, as well as the gas and railway industries.[64] In Bristol these ranged in 1884 from the minor amounts given by the Mangotsfield Pennant Stone Co., to £20 from C Division City Police, to large subscriptions such as the £88 from Bristol Wagon Works Co.[65] This long-run shift towards the support of hospitals by businesses, whether from annual profits or from the organised workers' collections, reflected the employers' perception that hospitals had both social utility and industrial value. In the years before industrial injury legislation (1897), collective contribution gave workers some security, while employers gained protection for their workforce. Such paternalistic involvement in welfare was similar to employer sponsorship of friendly societies. For example, many coal-owners supported pit clubs that provided life and accident assurance, both by direct contributions and by compulsory deductions from wages.[66] In industrial areas similar processes operated, as in Wigan, where the 'quasi-feudal bonds' between coal- and iron-owners and their employees accounted for the scale of mass collections in that town: they provided 40 per cent of hospital income in the 1870s.[67] In practical terms, encouragement might operate through businesses keeping their 'Infirmary box' in their counting house, so that employees might conveniently contribute when they received their pay.[68]

However, it is unlikely that the impetus for workers' contributions came entirely from above. Trade unions and friendly societies increasingly numbered among hospitals' institutional subscribers, as Birmingham General again demonstrates: in 1861 it was supported by four trade clubs (journeymen curriers, operative masons and two tailors' societies) and thirty-nine friendly societies, including thirteen Odd Fellows lodges, two Druids, four United Brothers and several independent clubs, like the Tipton's Amicable Society or Walsall's Queer Fellows.[69] This suggests an affinity between hospital contribution and the mutual health insurance developed by benefit clubs. Indeed, the appearance of workers' subscriptions coincides with the mid-century consolidation of the friendly society movement, when local clubs gave way before the national affiliated orders, notably the Foresters and the Odd Fellows, which attracted extensive working-class support; total friendly society membership was around 2,940,000 by 1876.[70] A monthly payment typically insured members for a weekly benefit during sickness and a lump sum payable at death; medical attendance by doctors who certified and treated the illness increasingly became the norm.[71] At the same time, new model trade unionism shifted the interests of organised labour towards the collective provision of health benefits.[72]

This parallel development of collective welfare structures may have encouraged workers to respond favourably to proposals for hospital contributions. First, friendly society discourse emphasised the need for respectable workers to achieve independence from the poor law; similarly, contribution offered access to hospital without the demeaning recourse to a charitable patron.[73] Second, with its grounding in the new actuarial science of the risks of morbidity and mortality, mutual insurance effected a cultural shift in attitudes to the body. For the first time working people were encouraged to take a long-term view of their own future health and well-being, and to adopt new norms of social responsibility for addressing individual risk.[74] Hospital contribution may therefore have reflected the internalisation of these norms, and the implanting in British society of the 'hospital habit' – the popular demand for institutional medical treatment. Third, by promising democratic structures of organisation and representation, the new hospital funds drew on existing models of friendly society and cooperative working.[75] Finally, a more prosaic factor underpinned the expansion of working-class mutuality: from mid-century, rising real incomes permitted greater numbers to include a prudential element within their family budgets.[76]

Patterns of development before 1914

What was the impact of this new form of funding on hospital finances? One approach is to document this in individual hospitals, and Figure 2.1 illustrates the growth of mass contribution relative to philanthropic subscriptions to Glasgow Royal Infirmary from 1833. Contribution remained the lesser of the two income sources, remaining at a fairly low level before 1850, then rising markedly up to 1873, reflecting a booming local economy; after this, competition from neighbouring hospitals and trade recession halted expansion.[77] Growth recommenced in the mid-1880s, yet by the start of the twentieth century it still yielded less than subscription and provided only about 15 per cent of the hospital's income in 1901.[78]

Nationally, the proportion generated by contribution may be viewed through the summary statistics published from 1889 in Burdett's annual hospital yearbooks (see Figure 2.2). These are not comprehensive, though they are representative of the larger voluntary hospitals, for which a full breakdown of income was recorded. In 1911, for example, a breakdown of income sources is available for 159 out of 752 institutions in England, Scotland and Wales, but these large hospitals accounted for 58 per cent of all beds and 69 per cent of income.[79] The expansion of contributory income is clear. In 1889, total income from the Saturday and Sunday funds, along with the 'contributions from workpeople', amounted to £73,156. This had risen to £215,548 by 1901 and to £290,341 by 1913. Figure 2.2 illustrates the changing income composition. Charitable subscriptions gradually declined in significance from their peak of 20 per cent, though, taken alongside 'other charity' (donations, collecting boxes, legacies), it is clear that hierarchical philanthropy remained the dominant component. Money from organised collecting funds, including the King's Fund, the Saturday and Sunday funds, and other workpeople's schemes, rose from 5.7 per cent of all income in 1889 to a high of 15.7 per cent in 1911, while a smaller proportion, 5.9 per cent by 1913, came from direct payment by patients.[80] The other major category was interest earned from investments.

Table 2.1 traces the growth of income from contributions and direct payments. It shows that approximately half of all income from collecting funds (column A) can be attributed to working-class contributions (column B), which at their peak in 1911 accounted for 7.7 per cent of hospital receipts. None the less, the annual sums from workers' contributions were frequently exceeded by earnings from direct payments by patients and fees for nursing services (column C), which also peaked at 7.7 per cent of all income, in 1913. On the eve of war, then, it was by no means evident that British hospitals were not set to follow the North American route of securing their finances by

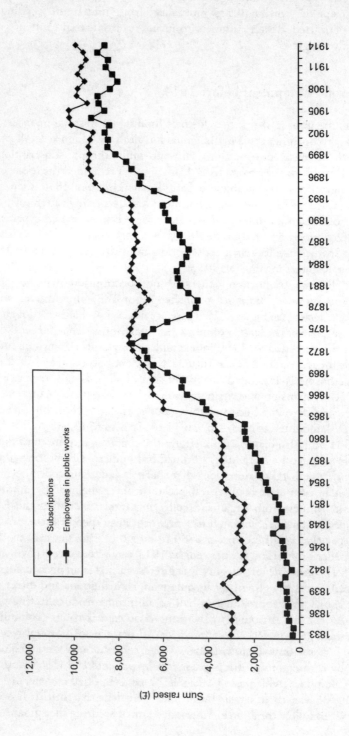

Figure 2.1. Comparison of subscriptions from philanthropists and employees' contributions to Glasgow Royal Infirmary, 1833–1914.

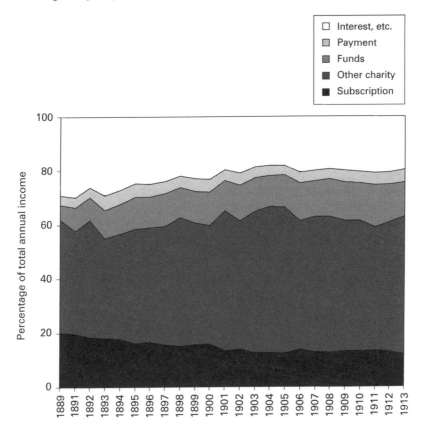

Figure 2.2. Composition of British voluntary hospital income, 1889–1913. (Note that no data are available for 1890.) Data from *Burdett's Hospitals and charities: the yearbook of philanthropy and hospital annual* (London, annual publication).

opening beds and services to paying patients, rather than by developing mass funding arrangements.[81]

These national aggregates conceal some marked regional variations in workers' contributions. Data in Burdett's yearbooks permit the differentiation of London from both the remainder of England and Wales and from Scotland (columns D, E and F). It is striking that London had lower levels of workers' contribution, attributable both to the persistence of traditional charity in the capital, which was home to so many wealthy patrons, and to the demands which the sheer number of competing institutions placed on a single fund.[82] The metropolitan Hospital Saturday fund appears to have had an uneasy relationship with hospital managers.[83] Further, London hospitals developed pay beds with greater enthusiasm than elsewhere: their income from this source more than doubled between 1905 (£29,334) and 1913 (£67,795), while workers' contributions rose more modestly (from £14,332 to £18,198). By 1914 there were 622 full paying beds in metropolitan hospitals.[84]

Table 2.1. Contribution and direct payment as a percentage of British voluntary hospital income, 1889–1913

	A	B	C	D	E	F
	All funds/ contributions[a]	Workers' funds[b]	Patients' payments	Workers' funds as a percentage of all income		
				London	England and Wales	Scotland
1889	5.7	1.9	3.3	1.0	4.0	
1891	8.8	3.3	3.8	1.5	6.8	
1892	8.5	3.3	3.6	1.3	7.3	
1893	10.5	6.0	7.0	0.7	10.5	11.2
1894	10.9	6.6	6.8	1.9	11.1	11.9
1895	12.1	6.7	6.6	1.7	11.4	12.4
1896	11.4	6.7	6.3	1.9	11.7	7.5
1897	12.2	6.2	6.6	1.6	11.6	10.8
1898	11.2	5.9	6.8	1.4	11.5	7.6
1899	11.8	6.2	7.1	1.3	13.1	8.6
1900	12.5	6.4	7.2	1.5	12.2	8.6
1901	11.2	5.5	6.7	1.2	9.6	9.5
1902	13.1	6.1	7.0	1.0	11.8	12.9
1903	12.3	5.7	7.1	1.0	10.6	10.6
1904	11.5	5.7	6.8	1.0	11.7	9.6
1905	12.0	5.9	6.2	1.1	9.6	12.5
1906	13.9	6.9	6.3	1.2	12.6	12.6
1907	13.3	6.4	6.3	1.3	11.7	10.8
1908	13.8	6.4	6.5	1.4	10.9	9.4
1909	14.2	6.7	6.9	1.4	11.4	10.1
1910	14.0	6.8	6.9	1.4	13.0	10.2
1911	15.7	7.7	6.7	1.5	14.6	12.3
1912	14.0	7.4	7.1	1.5	13.8	10.6
1913	12.7	6.5	7.7	1.1	13.3	8.8

[a] Prince of Wales (later King's) Fund, Hospital Sunday Fund, Hospital Saturday Fund, contributions from workpeople.
[b] Hospital Saturday Fund, contributions from workpeople.
Source: *Burdett's Hospitals and charities: the yearbook of philanthropy and hospital annual* (London, annual publication).

Beyond London the fundamental distinction was between the southern part of the country, where few hospitals relied heavily on contributions, and the industrial centres of the Midlands, the North East, the North West and Scotland.[85] Institutional experience could vary markedly, according to the wealth base which sustained traditional charity and the structure of the local economy. In the towns of industrial Lancashire, such as Preston, Bolton, Blackburn and Wigan, workers' funding was essential to the extension of general hospital provision outside the larger urban centres.[86] Other cities saw traditional modes of charity retain their significance in the income mix. Workers' contributions to

Bristol Royal Infirmary rose from a mere 0.1 per cent of total income in 1847 to 7 per cent by 1884, and to 13.5 per cent by 1911.[87] In contrast, workers' gifts in Wolverhampton were worth only 3.6 per cent of total income in 1851, but rose to 20 per cent by 1874, the first year of the Saturday fund, and 36 per cent by 1911.[88]

The changing basis of admission and representation

The new funding mechanisms gradually undermined the social hierarchies implicit in the administrative and operational procedures of the voluntary hospitals. One effect was the erosion of the practice of admission by subscriber's letter. An early example is Ancoats Hospital, where the establishment of a workers' 'provident scheme' in the late 1870s permitted members' admission without a recommendation.[89] In Newcastle upon Tyne, the Royal Victoria Infirmary took the decision in 1888 to become an 'open' hospital: 'The labour of seeking for letters of admission is now entirely done away with. "Suffering" accompanied by inability to procure medical assistance privately commands at once admission to the Infirmary'.[90] The catalyst for this was a financial crisis following the opening of new wards, and the desire to emulate Sunderland's success in tapping fresh sources of income; moreover, the economic rationale for the ticket system had disappeared, as treatment costs per patient now exceeded the cost of each ticket and subscriber numbers remained static.[91]

In Sunderland itself the Royal Infirmary's early introduction of workers' contributions began to overturn the principle of hierarchical charity from the 1860s. Initially contributing workplaces received admission tickets that entitled people to up to one month's in-patient care.[92] However, the hospital's medical staff soon began to complain that there were insufficient beds for acute patients, because contributors or their dependants occupied the available accommodation, insisting on their entitlement to stay to the maximum time allowed. Moreover, they did not display due deference to the nurses, 'thinking everyone in the house are their servants' and claiming their care as a right 'on account of giving a halfpenny a week'.[93] Worse still, there were rumours of tickets changing hands for cash. The governors responded by making the medical staff the sole arbiters of entry and discharge, and by 1878 they abandoned the ticket system entirely, trusting that the admission rights of philanthropic subscribers would be 'gracefully waived'.[94] The replacement of ticketing by free access meant that medical criteria for admission were applied, rather than social ones, but it also curbed claims to treatment as an entitlement based on financial contribution and reasserted professional authority over the wards.

Table 2.2 suggests, however, that open access remained the exception. This is based on a consistent set of hospitals which recorded admission details in Burdett's yearbooks in 1901 and 1928 (its final year of publication).[95] There is a certain amount of double-counting within table 2.2, as some hospitals recorded more than one method of admission. However, most institutions (66 per cent in 1901) retained a subscriber's ticket system, presumably for fear that

Table 2.2. Numbers of British voluntary hospitals operating particular types of admission regime, 1900 and 1928

	General hospitals (*n* = 539)		Special hospitals (*n* = 170)	
	1901	1928	1901	1928
Subscriber's ticket	346	323	80	79
Patient's payment	170	245	29	62
Means tested payment	20	114	12	52
Free, open access	91	125	69	98
Provident scheme	6	5	2	0

Note that some double counting arises with hospitals concurrently running more than one admission system.
Source: Burdett's *Hospitals and charities* (1901, 1928).

charitable subscribers would desert if this privilege were removed. Some workplace contributors were included in the category of corporate subscribers, thus subverting the hierarchical nature of ticketing. For example, in Nottingham any workplace providing at least two guineas per annum from worker subscriptions was entitled to recommend one in-patient and three out-patients for each two guineas subscribed.[96] The most marked change between 1901 and 1928 was the growth in the arrangements for patients' payments, whether at a fixed rate or means tested, while only a minority operated free admission (though a rather higher proportion of special than general hospitals did so).

This disruption of traditional financial hierarchies was paralleled by change in the social composition of hospital management, with the appearance of worker representatives. In Glasgow, for example, this began in 1888, when the constitution of the new Victoria Infirmary stated that the governing body should include three workers elected by the representatives of 'every shipyard, factory or workshop' that donated at least £50 or subscribed at least £5 annually.[97] The Glasgow Royal Infirmary followed suit in 1901 with a supplementary charter empowering it to add two women and two workmen to its board of management.[98] In Nottingham the minimal two guineas per annum subscription permitted firms to have a delegate join the board of governors, which selected the managers.[99] Workers' representation in Sunderland followed the removal of admission rights and was perhaps a *quid pro quo* to ensure continuing support. Here approaches were made to the hospital governors by workplace representatives, the trades council and a local vicar, and in 1881 four workers' nominees joined the twenty-strong general committee.[100]

1918–23: the post-war expansion of mass contribution

The wartime emergency of 1914–18 demonstrated the resilience of workers' contributory funds and left them poised for expansion thereafter. Some initially suffered from the disruption caused by mobilisation, and the proportion of hospital income received from workers' schemes and Saturday funds fell from 13 per cent in 1914 to 11 per cent in 1916, before regaining pre-war levels in 1919.[101] In Nottingham, for example, fund income fell substantially in 1915 as contributors joined the armed forces.[102] However, buoyant labour markets gave some hospitals a boost: thus, in Newcastle upon Tyne workers' contributions rose from £24,722 in 1915 to £29,409 in 1916, the increase coming from both the collieries and munitions workers, the latter notably those in the Armstrong Whitworth firm.[103] Nationally, of fifty-three hospitals consistently reporting income, workers' contributions rose from £112,055 in 1915 to £151,045 in 1917, although allowing for price inflation the real increase was very modest.[104] Thus, despite wartime mobilisation, contributions held up.

The importance of contributory schemes to hospital exchequers was more widely acknowledged in the difficult aftermath of war, when expenditure demands began outstripping income. By 1921, 68 per cent of London's hospitals were in the red, with the total deficit standing at nearly £400,000; for many this meant the need to increase borrowing.[105] Both short- and long-term factors contributed to the malaise. First, the war had temporarily postponed the impact on hospitals of national health insurance (NHI). This was introduced in Part I of the 1911 National Insurance Act (Part II covered unemployment insurance) and provided manual and other workers with sickness benefit when ill, along with medical attendance by doctors. In some places this increased pressure on hospitals, as general practitioners referred greater numbers of difficult cases.[106] It also raised popular expectations of standards of care and enhanced notions of entitlement to good health care.[107] However, hospitals were ill-equipped to meet patients' demand for services. The wartime emergency had destabilised existing arrangements, with over half of all nurses and many consultants seeing active service abroad, with building works and physical improvements suspended, and with some 16,000 beds allocated for military requirements.[108] Moreover, wartime state subventions were pro rata maintenance payments, which the voluntary hospitals claimed fell far short of actual expenditure.[109] Then in 1918 the global influenza pandemic reached Britain, overwhelming services and afflicting staff, sometimes fatally.[110] Finally, the immediate post-war years saw high price inflation affecting the costs of essential items such as food and coal.

Government responded with a special committee chaired by Viscount Cave to consider the voluntary hospitals' financial predicament and to recommend solutions. It originated in the debates surrounding the newly established Ministry of Health's proposals for local authority funding of general hospitals; objections from the voluntary lobby led to the withdrawal of this scheme and appointment of the committee.[111] Supporters of the voluntary system dominated, and with evidence drawn largely from voluntary hospital administrators and from the King's Fund the policy option of sustained state assistance for hospitals was not central to the agenda.[112] Cave's 1921 report recommended a temporary Treasury grant to rescue the voluntaries from the immediate crisis, tax exemptions on gifts and contributions, a standing Voluntary Hospitals Commission (VHC) and local hospital committees to promote coordination.[113]

Cave also urged hospitals to take steps to achieve financial security through diversification of funding sources, including greater reliance on paying patients, the extension of NHI to include payments for hospital treatment, and the development of mass contributory schemes.[114]

The committee's support for contributory schemes reflected the recommendations of several witnesses.[115] Other options seemed less promising. Hospital administrators felt that traditional charitable sources could not provide long-term stability, given the extension of personal taxation that had occurred in the war years.[116] Indeed, the Order of St John, another fundraising body, pithily observed in 1923 that 'the Old Rich ... had become the New Poor'.[117] Some places already lacked a philanthropic middle class, such as Merthyr Tydfil, where miners' representatives commented on the small numbers of subscribers to the local hospitals and pointed out that the coal-owners and steel-owners were non-resident and 'spent their money elsewhere'.[118] Another option was opening spare capacity in the poor law infirmaries but this idea was dismissed on the grounds that patients would enter these hospitals only if they were 'dissociated entirely from the Poor Law'.[119] Equally problematic was the proposal to extend NHI benefits to include hospital treatment.[120] This had been championed in 1911 by Henry Burdett but was opposed by Lloyd George and his advisers, who feared the hospitals would be 'out for plunder'.[121] They were concerned above all with poverty, and the principal benefits were modelled on those offered by friendly societies; German-style hospital cover was rejected, though NHI did include the costs of treatment in tuberculosis sanatoria.[122] Consultants also opposed NHI hospital cover, fearing that state remuneration would lower their status and remove their control over admissions.[123]

Why, though, was the extension of NHI not pursued during the post-war funding crisis? Cave's interim report had recommended that payments to hospitals for insured persons should be made from the accumulated surpluses of £7,000,000 held by the 'approved societies' (these were friendly societies recognised by the state as agencies for the administration of the NHI scheme).[124] This was supported in the medical press and in the House of Lords, which argued that such grants could be made under the existing national insurance legislation.[125] Cave's final report, however, refrained from calling for a NHI hospital benefit. This might undermine the voluntary character of the system, which he sought to preserve, while direct payment to doctors treating insured patients would seem invidious and could lead to calls for a salaried consultant service.[126] Government, too, was wary of raising the state's contribution to NHI at a time of Treasury retrenchment; indeed, it rejected Cave's plea for a one-off grant of £1,000,000 to rescue the hospitals, and offered instead half that sum, and on condition it was matched from voluntary sources. Meanwhile the 1921 Public Health (Tuberculosis) Act terminated the NHI sanatorium benefit and passed responsibility for institutional care of people with tuberculosis to local authorities.[127]

Cave's recommendation therefore pulled back from compulsion. NHI payments to hospitals were classed as optional 'additional benefits' and, despite Ministry of Health exhortations, few such grants were made at a significant level. Thus, although the issue was periodically raised again, the overall income from this source remained low. In 1937, for example, out of a total £3,798,624 additional benefits paid in Britain, only £107,187 went to hospitals, against £216,878 to convalescent homes.[128] This was a trifling sum: the annual income of Guy's Hospital alone in that year was £296,181.[129]

Instead, Cave argued that if the voluntary system was to 'continue and prosper', it had to switch from charitable support to 'moderate and continuous contributions from all classes of the community'.[130] Practical support for the schemes came from the committee's successor organisation, the VHC. Chaired by Lord Onslow, this was set up principally to distribute the one-off Treasury grant, and in 1925 reported on hospital accommodation and waiting lists.[131] In 1922 the Commission held an enquiry into the contributory schemes, which, according to its secretary, were a 'new El Dorado offered by the patient class'.[132] Questionnaires were sent to existing contributory schemes, and the seventy-three replies were collated and summarised in a short publication which identified the range of administrative practices currently followed.[133] There was some internal deliberation as to the extent of guidance the Commission should give (for example on whether explicitly to warn against the 'over-representation of mass contributors' on hospital boards), but the final pamphlet merely provided a 'summary of facts'.[134]

The chronology of the foundation of further contributory schemes in the early 1920s suggests that many hospitals had initiatives underway indepen-dently of the Cave and Onslow reports. Oxford's Radcliffe Infirmary, for example, began its scheme in 1920 by urging local workers to match hospital supporters in Leicester, who had raised £30,000.[135] Financial crisis galvanised activity in Winchester from 1920, as the Royal Hants' burgeoning overdraft prompted the hospital's bankers to ask for title deeds and share certificates as collateral. With ward closures in prospect, treasurer Leonard Keyser addressed the local Labour Party and trades council proposing an 'insurance scheme', under which those covered would be excused a new maintenance charge for patients.[136] At Gloucestershire Royal Infirmary the managers in 1922 despaired of increasing the number of its charitable subscribers, since the 'altered condi-tions of living forbade hope of obtaining a permanent addition'.[137] They duly initiated a workmen's (*sic*) contributory scheme, building on the pre-existing Saturday fund and workplace contributions.[138]

Edinburgh Royal Infirmary also illustrates the importance of specific internal factors encouraging joint action by managers and labour leaders. Pressures for a greater working-class presence on the management board had built during the war, and in 1917 this representation was increased to include two members of the local trades council and four from miners' associations of Lothian, Fife and Kinross.[139] As a *quid pro quo* the trades council was asked to raise subscriptions and discussions began about organising 'groups of systematic contributors … in every workshop, factory, warehouse and business establishment in the city'.[140] Meetings held between the trades council and the Infirmary discussed running the scheme through the trades unions, before it was decided to establish a more broadly based 'League of Subscribers'.[141] The first collection was made in 1919, and it yielded £4,296 at a time when the Infirmary had a £12,000 overdraft and was selling reserves of stock.[142] By 1920 there were 50,000 contributors, representing, according to the annual report, a 'great awakening of the workers'.[143]

Such local initiatives, coupled with Cave and Onslow's approval, prompted other voluntary bodies to advocate contributory schemes as a route to salvation. In London the King's Fund moved quickly on Cave's recommendation, and in tandem with the local committee of the British Hospitals Association (BHA) it set up in 1922 a contributory scheme for London, the HSA. Sometimes erroneously titled the 'Hospital Savings Association', its purpose was to 'save' the hospitals, not to provide a vehicle for individual savings against the contingency of hospital admission. The depiction by the King's Fund's historian of its enthusiastic support for the formation of the HSA is not entirely accurate. Members of its general council feared it would undermine private practitioners by boosting hospital utilisation, and that by encouraging self-interested rather than altruistic motives for hospital support it would be a 'desecration of the memory of King Edward'. Indeed, the HSA was from the outset managed independently of the Fund.[144] The Joint Council of the Order of St John and the British Red Cross, which had a similar advocacy and information-gathering role for provincial hospitals, also endorsed the new movement, and urged in 1923 that any hospital governors still without a scheme should 'initiate one without delay and push it with all the power at their command'.[145] Sir Napier Burnett, its director of hospital services, suggested hospitals alter their publicity materials so that they might be 'revisualised by the public ... as the great health centre of the community'.[146] In a similar vein, the standard reference book for hospital administrators in the 1920s, Stone's *Hospital organization and management*, epitomised the new thinking. It was to the schemes, Stone urged, 'that hospitals must look more and more in the future for their ever-increasing needs'. And the sure result of mass contribution had been to alter 'the character of the voluntary system from the maintenance by the rich for the benefit of the poor to maintenance by the masses for their own good'.[147]

Conclusion

This chapter has examined the emergence of workers' contributory funds and charted their development into the inter-war period. Limited workshop collections occurred in the early nineteenth century, but it was in the mid-Victorian period that workers' funding became a significant aspect of hospital support. The establishment of organised collecting funds to address the financial shortfalls of the 1870s saw these unsystematic contributions formalised, most notably in the Hospital Saturday funds. However, before the First World War the sums provided from this source were, for most hospitals, not a large component of total income. This began to change from 1918, when the long-term tendency of hospital expenditure to grow faster than its traditional sources of charitable income was exacerbated by a short-term post-war funding crisis.

Although a greater role for state funding was proposed, either through local authorities or NHI, Britain's commitment to the ideology of voluntary welfare provision ensured its rejection. Instead, policy-makers encouraged the growth of contributory schemes as the salvation of the system, while concurrently hospital managers enthusiastically adopted this course.

The result was that in the 1920s and 1930s working-class contribution became an essential element of the hospital system, and in many institutions provided the core of their funding. This signified a major shift in the nature of the voluntary hospitals, which could no longer be regarded as charities for the poor. Now they were increasingly funded by those who expected to use them, and this raised expectations of entitlement and control. The schemes were also characterised by structural and procedural diversity, at a time when policy-makers were starting to consider the need for regional organisation of the health system.[148] Inherent in the growth of mass contribution, then, was a set of new problems, concerning entitlement, representation and the schemes' role within a national hospital system. It is to these issues that the next chapters turn.

Notes

1   B. Abel-Smith, *The hospitals 1800–1948: a study in social administration in England and Wales* (London, 1964); J. E. Stone, *Hospital organization and management (including planning and construction)* (London, 1927), pp. 11–12.

2   M. A. Crowther, *The workhouse system 1834–1929: the history of an English social institution* (London, 1981), pp. 156–67; J. Brotherston, 'Scottish health services in the nineteenth century', in G. McLachlan (ed.), *Improving the common weal: aspects of Scottish health services 1900–1984* (Edinburgh, 1987), pp. 26–7.

3   M. Daunton, *Progress and poverty: an economic and social history of Britain 1700–1850* (Oxford, 1995), pp. 452–3; A. Brundage, *The English poor laws, 1700–1930* (Basingstoke, 2002), pp. 75–81; S. Hussey, '"An inheritance of fear": older women in the twentieth-century countryside', in P. Thane and L. Botelho (eds), *Women and ageing in British society since 1500* (Harlow, 2001), pp. 186–206. In Scotland the Poor Law Amendment Act was passed in 1845.

4   A. Hardy, *Health and medicine in Britain since 1860* (Basingstoke, 2001), pp. 16–17; S. Sheard, 'Reluctant providers? The politics and ideology of municipal hospital finance, 1870–1914', in S. Sheard and M. Gorsky (eds), *Financing medicine: the British experience since 1750* (London, forthcoming, 2006); Brotherston, 'Scottish health service', pp. 5–34, at p. 28.

5   J. M. Eyler, 'Scarlet fever and confinement: the Edwardian debate over isolation hospitals', *Bulletin of the History of Medicine*, 61 (1987), pp. 1–24, at p. 8.

6   J. Pickstone, *Medicine and industrial society* (Manchester, 1985), p. 11; L. Granshaw, '"Fame and fortune by means of bricks and mortar": the medical profession and specialist hospitals in Britain, 1800–1948', in L. Granshaw and R. Porter (eds), *The hospital in history* (London, 1989), pp. 199–220; R. Porter, 'The gift relation: philanthropy and provincial hospitals in eighteenth-century England', in L. Granshaw and R. Porter (eds), *The hospital in history* (London, 1989), pp. 149–78, at pp. 159–61; S. Cherry, 'Change and continuity in the cottage hospitals c. 1859–1948: the experience of East Anglia', *Medical History*, 36 (1992), pp. 271–89; J. Woodward, *To do the sick no harm: a study of the British voluntary hospital system to 1875* (London, 1974), pp. 12–13, 17–18, 149–52.

7   A. Borsay, "'Persons of honour and reputation": the voluntary hospital in an age of corruption', *Medical History*, 35 (1991), pp. 281–94.
8   M. Fissell, *Patients, power and the poor in eighteenth century Bristol* (Cambridge, 1991), p. 74; Porter, 'The gift relation', pp. 154–5; M. Gorsky, *Patterns of philanthropy: charity and society in nineteenth century Bristol* (Woodbridge, 1999), pp. 198–9.
9   Gorsky, *Patterns of philanthropy*, p. 200; P. Shapely, 'Charity, status and leadership: charitable image and the Manchester man', *Journal of Social History*, 32 (1998), pp. 157–77.
10 G. B. Risse, *Mending bodies, saving souls: a history of hospitals* (Oxford, 1999), pp. 231–6; Woodward, *To do the sick no harm*, pp. 38–9.
11 Fissell, *Patients, power and the poor*, pp. 87, 113–15; F. B. Smith, *The people's health 1830–1910* (London, 1979), pp. 254–5.
12 Fissell, *Patients, power and the poor*, pp. 81–6; Risse, *Mending bodies*, pp. 233, 236; Woodward, *To do the sick no harm*, pp. 151–2.
13 H. Marland, 'Lay and medical conceptions of medical charity during the nineteenth century', in J. Barry and C. Jones (eds), *Medicine and charity before the welfare state* (London, 1991), pp. 149–71.
14 K. Waddington, *Charity and the London hospitals, 1850–1898* (Woodbridge, 2000), pp. 30–1; Fissell, *Patients, power and the poor*, pp. 74, 85, ch. 5; A. Digby, *Making a medical living: doctors and patients in the English market for medicine, 1720–1911* (Cambridge, 1994), p. 86.
15 Fissell, *Patients, power and the poor*, pp. 117, 136–7.
16 Hampshire Record Office (HRO), 5M63/199, County Hospital at Winchester, annual report, 1811; Birmingham City Archives (BCA), Birmingham General Hospital, annual report, 1810–11.
17 F. M. Eden, *The state of the poor*, abridged, ed. A. G. L. Rogers (London, 1928), p. 327; figures refer to the 1790s.
18 A. Berry, 'Community sponsorship and the hospital patient in late eighteenth century England', in P. Horden and R. Smith (eds), *The locus of care: families, communities, institutions and the provision of welfare since antiquity* (London, 1998), pp. 126–50.
19 S. Cherry, 'Hospital Saturday, workplace collections and issues in late nineteenth century hospital funding', *Medical History*, 44 (2000), pp. 461–88, at p. 471. Alannah Tomkins' discovery of an employees' scheme founded at the North Staffordshire Infirmary in 1815 came too late for inclusion in this chapter. See A. Tomkins, '"The excellent example of the working class": contributory schemes and the North Staffordshire Infirmary from 1815', paper given at the conference Apothecaries, Art and Architecture: Interpreting Georgian Medicine, Apothecaries' Hall, London, November 2005.
20 Tyne and Wear Archive Service (TWAS), HO/RVI, Newcastle Royal Infirmary, annual reports, 1801, 1811, 1821.
21 BCA, Birmingham General Hospital, annual report, 1826–27.
22 Mitchell Library, Glasgow (ML), HB 14/2/1, 'A list of the qualified contributors &c. to the Royal Infirmary Glasgow', 1 January 1812.
23 ML, Glasgow Royal Infirmary, annual report, 1830.
24 ML, Glasgow Royal Infirmary, annual reports, 1831, 1832.
25 ML, Glasgow Royal Infirmary, annual reports, 1830, 1832.
26 ML, Glasgow Royal Infirmary, annual reports, 1833, 1838.
27 Bristol Record Office (BRO), 35893(21)e, Bristol Infirmary, annual reports, 1846, 1847, 1852.
28 BRO, 35893(21)e, Bristol Infirmary, annual report, 1851.
29 ML, Glasgow Royal Infirmary, annual reports, 1833, 1838.
30 TWAS, HO/SRI/63/1, Sunderland Royal Infirmary, annual report, 1861.
31 TWAS, HO/SRI/1/4, General committee, 20 March 1861; TWAS, HO/SRI/63/1, Sunderland Royal Infirmary, annual report, 1902.
32 TWAS, HO/SRI/1/4, Special court of governors, General committee, special committee, 17 November 1864; TWAS, HO/SRI/1/5, Half-yearly court of governors, 24 February 1870.

33　*Sunderland Herald*, 19 July 1867.
34　TWAS, HO/SRI/1/4, General committee, 6 June 1872.
35　TWAS, HO/SRI/63/1, Sunderland Royal Infirmary, annual reports, 1873, 1875, 1881.
36　W. D. Rubinstein, 'The size and distribution of the English middle classes in 1860', *Historical Research*, 61 (1988), pp. 65–89, at pp. 83, 89.
37　TWAS, HO/SRI/63/1, Sunderland Royal Infirmary, annual reports, 1861, 1902.
38　TWAS, HO/SRI/1/4, Special court of governors, 17 November 1864.
39　*Sunderland Times*, 16 July 1875.
40　J. Benson, 'Coalowners, coalminers and compulsion: pit clubs in England, 1860–80', *Business History*, 44 (2002), pp. 47–60.
41　Risse, *Mending bodies*, p. 234; Stone, *Hospital organization*, p. 599.
42　K. Waddington, *Charity and the London hospitals*, pp. 51–6; K. Waddington, 'Bastard benevolence: centralisation, voluntarism and the Sunday Fund 1873–1898', *London Journal*, 19 (1995), pp. 151–67.
43　H. C. Burdett, *Hospital Sunday and Hospital Saturday: their origins, progress and development* (London, 1884), pp. 7–10; Stone, *Hospital organization*, pp. 598–9.
44　H. C. Burdett, *Burdett's hospitals and charities, 1926* (hereafter *Burdett's*) (London, 1926), pp. xxiv–xxv.
45　Waddington, *Charity and the London hospitals*, pp. 56, 67–8.
46　*Ibid.*, pp. 50–1.
47　*Ibid.*, p. 68.
48　A. T. Page, *Pennies for health: the story of the British Hospitals Contributory Schemes Association* (Birmingham, 1949), pp. 36–44; *Burdett's* (1914), pp. 137–8; where these two sources differ on foundation year the earlier is recorded, on the assumption that later dates might represent the reconstitution of existing bodies.
49　H. C. Burdett, *Hospitals and asylums of the world, vol. III: Hospitals – history and administration* (London, 1893), pp. 121–9.
50　A. Teebon, *The history of three Nottingham welfare schemes* (Nottingham, n.d. but 1970s), pp. 1–5.
51　BCA, General Hospital Birmingham, minute book no. 3, 1869–1925, annual board of governors, 17 September 1873.
52　Birmingham Local Studies Library (BLSL), LF4663, Hospital Saturday fund, Birmingham, collection of newspaper cuttings etc. 1873–1891; *Birmingham Daily Post*, 8 January 1873, 13 June 1873.
53　HRO, 5M63/155, Royal Hampshire County Hospital, annual report, 1882/83.
54　HRO, 5M63/156, Royal Hampshire County Hospital, annual report, 1895/96.
55　Wolverhampton Archives and Local Studies (WALS), Royal Hospital Wolverhampton, annual report, 1938.
56　WALS, Royal Hospital Wolverhampton, annual report, 1845/49.
57　WALS, Royal Hospital Wolverhampton, annual report, 1851.
58　WALS, Royal Hospital Wolverhampton, annual report, 1869.
59　WALS, Royal Hospital Wolverhampton, annual report, 1872; Mason, *For whom we serve: a brief history* (Wolverhampton, 1984), pp. 8–9.
60　*Midland Counties Evening Express*, 2 November 1874.
61　*Burdett's* (1914), p. 130.
62　S. Cherry, 'The role of the English provincial voluntary general hospitals in the 18th and 19th centuries', unpublished PhD thesis, University of East Anglia (1976), pp. 170–1; Smith, *The people's health*, pp. 278–82; K. Waddington, '"Grasping gratitude": charity and hospital finance in late-Victorian London', in M. Daunton (ed.), *Charity, self-interest and welfare in the English past* (London, 1996), pp. 181–202.
63　M. Gorsky, M. Powell and J. Mohan, 'British voluntary hospitals and the public sphere', in S. Sturdy (ed.), *Medicine, health and the public sphere in Britain, 1600–2000* (London, 2002), pp. 129–30.
64　BCA, Birmingham General Hospital, annual report, 1861/62.
65　BRO, 35893(21)h, Bristol Royal Infirmary, annual report, 1884.

66   Benson, 'Coalowners, coalminers and compulsion', pp. 47–60.
67   Pickstone, *Medicine and industrial society*, pp. 144–5, 154.
68   *Bristol Mercury*, 11 and 18 January 1868.
69   BCA, Birmingham General Hospital, annual report, 1861/62.
70   B. Harris, *The origins of the British welfare state: social welfare in England and Wales, 1800–1945* (Basingstoke, 2004), pp. 82–3.
71   P. Gosden, *The friendly societies in England 1815–75* (Manchester, 1961), pp. 138–49.
72   G. D. H. Cole, *A short history of the British working class movement 1789–1947* (1948 edn) (Watford, 1966 reprint), pp. 139–78; H. Southall and E. Garrett, 'Morbidity and mortality among early-nineteenth century engineering workers', *Social History of Medicine*, 4 (1991), pp. 231–52.
73   G. Crossick, *An artisan elite in Victorian Society: Kentish London, 1840–1880* (London, 1978), ch. 9; S. Cordery, 'Friendly societies and the discourse of respectability in Britain, 1825–1875', *Journal of British Studies*, 34 (1995), pp. 35–58.
74   N. Doran, 'Risky business: codifying embodied experience in the Manchester Unity of Odd-fellows', *Journal of Historical Sociology*, 7 (1994), pp. 131–54; A. Labisch, 'Doctors, workers and the scientific cosmology of the industrial world: the social construction of "health" and the "homo hygienicus"', *Journal of Contemporary History*, 20 (1985), pp. 599–615.
75   S. Yeo, *Religion and voluntary organisations in crisis* (London, 1976), pp. 211–17.
76   J. Benson, *The rise of consumer society in Britain, 1880–1980* (London, 1994), pp. 12–13.
77   J. Jenkinson, M. Moss and I. Russell, *The Royal: the history of Glasgow Royal Infirmary 1794–1994* (Glasgow, 1994), pp. 120–1.
78   Total income £56,315: *Burdett's* (1901), p. 171.
79   *Burdett's* (1911), pp. 82–5.
80   In addition to pay beds this includes a small amount earned through home nursing services and nurse training fees.
81   R. Stevens, *In sickness and in wealth: American hospitals in the twentieth century* (2nd edn) (Baltimore, 1989), pp. 18–39.
82   Cherry, 'Hospital Saturday', pp. 478–80.
83   Burdett, *Hospital Sunday*, pp. 18–19, 22–5.
84   King Edward's Hospital Fund for London, *Statistical report … for the year 1914* (London, 1915).
85   Cherry, 'Hospital Saturday', pp. 486–7.
86   Pickstone, *Medicine and industrial society*, pp. 142–5; Cherry, 'Hospital Saturday', pp. 472–3.
87   BRO, 35893 (21) e,h,k, Bristol Royal Infirmary, annual reports, 1847, 1884, 1911.
88   WALS, Wolverhampton Royal Hospital, annual reports, 1851, 1891, 1922.
89   Pickstone, *Medicine and industrial society*, p. 146.
90   TWAS, HO/RVI, Newcastle Royal Infirmary, annual report, 1888.
91   G. Haliburton Hume, *The history of the Newcastle Infirmary* (Newcastle upon Tyne, 1906), pp. 82–91.
92   TWAS, HO/SRI/1/4, General committee, 20 March 1861.
93   TWAS, HO/SRI/63/1, Sunderland Royal Infirmary, annual report, 1873; TWAS, HO/SRI/1/6, General committee, 1 March 1877; *Sunderland Times*, 25 July 1873.
94   TWAS, HO/SRI/63/1, Sunderland Royal Infirmary, annual reports, 1875, 1877, 1888.
95   Based on an electronic version of data from Burdett's yearbooks. For further details, contact John Mohan.
96   Teebon, *Nottingham welfare schemes*, pp. 6–7.
97   S. D. Slater and D. Dow (eds), *The Victoria Infirmary of Glasgow 1890–1900: a centenary history* (Glasgow, 1990), p. 17.
98   Jenkinson *et al.*, *The Royal*, p. 154.
99   Teebon, *Nottingham welfare schemes*, pp. 6–7.
100 TWAS, HO/SRI/1/6, General committee, 2 September 1875, 4 May 1876, 1 June 1876; TWAS, HO/SRI/1/6, Annual court, 24 July 1879; *Sunderland Times*, 25 July

1873, 16 July 1875; *Sunderland Daily Echo*, 3 August 1882; TWAS, HO/SRI/63/1, Sunderland Royal Infirmary, annual report, 1882.

101 *Burdett's* (1914, 1916, 1919).
102 Teebon, *Nottingham welfare schemes*, p. 16.
103 TWAS, HO/VIR/72/95, Royal Victoria Infirmary, annual report, 1916.
104 *Burdett's* (1915, 1917).
105 M. Gorsky and J. Mohan, 'London's voluntary hospitals in the inter-war period: growth, transformation or crisis?', *Nonprofit and Voluntary Sector Quarterly*, 30 (2001), pp. 247–75, at pp. 252–5.
106 TNA: PRO, MH/58/204, Evidence to the Cave committee, 5th day, Vernor Miles; *British Medical Journal*, 30 July 1921, p. 163.
107 E. Roberts, 'The recipients' view of welfare', in J. Bornat, R. Perks, P. Thompson and J. Walmsley (eds), *Oral history, health and welfare* (London, 2000), pp. 203–26, at pp. 214–15, 217, 223; *British Medical Journal*, 30 July 1921, p. 163.
108 W. Macpherson, *History of the Great War: medical services general history* (London, 1921), pp. 82–3.
109 F. Prochaska, *Philanthropy and the hospitals of London: the King's Fund, 1897–1990* (Oxford, 1992), p. 81.
110 S. Tomkins, 'The failure of expertise: public health policy in Britain during the 1918–19 influenza epidemic', *Social History of Medicine*, 5 (1992), pp. 435–54, at pp. 441–2; BRO, 35893(21)n, Bristol Royal Infirmary, annual report, 1918.
111 *Lancet*, 1 January 1921, p. 41–2; *Lancet*, 18 June 1921, p. 1311.
112 Prochaska, *Philanthropy and the hospitals of London*, pp. 92–3.
113 Ministry of Health, Voluntary Hospitals Committee, *Final report*, Cmd 1335 (London, 1921).
114 Stone, *Hospital organization*, p. 46.
115 TNA: PRO, MH/58/204, 'Evidence to the Cave committee', day 5, Vernor Miles (Hampstead General and North-West London Hospitals), day 15, Charles Irwin (Royal Victoria Infirmary, Newcastle upon Tyne), day 17, T. Ratcliff (Birmingham General Hospital).
116 *Ibid.*, Irwin.
117 F. Colchester-Wemyss, 'Contributory schemes', in F. Menzies (ed.), *The voluntary hospitals in Great Britain (excluding London): fifth annual report for the year 1923* (London, 1924), p. 101.
118 TNA: PRO, MH/58/204, Cave committee, evidence, days 12, 13.
119 *Ibid.*, Ratcliff.
120 Ministry of Health, Voluntary Hospitals Committee, *Interim report*, Cmd 1206 (London, 1921).
121 B. Gilbert, *The evolution of national insurance in Great Britain: the origins of the welfare state* (1966 edn) (Aldershot, 1993 reprint), pp. 389–94.
122 *Ibid.*, pp. 314–16; E. P. Hennock, *British social reform and its German precedents: the case of social insurance 1880–1914* (Oxford, 1987), pp. 173–8, 184–5, 190–1, 213; L. Bryder, *Below the magic mountain: a social history of tuberculosis in twentieth-century Britain* (Oxford, 1988), pp. 36–41.
123 Gilbert, *National insurance*, pp. 391–2.
124 Ministry of Health, Voluntary Hospitals Committee, *Interim report*. It was the perceived urgency of proffering this advice, before the approved societies formulated other schemes for utilising their surpluses, which prompted the issuing of the *Interim report*; *Lancet*, 25 April 1921, p. 867; *Lancet*, 18 June 1921, p. 1311.
125 Stone, *Hospital organization*, pp. 46–7; *British Medical Journal*, 30 July 1921, pp. 261–3; *Lancet*, 20 August 1921, pp. 293–4.
126 Stone, *Hospital organization*, pp. 206–7.
127 Political and Economic Planning (PEP), *Report on the British health services* (London, 1937), pp. 285–6.
128 *Ibid.*, p. 206. The bulk of the benefits were paid towards dental (£2,473,236) and ophthalmic (£613,254) costs.

129 London Metropolitan Archives (LMA), H9/GY/A94, Guy's Hospital, annual report, 1937.
130 Ministry of Health, Voluntary Hospitals Committee, *Final report*, p. 19, and see paras 29–35.
131 VHC, *Report on voluntary hospital accommodation in England and Wales*, Cmd 2486 (London, 1925).
132 TNA: PRO, MH 58/177, H. N. Crouch to Minister of Health, 20 November 1923.
133 VHC, *Contributory schemes* (London, 1923).
134 TNA: PRO, MH 58/200, Minute sheet, Brock to Onslow, 19 July 1923, Onslow to Brock, 22 July 1923.
135 Warneford Hospital Archives Room, Oxford, Radcliffe Infirmary and County Hospital Oxford, annual report, 1920.
136 B. Carpenter Turner, *A history of the Royal Hampshire County Hospital* (Chichester, 1986), p. 106; HRO, 5M63/155, Royal Hampshire County Hospital, annual report, 1921.
137 Gloucester Record Office (GRO), HO19/8/6, Gloucestershire Royal Infirmary, annual report, 1922.
138 GRO, HO19/8/6, Gloucestershire Royal Infirmary, annual reports, 1918, 1925.
139 Lothian Health Services Archive (University of Edinburgh Library) (LHSA), LHB 1/1/55, Royal Infirmary, Minute book, 22 October 1917.
140 LHSA, LHB 1/1/56, Royal Infirmary, Minute book, 22 July 1918.
141 LHSA, LHB 1/1/55, Royal Infirmary, Minute book, 25 February, 22 July 1918.
142 LHSA, LHB 1/1/55, Royal Infirmary, Minute book, 14 January 1918; LHSA, LHB 1/1/56, Royal Infirmary, Minute book, 23 December 1918.
143 LHSA, Edinburgh Royal Infirmary, annual reports, 1918–24, *passim*.
144 Prochaska, *Philanthropy and the hospitals of London*, pp. 103–4; King Edward's Hospital Fund for London, annual report, 1922, p. 7.
145 Stone, *Hospital organization*, p. 231; Colchester-Wemyss, 'Contributory schemes', p. 103.
146 N. Burnett, *Third annual report of the voluntary hospitals of Great Britain (excluding London) for the year 1921* (Joint Council of the Order of St John and the British Red Cross, held at the Museum and Library of the Order of St John), p. 6.
147 Stone, *Hospital organization*. Joseph Stone was accountant to St Thomas's Hospital and regularly lectured and wrote on hospital finance and management. See the *Hospital Gazette*, March 1921, p. 87; *ibid.*, June 1924, p. 123; the passages quoted, from his 1927 chapter on contributory schemes, are identical to those in a 1924 paper entitled 'The changing character of the voluntary system' by C. A. Mason, secretary to the Midland Eye Hospital, Birmingham, in the *Hospital Gazette*, July 1924, p. 137.
148 D. Fox, *Health policies, health politics: the British and American experience, 1911–1965* (Princeton, NJ, 1986).

Chapter 3

Mass contribution and hospital finance in inter-war Britain

This chapter traces the development of contributory schemes in the inter-war period and seeks to assess the overall impact that they had on hospital finances. First, the heterogeneous nature of the schemes is outlined: there were single-hospital schemes as well as multi-institutional or city-wide funds; contributory schemes can be distinguished from provident ones (the predecessors of private medical insurance); and those premised on user fees may be differentiated from those supporting an 'open door' policy. The growth of membership and of income, and the developing pattern of benefits paid and other expenditure, are then charted. In the case of the multi-hospital funds, an important issue is the criteria which were used in reimbursing hospitals, which raised questions about whether appropriate incentive structures were in place to stimulate efficiency. Finally, there is an assessment of the aggregate impact of the schemes on hospital finances, and of the extent to which the schemes both enabled hospitals to treat more patients and stimulated demand for hospital services. These various analyses permit a fuller evaluation of how successful the schemes were in enhancing the financial position of the hospitals.

The nature of the contributory schemes in the inter-war years

The sheer diversity of the hospital contributory schemes often attracted comment. Some schemes were administered directly by hospitals themselves, while others were operated by separate organisations, sometimes pre-existing Saturday funds, but also newly constituted bodies. There were in addition substantial variations with respect to internal organisation, subscriptions, representation on local hospital boards, expectations of treatment and attitudes to entitlement.

One key issue was whether contributions went to a single hospital or were pooled between those within a given locale. In theory the principle of a shared distribution between institutions had been the factor which originally differentiated Saturday funds from earlier contributory arrangements. However, it was still the case that both long-established schemes, such as that at Newcastle upon Tyne's Royal Victoria Infirmary, and newer ones (many founded in the early 1920s), such as that run by the Royal Hampshire Hospital in Winchester, were geared to only one hospital.[1] Judging by the names of the schemes recorded in the *Hospitals yearbooks* during the 1930s, the vast majority (over 90 per cent) were associated with a single hospital. Moreover, many schemes were very small; of 242 schemes in mainland Britain reporting membership figures for 1938, 126 had fewer than 10,000 contributors, and, of these, 86 had fewer than 5,000.[2] These schemes almost certainly depended on the voluntary effort of a small number of committed individuals, which was bound to set limits on their ability to expand beyond a certain size.

At the other end of the spectrum, much of the total membership is accounted for by multi-hospital funds, mostly established in the twentieth century, some of which had several hundred thousand contributors. Such developments reflected a trend towards collaboration between voluntary institutions, which had initially developed spontaneously, as in Glasgow for example, where the Joint Consultative Committee of the Royal, Western and Victoria Infirmaries was formed in 1910.[3] Such *ad hoc* developments began to be formalised in the inter-war period, following the constitution by the Cave committee of local voluntary hospital committees to act as distribution agents for the post-war state grant (see chapter 2). Other duties involved coordinating appeals, joint purchasing, systematising patient transfers and organising contributory arrangements.[4] Such committees, often known as hospitals councils, were often short-lived, but local elites in a few large cities saw the benefits of continuing with joint bodies.[5]

The most fully researched of these is the Sheffield Hospitals Council (SHC), developed by a group of doctors, academics and civic leaders,[6] but there were some similar organisations. Proposals for collaboration reflected several motivations: concerns at deficiencies in and the poor quality of hospital accommodation; a desire to overcome inter-hospital rivalries; and the promotion of medical teamwork and specialisation through greater integration of hospital services. The importance of obtaining a systematic and reliable source of funding provided a further motivation, not least because of plans for hospital reorganisation and reconstruction, such as the Birmingham Hospitals Centre. The result was the establishment of several city-wide coordinating bodies, with their associated multi-institutional contributory schemes governed by a contributors' association. For example, the Sheffield and Birmingham hospitals councils established associations of contributors which were responsible for fundraising, while the councils dealt with questions of relationships between hospitals. The Birmingham Hospital Contributory Association (BHCA) had 700,000 members by 1938. The Merseyside Hospitals Council (MHC), with 250,000 members, was slightly different, in that it was constituted primarily as a contributory scheme, though it also had a contributors' association, and a 'hospitals organisation committee' that dealt with service coordination. The largest multi-institutional scheme was the London-based HSA, though here contributors had only minority representation on the governing body and there was no controlling hospitals council.

The schemes formed the BHCSA in 1931, following the first national conference of contributory schemes in 1930. This was inspired by the Birmingham

Hospitals Council;[7] the first BHCSA president was Bertram Ford (managing director of Birmingham Newspapers) and its honorary secretary was T. W. Place, respectively chair and secretary of the Birmingham scheme, and its executive also included the secretaries of the Sheffield, Liverpool and Leeds funds.[8] Early discussion at the Association was dominated by the issues which these large schemes confronted.[9] The core problem was how to reconcile the local, voluntarist base of contribution with the need for a regional, and indeed national, hospital system; debate therefore covered issues such as territorial disputes between schemes, the development of reciprocal arrangements between schemes for reimbursement of hospitals, and the position to adopt towards the rapidly improving municipal hospitals.[10] The focus in the 1930s was therefore on the resolution of practical administrative concerns; the Association did not, at this stage, press the case for contributory schemes in the national policy arena. However, John Dodd, a leading figure in the movement (he became secretary of the BHCSA after positions in the Merseyside and Bristol funds) argued that even in this capacity the BHCSA had found it difficult to persuade its members to adopt recommendations, and that meetings had been dominated by small schemes, which had aired 'parochial grievances'.[11] There were also concerns that the BHCSA should not have been established as a separate organisation but should, instead, have been an integral part of the BHA, the representative body for the voluntary hospitals.[12] It is at least arguable that this left the BHCSA in a weak position when proposals for the NHS were being debated in wartime (see chapters 7 and 8).

In terms of the practicalities of scheme organisation, subscriptions were usually deducted from wages, while arrangements for the self-employed ranged from the provision of collecting boxes to the use of a card which was stamped on payment.[13] Contribution levels varied, with 2*d* or 3*d* per week a common sum payable, and many schemes operated a graded scale.[14] In Sheffield, workers gave 1*d* for each £1 of their weekly earnings (hence it was dubbed locally the 'penny in the pound' scheme); we do not have data on typical wage levels in individual industries in Sheffield at that time, but one estimate was that some 25 per cent of the city's labour force earned under £2 10*s* per week, while 62 per cent earned between £2 10*s* and £5 per week.[15] The self-employed were charged a flat rate of £1 per annum.[16] The London-based HSA required 12*s* per annum if paid in advance, or 13*s* per annum if paid weekly (3*d* per week), while members aged under eighteen years paid 2*d* per week, but there was no differentiation of contribution rates according to income.[17] The Royal Hampshire's scheme charged 2*d* per week for adult wage earners and 1*d* for their dependent children, while the 'small traders and those of moderate means' paid 10*s* 6*d* per annum for an adult and 5*s* for a child.[18] Differentials in levels of contribution to the North Riding Infirmary in Middlesbrough (either 2*d* or 3*d* per week) were justified because 'all works do not entail the same risks'.[19] At the upper end of the scale were the explicitly 'provident' schemes which specified particular benefits and were aimed at the lower middle classes. Thus the Sussex Provident Scheme asked £1 per annum from single subscribers, rising to £2 from married couples with children under sixteen.[20] Members

were entitled to free treatment in the most appropriate of eight general and
special hospitals in Brighton, Hove and Chichester, with X-rays, laboratory
work and vaccines also included, along with domiciliary visits by consultants.[21]
This was effectively an insurance scheme, although members were not entitled
to precedence over urgent admissions.[22] Indeed, immediate admission was a
rarity, offered by only three of the schemes examined by the VHC.[23]

What entitlements did scheme membership bring? It must be stressed that
it brought no automatic right to hospital admission; hospital doctors remained
in control of admission decisions, which were based purely on clinical need,
though some evidence implies that scheme members made above-average
use of hospital services (see below, 'Effect of the contributory schemes on
hospital finances and activity'). The standard 'privilege' was admission for
treatment without any charge being made.[24] Most hospitals had a standard
maintenance charge which patients would be required to pay if they were not
a contributory scheme member, though a sliding scale which took income
into account was typically operated.[25] Thus, on entry to the hospital, patients
would be quizzed by an almoner, who would excuse them from the charge on
production of evidence of either scheme membership or that they were on a
very low income. Others would pay. In Gloucester, for example, non-scheme
patients were charged 'in conformity with their means', up to 14s per week
for maintenance.[26] At the North Lonsdale in Barrow-in-Furness the rate for
non-contributors was 6d per day.[27] The Royal Northern in London aimed to
cater even more precisely to the social spectrum of its catchment. In 1923 it
opened private wards, in which the full cost of maintenance and treatment
was charged, at 18s per day, 'contributory wards', where patients paid on a
sliding scale from two to four guineas, and general wards, which were free
to the poor but otherwise cost between 1s and 20s, according to the patient's
circumstances.[28] At the same time, a system of contributors' certificates was
introduced, whereby scheme members received a certificate valid for ten years
to the full value of their contribution, which could then be presented in lieu of
payment.[29] Once again, there were many variations on this theme. In hospitals
which still used subscribers' admission notes the schemes were sometimes
issued with these to distribute to members as required: this was effectively a
'pre-vetting' system.[30]

In contrast, there remained some schemes which were committed to an
'open door' policy. These were mostly single-hospital funds in Scotland and the
North East of England, which had no fixed rate of contribution and resolutely
refused to adopt means testing. We show in chapter 5 how such schemes
rejected the standard English model and were able to ensure that all patients
would be admitted without charge.[31] Finally, in addition to hospital benefits,
some schemes offered dental treatment and access to convalescence care as
extra incentives.[32]

With respect to coverage of dependants, some two-thirds of the schemes
surveyed in the early 1920s included the free maintenance of wives and children,
while the remainder levied some additional payment.[33] The HSA, which had
comparatively high contribution rates, illustrates the former approach: it

extended its benefits to wives and children and to any other co-resident and dependent kin.[34] By contrast, in Gloucester contributors paid 2*d* per week, but they could secure coverage for their wives by increasing this to 3*d*, while the children of contributors were treated at half the charge which was set by the almoner according to means.[35] The Oxford scheme allowed free treatment for old age pensioners and children, though as soon as children became wage earners they were expected to contribute, initially at half the adult rate.[36] Several schemes offered lower rates of contribution to widows, pensioners and people with a disability.[37]

The schemes were designed to attract those on low incomes but the medical profession was concerned that doctors' earnings would be threatened if people enrolled in the schemes who were wealthy enough to afford to purchase medical services privately. The response was to specify a maximum income limit for membership. The upper end is illustrated by the Sussex Provident Scheme, which was open to single people earning up to £260 per annum, and to families with children up to £500; clearly, this brought hospital insurance well within the reach of the lower middle class.[38] The HSA pitched its maximum lower, at £208 for adults and £312 for families. However, it also allowed those earning above these sums to become 'honorary contributors', at the cost of £1 per annum, which conferred the right to reimbursement of hospital costs up to a maximum of £10, as well as the standard dental, ophthalmic and convalescent home benefits.[39] A few schemes used the NHI or income tax thresholds, but more commonly (in 67 per cent of cases) no precise limit was imposed, and it seems that the better-off were simply trusted not to exploit the situation.[40]

As income levels rose, schemes had to consider the question of how best to address the needs of those deemed 'middle-class patients'. The Birmingham fund is illustrative. Initially, the scheme had accepted that better-off white-collar workers were bound to enter under the 'general section', but that it remained the hospitals' right to make an additional charge on contributors they considered able to afford it. In such cases members entering pay wards were allowed a rebate on their hospital bills from the fund.[41] Clearly, this approach still relied on the goodwill and honesty of better-off patients, and it was not long before the local branch of the British Medical Association (BMA) was complaining that the scheme's trust was being abused. In 1931, for example, doctors complained that patients who could well afford private practice were using the BHCA to obtain treatment at the dispensary and at out-patient departments.[42] More seriously, Birmingham Dental Hospital objected in 1932 that erstwhile private patients were now receiving their dental care under the scheme: it claimed to have had 7,000 new patients a year before the scheme began and 1,400 afterwards, and to have lost £2,000 per year in subscriptions as local firms had moved into the BHCA.[43] Birmingham's 'extended benefits' scheme did not precisely address these concerns about out-patients but it did signal to 'professional and business men and women' that there was an appropriate alternative to the main scheme.[44] It permitted members who paid a slightly higher rate to insure against charges of nursing homes or hospital pay wards, and by 1940 it had nearly 7,000 members.[45] The extended benefits scheme became one of the founder members of the British United Provident Association (BUPA), a new organisation formed to offer provident health insurance for those who wished to purchase medical care outside the NHS (see chapter 8).

Membership trends and income

Mass subscription became an essential element of hospital funding in the inter-war period. Figure 3.1 continues the earlier analysis (figure 2.2, p. 29) of the composition of hospital income up until 1935, at which point the data source merged contributory income with patients' payments for services. The London hospitals are excluded because the statistics collated by the King Edward's Hospital Fund for London failed to disaggregate Hospital Saturday income from other voluntary gifts. Given the comments on London made in chapter 2, the capital's omission here probably slightly inflates the overall significance of contributory schemes in comparison with charity and patients' payments. Note that the number of hospitals whose financial details were recorded in the *Hospitals yearbooks* changed over the sequence, from around 160 in 1914 to over 300 in the 1930s, but this does not affect the overall trends. Figure 3.1 is arranged slightly differently from figure 2.2: the comparatively minor sums from the King's Fund and Sunday collections are now included in the 'Other charity' category, along with donations and legacies; the 'Contributory' category includes sums recorded as either Hospital Saturday or workers' contributions. Patients' payments are presented separately from receipts for public services, effectively to show the hospitals' earnings from selling their services.[46]

Contributory income grew appreciably, rising from 12 per cent of all income in 1914 to 25 per cent by 1935. Indeed, figure 3.1 graphically depicts Burnett's image of the hospital in transition from charitable institution to 'health centre of the community'. By the mid-1930s the traditional forms of philanthropy

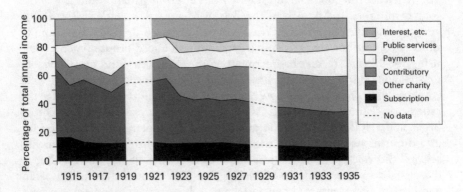

Figure 3.1. Composition of British voluntary hospital income (excluding London), 1914–35.

accounted for only one-third of all income, interest on capital supplied a further 10–15 per cent and the remainder was elicited in the form of various payments by users – local authority subventions, direct fees from patients or from contributory schemes, which one might see as a pre-payment plan (though this was disputed: see chapter 5). Finally, figure 3.1 also suggests that the early 1920s were a time of particular expansion; hospital income in general was increasing and the schemes were providing a growing proportion of it. Many new schemes were established and this trend continued in the inter-war years; in 1932, the *Hospitals yearbook* recorded 259 active contributory schemes in mainland Britain; by 1938 there were 388, and it appears that new formations were still occurring in wartime, as the 1942 *Hospitals yearbook* recorded 420 schemes.[47]

A different perspective on this expansion is offered in table 3.1, which draws on the income statistics of a consistent set of sixty-three large general hospitals which reported to the *Hospitals yearbook* in each year between 1926 and 1936, thereby overcoming the problem that the national summary totals did not always include the same institutions from year to year. The underlying data are the detailed income tables which only hospitals of a substantial size provided,[48] and all figures are adjusted to constant (1936) prices. In large general hospitals the significance of contributory schemes was much greater than the national totals would suggest: by 1926 scheme income far exceeded that from subscriptions, by 1936 it accounted for 34 per cent of total income, and over the eleven-year period it almost doubled in real terms. Receipts from patients' payments grew at a faster pace, but these began from a much lower base and even by the mid-1930s provided less than half the amount furnished by mass contribution, income from which assumed particular importance in

Table 3.1. Principal sources of income in a consistent set of large hospitals, England, Scotland and Wales, 1926–36

Year	Subscriptions	Other charity	Patients' payments	Contributory schemes	Interest	Public services	Total income
1926	293,777	718,404	181,577	685,395	339,521	178,632	2,404,665
1927	308,200	828,107	200,360	785,416	349,153	191,357	2,788,461
1928	302,957	767,771	213,918	850,228	366,697	179,344	2,709,517
1929	306,796	786,049	245,583	908,105	381,437	179,879	2,863,826
1930	313,778	809,053	278,957	944,847	400,008	193,608	2,980,126
1931	330,182	868,435	342,186	941,707	447,674	193,403	3,145,289
1932	325,498	931,437	386,272	1,045,174	467,600	183,477	3,402,018
1933	328,023	899,930	438,659	1,136,898	459,495	179,041	3,514,118
1934	331,132	934,879	473,319	1,215,425	470,312	172,059	3,652,900
1935	332,911	909,964	525,817	1,262,572	470,248	163,402	3,745,157
1936	329,582	895,575	556,702	1,316,697	464,345	145,469	3,832,221

Figures rebased to constant (1936) prices. Some minor sources of income are excluded.
Source: *Hospitals yearbooks*, 1926–36.

large provincial general hospitals. For general hospitals, on average, 33 per cent of their income was derived from contribution in 1936, compared with 11 per cent for specialist institutions. We cannot take this time series on beyond 1936 because of changes to the categorisation of income sources, but there is evidence that income from patients' payments (which, from 1936, included contributory schemes) continued to increase into the wartime years, although the impact varied for individual hospitals, presumably reflecting the effects of wartime relocation of firms and of mobilisation (serving soldiers were often permitted to retain membership but excused contribution).

As these income data imply, scheme membership grew rapidly in the inter-war years. The most reliable figures are probably those presented in the *Hospitals yearbooks*, which draw on returns made by the schemes themselves. There are also reports of the major schemes we have studied in more detail, though as contribution was organised mostly by workplace, it was unusual for the scheme administrator to know the precise total membership. The best available esti-mate of the peak level of total membership is around 11 million in 1942, the last year for which data were presented in the *Hospitals yearbooks*, although the BHCSA arrived at a similar figure for 1946.[49] Membership trends were dominated by the expansion of the large multi-hospital schemes; illustrative figures for five of the largest schemes (figure 3.2) are based on discontinuous data, but the general upward trend is clear enough (note that because of its size, the membership figures for the HSA are shown on the right-hand scale in figure 3.2). The main exception, a reduction in HSA membership in 1938–40, almost certainly reflects evacuation (not call-up: combatants continued to be treated as members, even if they were not in a position to pay subscriptions).

The resources generated by the schemes did not depend solely on the membership, because it was hoped that employers would recognise their

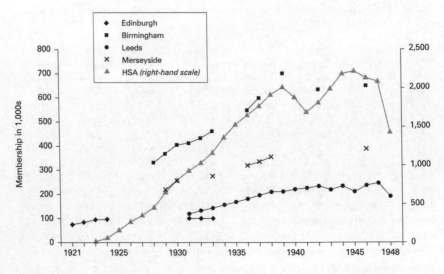

Figure 3.2. Growth in membership of major contributory schemes, 1921–48.

obligations to the community by making matching contributions. The Cave committee noted that though some employers gave generously, the majority were generally content with a small yearly subscription, which contrasted sharply with the enthusiasm of their workers.[50] Good examples of employer contribution included Sheffield, where employers (in theory) added one-third to their employees' subscriptions, and the 'Braime Scheme' in Leeds, an employers' fund which raised 2s per annum for each employee covered.[51] The Birmingham fund soon persuaded the city council to make matching contributions of 25 per cent, and it was hoped that this 'faith' in the scheme would 'not be without influence' on private employers. The recruiting slogan used – 'Poor health means poor service' – reminded employers of the effect on productivity of avoidable absenteeism.[52] By 1930, 3,200 Birmingham employers added 25 per cent or more in matching funds, and a total of 6,700 employers were contributing.[53] In 1933 nearly all the 'large' firms and the 'majority of the remainder' were supporting the movement, but employer participation apparently reached a plateau, because in 1936 the annual report suggested that the scheme still 'falls short of that complete cooperation' which would maximise the resources available.[54]

This favourable experience was also evident on Merseyside and in Sheffield. On Merseyside, employers' contributions were, untypically, differentiated in the annual reports from those of the workforce. In the fund's early years, employers gave approximately 27 per cent of the value of employees' contributions, though by 1947 this had fallen to 23 per cent. In Sheffield, employers' giving was never shown separately, and there was a reporting convention that the actual amounts given by individual establishments would not be shown. However, in 1926, at the request of the contributors' association, the annual report listed all contributing firms and businesses, dividing them into those which operated the scheme in full, that is, where employers contributed a third of the sum raised from employees (the majority), those where they contributed less than a third (a small minority) and those where only employees contributed (a larger minority).[55] The corporation was held up as a model; for example, in 1937 its employees gave £8,967 and the employers £2,732 (i.e. 30 per cent).[56]

In contrast, the HSA was rather less successful in extending employer cooperation beyond assistance with payroll deduction of contributions. In December 1927 its president, Viscount Hambleden, wrote to *The Times*, appealing publicly for greater support from employers.[57] The idea of matching contributions of a penny a week was mooted; Sir Alan Anderson (the chairman) suggested that this should be a matter of 'civic pride' for every employer.[58] Some companies looked upon the HSA as an 'important feature of their welfare work' but there were others in which 'employers will not recognise us.'[59] Of forty-eight firms where payroll deduction had been established by late 1929, only three made matching contributions and one of these had then ceased its previous practice of *ad hoc* donations to hospitals.[60] Complaints about the lack of employer contributions were a constant refrain in the 1930s; London was compared unfavourably with unnamed 'cities of the industrial north', in which it seemed almost a 'rule of self-respect' to make such contributions.[61] In 1941

Anderson referred to the 'lack of corporate spirit in the sprawling mass of the London area'.[62] This was demonstrated by a survey of fourteen representative schemes, which showed that in Sheffield and Merseyside, respectively, 19.7 per cent and 16.3 per cent of funds were generated by employers' contributions, followed by Birmingham at 11.1 per cent, but schemes such as the HSA, the Norfolk Hospital contributors' association, and the Radcliffe Hospital's contributory scheme attracted minimal employer support (less than 2 per cent of the total).[63] Such variations could reflect the size distribution of employers; in London the labour market was less likely to have been dominated by large employers. Nevertheless, Birmingham and Sheffield had support from several thousand businesses, and they cannot all have been large employers. Another possibility is the resilience of donations and subscriptions in the funding mix of London's hospitals; perhaps employers supported the hospitals in this way (rather than through matching contributions) because of the social networks to which it gave access.[64] Without investigating the records of individual companies we have no access to the thinking which underpinned such decisions. But the key point is that employer contributions and partnerships were far from ubiquitous, and even where successful, this form of joint funding was a long way from the uniform and systematic risk-sharing embodied in NHI. Insofar as we can generalise, then, large employer contributions were a feature of large, multi-hospital schemes in major industrial cities, in which the formation of city-wide joint hospital planning structures meant that questions of hospital finances were constantly in the public domain. Elsewhere, these sources did not provide substantial additional revenue for the hospitals.

To what extent were the schemes a reliable source of income for the hospitals? A criticism of social insurance as a funding mechanism has been that it is dependent on the state of the labour market and that, as a consequence, the resources raised in this way are somewhat unpredictable. Given the significance of unemployment (whether cyclical or structural) in the inter-war years, it is appropriate to investigate its effect on scheme revenue. Our argument is that while schemes could provide impressive proportions of hospital funds, this could also create risks of dependency on one source of income.

There are occasional reports in *The Hospital* (a managerial rather than a medical publication) concerning the impact of unemployment on income from mass contribution,[65] but here we focus on the experience of individual funds. In some places workers' contributions were practically the sole source of hospital income; the absence of a philanthropic middle class left industrial communities with no realistic alternatives.[66] Communities reliant on industries vulnerable to the trade cycle were bound to be exposed to the vagaries of rising unemployment, as is confirmed by the experience of several small hospitals in locations such as Jarrow (Palmer Hospital), Durham (County Hospital), Sunderland (Monkwearmouth) and Bishop Auckland (Lady Eden), where, in some cases, workers' contributions almost dried up completely as a result of short-time working, unemployment or plant closures. As a consequence, these hospitals were forced to liquidate assets, expand overdrafts or, *in extremis*, cease to treat patients.[67]

Such institutions carried out only a small proportion of the total hospital workload, but even major general hospitals, such as the Sunderland Royal Infirmary, were sometimes vulnerable to fluctuations in income from workers' contributions, though the number of workplaces taking part in the contributory schemes reduced dependency on single large firms. The reports of the Sunderland Royal Infirmary reveal that, in 1926, the 'stoppage in coal and industrial depression [had] depleted funds to a greater extent than ever previously', and this was followed by several difficult years; to cope with such problems the Infirmary therefore ran a substantial overdraft for much of the inter-war period.[68]

The multi-hospital schemes, as in Birmingham, Sheffield and Liverpool, were not immune to these difficulties. In Birmingham progress was considered 'satisfactory' despite the 'trade depression' in the early 1930s, but the effects of unemployment were noted none the less.[69] In Merseyside the need to attempt to include casual and seasonal staff in the scheme was stressed and the 'relatively poor' showing of the scheme in 1936 was attributed to the scale of unemployment.[70] In Sheffield, in 1926 membership grew but income fell by over 10 per cent; payments to the city's hospitals then dropped from £72,500 in 1927 to £62,000 in 1929, before resuming growth during the 1930s.[71] The League of Subscribers of the Edinburgh Royal Infirmary also noted the adverse effects of 'prolonged trade depression and consequent unemployment', though these were partly offset by the establishment of new groups.[72] It might be thought surprising that unemployment does not feature more frequently in reports of the schemes, but Edinburgh's experience suggests that recruitment of new members tended to outweigh the effects of labour market fluctuations.

If we examine trends in income per contributor for a range of schemes, there is some evidence of variations in the average amount raised per contributor per year, but these annual fluctuations are far smaller than the variations between schemes.[73] It was also suggested that while the attractions of the schemes were obvious, they represented a heavy additional burden on household finances for workers in occupations where short-time working was a frequent occurrence. As a Mr Hogg of the Durham Miners put it, referring to the effect of short-time working on weekly wages, you 'can't build a marble palace with slates'.[74] It was unrealistic to place too much faith in the schemes in communities where this was the case.

To summarise, this analysis confirms the steady upward trend in scheme membership and income. It is also clear, however, that local labour market circumstances could adversely affect the funds raised by the schemes. The experience of individual hospitals indicates clearly the risks of dependence on workers' contributions as the main or sole source of income.

Benefits and expenditure

A consideration of how the substantial funds raised by the schemes were spent requires, first, a discussion of the balance between expenditure on voluntary and that on municipal hospitals, and between hospital and non-hospital benefits. This is followed by an examination of the criteria used in devising methods of hospital reimbursement by multi-hospital funds. Third, there is an exploration of issues of dispute and principle which came up in the context of developing arrangements for the treatment of scheme patients in municipal hospitals. A general theme of this section is the effect on incentive structures of the development and expansion of contributory schemes as a major source of hospital funding.

The following comments draw on analyses of expenditure data for the HSA and for the Sheffield, Leeds and Merseyside schemes, though the different categorisations of expenditure prevent combining the datasets. The bulk of expenditure went on grants to hospitals towards the cost of treating scheme members. The HSA insisted that at least 75 per cent of its income went on hospital services and, although we have no definite statement of policy for the other funds referred to here, they all expended similar proportions on hospital services. Most of this went to the voluntary hospitals, but use of the public sector grew steadily. The context for this was the 1929 Local Government Act, which had signalled the upgrading of the original poor law infirmaries and their transfer to the administrative control of the counties or county boroughs. The pace of development varied,[75] but many hospital authorities were anxious to improve their image and the quality of treatment offered, and they made efforts to make public hospitals available to all citizens, and not just those sent by the relieving officer. Technically, however, patients not in receipt of public assistance were supposed to make payment according to their means, and it was this obligation which was lifted by arrangements between contributory schemes and municipal hospitals.[76] In 1935 it was estimated that 8.6 per cent of scheme expenditure went to municipal hospitals, and by 1947 nearly 20 per cent of the MHC's expenditure went on municipal hospital services.[77] In Birmingham, at first, this amounted to 9 per cent of all institutional spending, but by the war years was as much as £50,000, or 14 per cent. The MHC also earmarked sums to go to the medical staff fund. This was an acknowledgement that, although voluntary medical staff continued to give their services *gratis*, they had some claim for a share in the increase in hospital income.

Two other benefits featured significantly. First, ambulance services received some funding. On Merseyside the ambulance service was run by the MHC; in Sheffield the town's Central Ambulance Service drew together vehicles from the Joint Hospitals Council, the St John's Ambulance and the city council; in Leeds there is evidence of grants to patients for conveyance to and from Leeds hospitals, as well as payments to ambulance services in outlying areas. The Birmingham contributory scheme spent up to 6 per cent of annual revenues on its own ambulance fleet.[78] These developments meant that the schemes played a very direct role in the integration of health services. Second, the schemes funded convalescence care, either in homes which they owned or through contractual arrangements. In the 1890s, for instance, the Birmingham Saturday fund had opened 'Tan-y-coed' convalescent home in Llandudno, free to all fund members who were Birmingham residents, provided they could pay their own fare to the coast.[79] The Sheffield fund had contractual arrangements with convalescent homes in moorland or coastal locations, such as Ilkley, Matlock, Rhyl and Southport; it also reimbursed voluntary hospitals (including institutions in Buxton, Droitwich, Harrogate and Woodhall Spa) which provided spa treatment, including the cost of transport to these.[80] In Sheffield the convalescence service also coordinated the efforts of the home help department, through which sick members could be referred to the Public Health Department, the Women's Service Bureau, the Red Cross and several other voluntary agencies.[81]

There were consumer pressures to expand the scope of benefits covered by the schemes. In the annual meetings of the HSA's group secretaries, expenditure on non-hospital benefits was frequently criticised as an irrelevant distraction from the core mission, which was to 'save' the hospitals. The HSA insisted on an upper limit for the proportion of such expenditures, in this case 15 per cent of benefits. But there were occasional demands to relax this restriction. One proposal was to extend coverage of dental benefits for the individual contributor by allowing one dental benefit per family (thus, if a husband were covered by NHI, his wife could benefit from his HSA coverage).[82] Another proposal was to support district nursing associations. Both of these were declined.[83] Concern about the cost of extra-hospital benefits led the HSA to establish its own optical service, to take advantage of scale economies in purchasing.[84] These 'fringe benefits' were useful as inducements to recruitment, but the risk was that such 'sidelines' could detract from the central purpose of the schemes.[85] One view was that it was 'grotesque' that schemes might, on the one hand, pay only a small proportion of the cost of hospital maintenance yet simultaneously advertise a 'long list of additional benefits'. On the other hand, it was suggested that such additional benefits were not 'window-dressing' but were integral to the efficient operation of the hospital service (e.g. ambulance services, because of their role in ensuring prompt treatment of casualties).[86]

Table 3.2 presents a summary of extra-hospital benefits offered, drawing on a survey conducted in 1936, which included schemes covering half the total membership in England and Wales. The fact that schemes sought to limit the

Table 3.2. Additional benefits provided by contributory schemes

Benefit	No. of schemes	No. of contributors	Percentage of total memberships surveyed[a]
Convalescence care	39	3,975,672	75.8
Ambulance	46	3,812,295	72.7
Private ward patients	48	3,141,035	59.9
Surgical aids	31	3,088,125	58.9
Ophthalmic treatment	32	2,152,120	41.0
District nursing	26	1,407,479	26.8
Dental care	19	687,086	13.1
Allowance for maternity	8	587,220	10.4

[a] In total the schemes responding to this survey had 5.4 million members and the percentages relate to this.
Source: *The Hospital*, 33 (1937), p. 25.

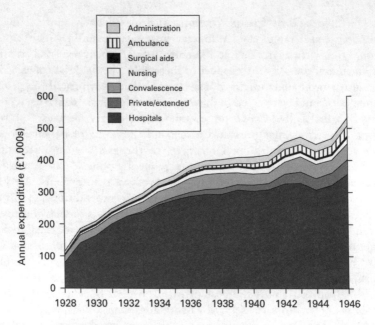

Figure 3.3. Composition of expenditure, Birmingham Hospitals Contributory Association, 1928–46.

proportion of funds allocated to such benefits indicates that they were seen as of secondary importance to the paramount objective of funding the hospitals. In contrast, in the post-war period these benefits came to form the core business of those schemes which reinvented themselves as providers of low-cost health insurance (see chapter 9). What had been irrelevances, in the view of some scheme officials, therefore subsequently took centre stage as the schemes moved into new markets.

Trends in the overall pattern of expenditure and of benefits are exemplified with evidence from the BHCA, the second-largest scheme (see figure 3.3). The bulk went to hospitals, whether voluntary or municipal. Most of these were local institutions but some were outside the city. The popularity of convalescent home benefits is evident; these absorbed, on average, 11 per cent of the total. The 'private/extended' category in figure 3.3 represents claims under the 'extended benefits' scheme (see above), along with the rebates made to contributors in pay wards – effectively the payments to middle-class members. This was a clear growth area, rising from 3 per cent in 1935, when the new scheme began, to 9 per cent in 1946. In addition to institutional support, a small amount, averaging about 7 per cent of the total, went towards other health services. One beneficiary was the district nursing service, which used funding to extend nurse visiting into newer suburbs of the city where it was not yet established. Another very minor service was the provision to members of 'surgical aids' (prosthetic devices and the like), a facility initially offered by the Saturday fund. The steady growth of extra-hospital benefits indicates that providing funds for the hospitals alone was not enough to attract new members, or even to sustain membership.

The criteria by which funds were allocated to hospitals are also of interest, because they show how the availability of a source of income, in which money, to some extent, followed the patient, affected the incentive structures confronting hospitals as well as donors. Most schemes were affiliated to individual hospitals, and so funds were simply transferred to the hospital in question. However, multi-hospital funds had to devise criteria for reimbursing those hospitals which treated scheme members. This raised the question of how to create appropriate incentive structures.

The operation of the MHC illustrates the potential problems. It was acknowledged that the gains from mass contribution might be offset by reductions in subscriptions and donations. The MHC therefore initially sought to compensate hospitals for the loss of income from other sources and to 'enable the hospital to pay its way after taking credit for all free legacies.'[87] This was subject to the proviso that the hospital was 'efficiently and economically administered', and the maximum grant available was not to exceed the amount required to balance the books.[88] As was soon pointed out, these conditions 'encouraged the hospitals to make their deficit as large as possible', which hardly seemed conducive to efficiency.[89] Similar views were expressed in Birmingham.[90]

Hospitals persistently made representations to the MHC concerning the inadequacy of their grants, but no new method of distribution was implemented. Reflecting dissatisfaction with their allocations, the Waterloo and District General Hospital withdrew cooperation, while the Royal Southern launched an appeal, in contravention of MHC byelaws. Its grant was therefore suspended; although it initially returned to the fold, it soon resumed its independent fundraising, and its grant was again suspended.[91] A formula for allocating funds was eventually devised in 1934. It was agreed that 75 per cent of MHC funds would be distributed in proportion to the work done at individual hospitals. In addition, there was a weighting for the complexity and cost of the workload of particular hospitals. In-patient days at the principal general and maternity hospitals in Liverpool and Birkenhead received a weighting of 1; in various cottage and specialist hospitals it was 0.8; and in four convalescent homes the weighting was 0.6.[92]

In contrast, the HSA paid hospitals a flat rate per in-patient day. The HSA council felt that there was an element of 'rough justice' in this system. If hospitals were reimbursed in proportion to the actual cost of the work they carried out, the net effect would be to the benefit of central London general hospitals, at the expense of suburban institutions. The risk of such a change in reimbursement procedures was that if funds were taken away from suburban hospitals, they might withdraw their cooperation and, conceivably, establish contributory schemes in competition with the HSA. There was a proposal to adopt (like Merseyside) a tiered system of reimbursement rates relating to the relative costs of hospitals,[93] but this was put on hold pending completion of the government's hospital surveys which were being undertaken during the wartime years as a basis for future planning.[94]

The question of reimbursement rates and incentive structures had occasionally been aired in *The Hospital*. The risk of flat-rate reimbursement was that it provided no incentive for increased efficiency. Depending on the resources generated by schemes, their daily reimbursement rates and the comparative costs of hospitals, institutions might receive highly divergent proportions of their maintenance costs; this was to the benefit of inefficient hospitals.[95] The schemes were therefore forced to confront the issue of how to develop incentive structures that would neither penalise efficient hospitals nor discourage other sorts of fundraising, and some tentative steps were taken, as the Merseyside example shows. There is some evidence that, consistent with their mutualist origins, the schemes did not wish to embrace competition between hospitals as a means of stimulating efficiency. For example, in considering possible changes in 1942, the members of the HSA's contributory schemes committee indicated that they 'had hoped to remove competition, removing the necessity to bargain with hospitals for service'.[96] We have found only one example of funds being positively withdrawn from a hospital on the grounds of its quality or inefficiency. This was the Lady Eden Hospital, Bishop Auckland. The miners' lodges of South West Durham had decided, 'quite correctly' in the opinion of the hospital surveyors, to transfer their funds from this hospital to the Newcastle Royal Victoria Infirmary, where they believed that serious injuries and accident cases would receive better treatment.[97] One reason why such action was exceptional can be found in the ambiguous nature of the schemes. Technically, the resources generated constituted a voluntary gift to the hospitals, and the schemes did not, therefore, act as what would now be recognised as 'purchasers' of health care on behalf of a defined population. They could not enforce hospital rationalisation through competitive mechanisms; at most they could devise some limited mechanisms which would go some way towards reflecting the comparative costs of institutions.

The issue of incentive structures and contractual obligations also arose in the context of arrangements for treatment of scheme members in the public sector, because the growth of the schemes outstripped the capacity of voluntary hospitals to accommodate additional patients. Concerns about the allocation of costs and liabilities between the contracting parties can be illustrated with examples from Liverpool, Birmingham and London. From the contributory schemes' perspective, any payments they made were diversions from their main object, namely support of the voluntary hospitals, and an additional burden on contributors who were also ratepayers. However, from the viewpoint of municipal public health committees, any work they did which relieved the waiting lists of the voluntary hospital was effectively a public subsidy for the voluntary sector, and the cost should therefore be recouped, because they were giving treatment while recovering only a small proportion of expenses.[98]

An illustration is provided by discussions between the HSA and several boards of guardians and municipal authorities. In 1927, the Stepney board of guardians terminated an agreement with the HSA on the grounds that its reimbursement was inadequate, even though the HSA believed that the reimbursement rate exceeded the average cost per case.[99] It was reported that some boards of guardians were attempting to charge HSA contributors at a higher rate than non-contributors. The HSA argued that this policy meant voluntary contributions were being used to relieve the rates, and that it involved discrimination against one set of ratepayers, 'not because they are richer, but because they looked ahead and saved money in advance of illness'.[100] As was pointed out in a discussion in the pages of *The Hospital*, municipal authorities had to remember that scheme members were also ratepayers and thereby entitled to municipal services. If they were discriminated against on account of their generosity to voluntary hospitals, this would be a 'startling innovation which would merit unanimous disapprobation'.[101] For this and for a number of other reasons, notably the savings to the municipal budget accruing from voluntary provision, the writer suggested that local authorities ought to 'err on the side of generosity' in order to sustain the voluntary hospitals. From the perspective of the HSA, this meant that payments to municipal authorities were based on the average amount recouped from people within their income limits, but payments to voluntary hospitals were less constrained: the voluntary hospitals 'are our shareholders [and] we pay them the highest dividend we can'.[102] Even so, there were still reports that some local authorities sought to extract more from patients who were members of contributory schemes than a 'strict assessment of means would justify'. This would in effect subsidise the local authority, turning the scheme into 'an insurance for the authority against the poverty of its residents'.[103]

Discussions of public–private contractual arrangements were therefore characterised by defensive haggling. Schemes typically reimbursed the municipal hospitals at an agreed rate below the actual cost, but as the quality of care in public infirmaries rose after the passing of the Local Government Act, these contracts were regularly, and sometimes acrimoniously, revisited.[104] Efforts to raise the reimbursement rate were deemed an 'unbearable burden' in Birmingham, where there was an 'absence of friendly and mutual discussion', while on Merseyside there was a 'somewhat difficult negotiation'.[105] Schemes would make efforts to limit their liabilities, as in Wolverhampton, where the Royal Hospital's contributors' association reduced to three months the maximum length of stay in public hospitals which it would cover, presumably because rising numbers using public institutions threatened to siphon money away from the Royal.[106] There is no sense that workers' representatives inclined more to the municipal side in these arguments, nor was it in their financial interest to do so. There also remained, not least in progressive authorities, the feeling among contributors that municipal institutions bore the 'taint of pauperism'; the Birmingham Saturday fund could observe even in 1936 that 'it would have been so much more satisfactory if the patients could have been treated at our own Voluntary Hospitals'.[107]

The schemes thus had to tread cautiously in developing links with the municipal sector. Surplus capacity in public hospitals offered a way of satisfying demands for institutional treatment, but if too many scheme members were treated in municipal hospitals or if a high proportion of revenues went to municipal hospitals, there was a risk of alienating contributors. From the perspective of the local authority, demanding an excessive level of reimbursement from schemes would also be counterproductive; local authorities would be sequestering funds from the voluntaries, thereby undermining their capacity to treat patients and throwing a greater burden onto the public sector. As a result, the general level of reimbursement from schemes to local authorities for the treatment of contributors in 1934 was low when compared with their payments to voluntary hospitals; nine schemes paid 3s a day, only two exceeded that figure and most of the remainder provided 2s a day or less.[108] This suggests that local authorities and contributory schemes were well aware of the balance that had to be struck.

The development of the schemes therefore illustrates not only some of the problems which confront social insurance systems, but also the generic problems of incentive structures in health care systems. The temptation to expand the range of benefits risked detracting from the primary purpose of the contributory schemes, namely raising money for hospitals. The reimbursement procedures carried with them the possibility of perverse incentives, with the concomitant possibility of rewarding inefficient hospitals. Finally, in developing contractual arrangements with municipal hospitals, the schemes were aware that, on the one hand, treating members in municipal hospitals could help relieve voluntary hospital waiting lists but, on the other hand, they ran the risk of antagonising their supporters, who were already, in their capacity as ratepayers, supporting the municipal service.

Effect of the contributory schemes on hospital finances and activity

Having established the principal features of the operation of the schemes in the inter-war years, what was their impact? This question is explored through an examination of the share of hospital income which they provided, the impact on patient throughput (the numbers of patients treated in hospital) and the effect on hospital utilisation rates (the proportion of the population making use of hospital services). Playing on the ambiguity in the title of the largest fund, in what sense could they be said to have contributed to 'saving' the hospitals?

On the first of these points, Cherry identified small numbers of institutions which, in the mid-1930s, drew over 60 per cent of their income from contributory insurance.[109] His analysis is extended considerably here through use of our database on pre-NHS hospital provision, which gives a breakdown of income sources for the largest general and specialist hospitals (those with over 100 beds). This is used to identify hospitals where mass contribution generated the greatest proportion of income. Typically, for each of the years 1926–36 there are between 70 and 160 hospitals for which an income breakdown is available (after 1936 income from contributory schemes is not recorded separately in the primary source for the database, the *Hospitals yearbook*).

In St Helens, contributions accounted for over 70 per cent of the hospital's income in five of these years, peaking at 77 per cent in 1936. North Ormesby (in Middlesbrough) experienced four years in which contributory schemes provided over 70 per cent of its income. Mansfield and District Hospital had two such years. Hospitals where contribution consistently provided at least 60 per cent of income included North Ormesby (on eleven occasions; the lowest proportion was 59.5 per cent), St Helens (ten occasions), Mansfield (seven), Barrow, the North Staffordshire Infirmary (Stoke-on-Trent) and the North Riding Infirmary (Middlesbrough) (six each), and Stockton and Thornaby, and Coventry and Warwickshire (five). In some localities, then, mass contribution was playing a very substantial role in hospital finance. Teesside is the best example; in almost every one of these years at least 60 per cent of the income of its three main general hospitals was generated in this way. Indeed, contributory schemes generated at least 60 per cent of income in several major provincial voluntaries, such as the Sheffield Royal Hospital, Sheffield Royal Infirmary and various important institutions in the Midlands (Wolverhampton, North Staffordshire, Coventry and Warwick). If one were to generalise, it could be said that these were all freestanding industrial centres, in which high proportions of the population had incomes of less than £5 per week.[110]

Because contributory schemes were merged in the statistical record with other patient payments from 1936, obtaining a true picture of the impact of mass contribution after that date would arguably require use of the accounts of individual hospitals. However, the *Hospitals yearbooks* identify contributory schemes which were associated with an individual hospital, so (making the assumption that no payments were made from schemes to other institutions) we can compare the income of these schemes with the income of the hospitals with which they were associated. This shows that in 1939 contributory schemes provided some hospitals with over 70 per cent of their ordinary income.[111] Six of these were in South Wales: at Llanelly (82 per cent), Porth and Maesteg (75 per cent), Mountain Ash, Caerphilly and Pontypool. Note that they were comparatively small, Llanelly and Pontypool having eighty beds and others around fifty beds. Thompson emphasises that several of these hospitals were founded by their potential users; these data show that they were being almost wholly funded by their users as well.[112]

An assessment of the effect of the schemes therefore draws very positive conclusions if stress is placed on the proportion of hospital income which they provided, and this is certainly consistent with the views of Doyle, based on his work on Teesside.[113] But if the schemes generated substantial proportions of resources for hospitals, the levels of provision that could be financed in this way depended on the absolute amounts raised. An investigation of whether the schemes had a demonstrable effect on hospital throughput and utilisation requires that variations in hospital finances, and the composition of income, are related to variations in hospital throughput.

The proportion of income from mass contribution and patients' payments, though impressive, might bear no relation to hospital income per bed. For 1938, of 101 English provincial general hospitals giving a breakdown of income sources, there were nine where the proportion of income from payments and contributions exceeded 75 per cent, but for these hospitals income per bed ranged from around £106 (St Helens) to £288 (West Bromwich).

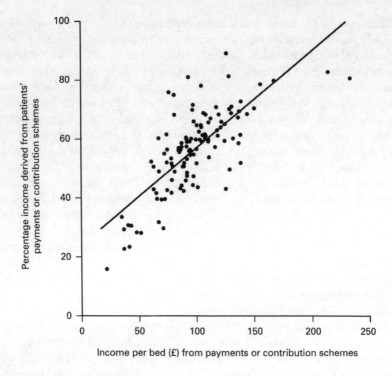

Figure 3.4. English general hospitals, 1938: income from payments and contributions, plotted against the proportion of income from those sources.

These institutions were all in industrial towns in the Midlands or the North. Many other hospitals clearly had a much more diverse funding mix. This point is underlined by figure 3.4, which focuses on the relationship between income per bed from payments and contributions combined, and the proportion of hospital income derived from this source. Generally, the greater the income per bed from contributory schemes and patients' payments, the greater was the share of total income, but there are hospitals which can be regarded as outliers in that the proportion of income generated by mass contribution was higher or lower than one would expect from the absolute amount. Thus, for five hospitals – in St Helens (two institutions), Scunthorpe, Darlington and Barrow-in-Furness – the proportion of income from contributions and payments (between 75 and 89 per cent) was substantially greater than one would expect from the absolute amounts per bed (between £80 and £130 in these cases). Conversely, there are several institutions (below the best-fit line on the graph) where the proportion was rather lower than would be expected (between 30 and 43 per cent) given the income per bed (between £43 and £75). These hospitals were in contrasting locations (Peterborough, Brighton, Bury, Bristol and Salford). The former group of hospitals were, relatively, much more dependent on contributions and payments than the latter, which clearly had a more diverse mix of income sources.

If the contributory schemes had genuinely improved the financial position of hospitals in the inter-war period, one would expect a positive relationship between growth in this source of income and throughput of patients. For a consistent set of provincial hospitals for the years 1926–36, the relationship between growth in income from contributory schemes and changes in patient throughput is analysed here. Simple percentage changes in hospital income from schemes cannot easily be calculated, because they were often starting off from a low base; change is therefore calculated not as a percentage increase on a base year of 1926, but as a proportion of the sum of the values of contributory scheme income, at constant prices, for 1926 and 1936 combined.[114] Growth in in-patient numbers was most closely associated with growth in total income; with a correlation coefficient of 0.54, this is statistically highly significant. For growth in income from mass contribution, the correlation coefficient (0.22) does not attain statistical significance. An interpretation would be that while growth of total income determines the capacity of a hospital to treat patients, there is a weaker relationship with individual components of income, such as that from contributions. Regional variations in the 'contribution of contribution', and reductions in income from other sources, could also account for these results. For example, in approximately one-third of the sixty-five hospitals whose finances were analysed for 1926–36, income from subscriptions declined in real terms (this may, though we cannot determine it from the data, suggest that employers who made matching contributions then reduced other forms of giving). Overall, the schemes undoubtedly increased the resources available to hospitals but they were not the sole source of growth in income and not all hospitals benefited from them to the same extent.

Concerns were also periodically expressed that the schemes would unleash suppressed demand for services. In the case of the HSA, utilisation rates rose steadily right from the inception of the scheme. In 1924 and 1925 the proportion of HSA contributors and dependants treated as in-patients was around 4.5 per cent, but by 1932 it had risen to 8.9 per cent, a ratio which was maintained throughout the 1930s.[115] Assuming an average of one dependant per member, this would imply that around 4.5 per cent of HSA contributors and their relatives received in-patient treatment in any one year in the 1930s. For the Birmingham scheme, in 1928 the ratio of in-patients to contributors was 7.3 per cent, rising to 9.5 per cent in 1930 and to 11.9 per cent in 1938,[116] implying a utilisation rate of nearly 6 per cent of the population. Finally, a Ministry of Health paper which gathered data for several schemes showed that the proportion of contributors and dependants treated was between 5.5 and 12.4 per cent.[117] For comparison, some 2.9 per cent of the population were in-patients in the English voluntary hospitals during 1938.[118] This suggests that hospitals were indeed experiencing higher levels of demand for their services as a result of the growth in membership of the contributory schemes. It is plausible that contributors saw their membership as conveying an entitlement to treatment, though it is also plausible that membership enabled contributors to obtain treatment which they might otherwise have foregone.

So, while mass contribution clearly generated additional resources, it also stimulated additional demand, and the success of the schemes in attracting new members may therefore have been part of the problem facing the voluntary hospitals in the late 1930s. At least one hospital – Enfield War Memorial – expressed the view in 1934 that it would have to expand in order to meet the growing liability to contributors (presumably there was a perception that excessive demand was being placed on the hospital), which suggests that this problem was acknowledged.[119] There are also occasional hints that the schemes were aware of this problem. If the HSA's journal, *The Contributor*, is a guide, concerns were expressed about excessive utilisation of services. Early issues of this publication included figures of the membership of individual groups, and the number of 'green vouchers' issued; in some groups, nearly 40 per cent of members had availed themselves of in-patient treatment. This suggested that some were joining in full knowledge that they were in need of treatment. In addition to the publication of statistics on usage rates for individual groups, the pages of *The Contributor* regularly drew attention to concerns about the difficulty of monitoring the use of services by 'singletons' – individual members not affiliated with a particular workplace. There were also comments that the accessibility of services in London led to a higher propensity to use them ('the hospitals are around the corner').[120] Such publicity kept the issue of responsible use of the hospitals before the scheme members, but there is no evidence of more active efforts to restrain use of services by contributors; to do so would have risked alienating the schemes' supporters.

Conclusion

In the inter-war years, working-class contribution became an essential element of the British hospital system. Membership expanded significantly, albeit with substantial regional variations (see chapter 4), although growth in revenues was not uninterrupted, and the hoped-for matching contributions from employers generally failed to materialise. For many institutions the schemes provided the core of funding, which underpinned the expansion of in-patient treatment; for some hospitals it offered the only significant source of revenue. This confirms the findings of previous scholarship, albeit for a larger sample of hospitals and a later date, but our analyses of scheme finances and hospital use add to the existing literature in two further respects.

First, mass contribution introduced new incentive structures and dilemmas into the hospital system. Reimbursement procedures, for example, took no account of the comparative costs or relative efficiency of individual hospitals, and this prompted threats of withdrawal of cooperation. As a result, there were efforts to devise more sophisticated methods of reimbursement. And once contracts were developed with the public sector, both contributory funds and local authorities had to tread carefully to avoid penalising the prudent, responsible citizens whose contributions were becoming the mainstay of hospital income. Finally, in order to boost recruitment, some schemes extended the range of benefits offered; they were criticised because, while they boosted recruitment, they were a diversion from the primary purpose – of financing the hospitals. The schemes thus provide a useful historical example of the difficulty of devising incentive structures which do not have unintended, and negative, consequences.

Second, a further (and no doubt unintended) effect was to raise expectations and therefore demand for hospital treatment. Does this imply that the schemes were subject to the problem of moral hazard, familiar to health economists, in which the availability of insurance prompts greater (and perhaps unnecessary) use of services? As Gray points out, it is difficult to detect evidence of moral hazard[121] for this period (use of health services was rising steadily, but this may only suggest that unmet need was being accommodated) but it seems clear that the use made of hospitals by scheme members was in excess of national utilisation rates. This suggests two possibilities. One is that the schemes were perceived by their members as having the character of insurance, even though this was not the legal position (and we discuss this more fully in chapter 5); therefore, despite the original aims of the schemes, their members began to adopt an instrumentalist attitude, demanding higher levels of service in return for their commitment. An alternative is that the schemes gave effect to demand which otherwise would have been suppressed. We cannot determine which of these is correct. It is nevertheless clear that the schemes both enhanced the capacity of hospitals to treat patients and also stimulated additional demand for treatment; thus, they proved only a partial solution to the problem of hospital finances.

Notes

1 F. Colchester-Wemyss, 'Contributory schemes', in F. Menzies (ed.), *The voluntary hospitals in Great Britain (excluding London): fifth annual report for the year 1923* (London, 1924), p. 103; TNA: PRO, MH 58/200, Voluntary Hospitals Commission, Lord Onslow contributory schemes memo, Notes on responses to questionnaires, 1923.

2 The annual *Hospitals yearbook* series was produced by the Central Bureau of Hospital Information, and was 'issued under the auspices of the Joint Council of the Order of St John and the British Red Cross Society and the British Hospitals Association'. The *Hospitals yearbooks* were subtitled *An annual record of the hospitals of Great Britain and Ireland incorporating 'Burdett's Hospitals and charities'* founded 1889 and, like *Burdett's*, presented statistics from two years before the year of publication. The annual series was broken in the 1943–44 *Hospitals yearbook*, which contained the 1941 statistics, and from 1944 it was produced by the BHA alone. The editor was either the secretary or the assistant secretary of the BHA; in the 1930s this was R. H. P. Orde, from 1942 A. E. Ceadel, and from 1947 J. P. Wetenhall.

3 ML, HB14/1/25, Glasgow Royal Infirmary minutes, Monthly meeting of managers, 1 June 1910.

4 J. E. Stone, *Hospital organization and management (including planning and construction)* (London, 1927), pp. 49–50.

5 *Ibid.*, p. 52.

6 S. Sturdy, 'The political economy of scientific medicine: science, education and the transformation of medical practice in Sheffield, 1890–1922', *Medical History*, 36 (1992), pp. 125–59; S. Cherry, 'Regional comparators in the funding and organisation of the

voluntary hospital system, *c.* 1860–1939', in M. Gorsky and S. Sheard (eds), *Financing medicine: the British experience since 1750* (London, forthcoming, 2006).

7 A. T. Page, *Pennies for health: the story of the British Hospitals Contributory Schemes Association* (Birmingham, 1949), p. 9.

8 *Ibid.*

9 BLPES, BHCSA 7/1, BHCSA general meetings 1931–41, 19 September 1931.

10 BLPES, BHCSA 7/1, Report of 3rd annual conference, 1933, pp. 18–19; BLPES, BHCSA 7/1, Report of the 4th annual conference, 1934, pp. 20–31.

11 J. Dodd, 'The present position of the contributory scheme movement', *The Hospital*, 33 (1937), p. 257.

12 *The Hospital*, 30 (1935), p. 19, 32 (1936), pp. 202–3, 32 (1936), p. 256.

13 TNA: PRO, MH 58/177, Summary of a number of contributory schemes: Bourne-mouth, Merthyr.

14 TNA: PRO, MH 58/177, Contributory schemes, 1923, p. 4.

15 C. Chisholm, *Marketing survey of the United Kingdom* (London, 1938), p. 112.

16 TNA: PRO, MH 58/200, Notes on responses; Stone, *Hospital organization*, p. 225.

17 Stone, *Hospital organization*, pp. 222–3.

18 HRO, 5M63/161, Royal Hampshire County Hospital, annual report, 1921.

19 TNA: PRO, MH 58/177, Summary of a number of contributory schemes: Middles-brough.

20 *Lancet*, 15 January 1921, p. 153.

21 *Ibid.*

22 Stone, *Hospital organization*, p. 221.

23 VHC, *Contributory schemes* (London, 1923), p. 5.

24 *Ibid.*, p. 6.

25 See, for example, Warneford Hospital Archives Room, Oxford, Radcliffe Infirmary and County Hospital Oxford, annual report, 1920; HRO, 5M63/161, Royal Hampshire County Hospital, annual report, 1921.

26 GRO, HO 19/8/6, Gloucestershire Royal Infirmary, annual report, 1922.

27 TNA: PRO, MH 58/177, Summary of a number of contributory schemes: Barrow-in-Furness.

28 LMA, Royal Northern Hospital Group, annual report, 1923.

29 LMA, Royal Northern Hospital Group, annual report, 1920.

30 TNA: PRO, MH 58/177, Summary of a number of contributory schemes: Blackburn.

31 See LHSA, LHB 1/18/2, Edinburgh Royal Infirmary, Minutes of meetings of the League of Subscribers to the Royal Infirmary of Edinburgh, 1930–1937; TWAS, HO/RVI/60 AM 21, Royal Victoria Infirmary, Minute book: workmen governors annual meetings, 21 March 1931, 12 March 1932; TWAS, HO/RVI/2/54, Minute book house com. no. 12, 16 February 1932.

32 TNA: PRO, MH 58/177, Summary of a number of contributory schemes: Leeds.

33 Stone, *Hospital organization*, p. 237. The 'contributor' was typically construed as male by contemporaries.

34 *Ibid.*, pp. 222–3.

35 GRO, HO 19/8/6, Gloucestershire Royal Infirmary, annual report, 1922.

36 Radcliffe Infirmary and County Hospital Oxford, annual report, 1920; Stone, *Hospital organization*, p. 220.

37 Political and Economic Planning, *Report on the British health services* (London, 1937), p. 235.

38 *Lancet*, 15 January 1921; F. Bedarida, *A social history of England 1851–1990*, trans. A. S. Forster and J. Hodgkinson (2nd edn) (London, 1991), p. 216.

39 Stone, *Hospital organization*, pp. 222–3.

40 *Ibid.*, p. 238.

41 BLSL, BHCA, annual report, 1932.

42 BCA, MS 1576/3, BHCA, Minutes of the management committee (MMC), 13 January 1932.

43 BCA, MS 1576/4, BHCA, MMC, 11 May 1932.

44 BLSL, BHCA, annual report, 1944.

45 BLSL, BHCA, annual report, 1940.

46 A separate category for public services was not introduced until 1923, hence the necessity of combining them with patients' payments through the sequence.

47 *Hospitals yearbooks*, 1934, 1940, 1944.

48 In 1935, for example, the minimum bed numbers for inclusion were 125 for general and 100 for special hospitals. *Hospitals yearbook*, 1937.

49 *Hospitals yearbook*, 1944, pp. 204–16; BLPES, BHCSA, 15/6, Analysis of replies to questionnaire, March 1946. Our 1942 estimate is higher than that recorded by B. Harris, *The origins of the British welfare state: social welfare in England and Wales, 1800–1945* (Basingstoke, 2004), p. 193, because we have imputed membership figures from those schemes which gave a figure for income but not for membership.

50 Ministry of Health, Voluntary Hospitals Committee, *Final report*, Cmd 1335 (London, 1921), p. 22.

51 TNA: PRO, MH 58/177, Summary of a number of contributory schemes: Leeds, Sheffield.

52 Birmingham Hospitals Saturday Fund (BHSF), annual report, 1928.

53 BCA, BHSF, annual report, 1930.

54 BCA, BHSF, annual reports, 1933, 1936.

55 Westfield Health Scheme Archive (WHSA), SHC, annual report, 1926.

56 WHSA, SHC, annual report, 1937.

57 *The Times*, 6 December 1927.

58 *The Contributor*, January 1929, p. 35.

59 *The Contributor*, October 1929, pp. 650, 652, April 1928, pp. 338–9.

60 *The Contributor*, September 1929, pp. 638, 636.

61 *The Contributor*, January 1936, p. 9, May 1937, p. 137.

62 *HSA Contributor*, 4(2) (1941), p. 26.

63 LMA, A/KE/11/1b, Comparative statement of contributory scheme results, 1938–39.

64 K. Waddington, 'Subscribing to a democracy? Management and the voluntary ideology of the London hospitals, 1850–1900', *English Historical Review*, 118 (2003), pp. 357–79, at p. 359.

65 For example, *The Hospital*, 27 (1931), p. 226, and 31 (1935), pp. 266–8.

66 S. Thompson, 'To relieve the sufferings of humanity, irrespective of party, politics or creed? Conflict, consensus and voluntary hospital provision in Edwardian South Wales', *Social History of Medicine*, 16 (2003), pp. 247–62.

67 J. Mohan, *Planning, markets and hospitals* (London, 2002), pp. 32–5.

68 TWAS, 1381, Sunderland Royal Infirmary, annual reports, 1926, 1931, 1932, 1923.

69 BCA, BHSF, annual report, 1930, 1938.

70 Merseyside Record Office (MRO), M610 MED 4/1, MHC, annual report, 1936.

71 WHSA, SHC, annual reports, *passim*.

72 LHSA, LHB, 1/18/2, Edinburgh Royal Infirmary, Meetings of League of Subscribers, 29 November 1931, 21 June 1932; for similar evidence in Glasgow, see LHSA, HB 14/1/37, Glasgow Royal Infirmary, Meeting of delegates of working-class contributors, 13 January 1923, 10 January 1925, 14 January 1933.

73 This comment is based on data on income and membership for the Leeds, Birmingham, Merseyside and Sheffield schemes and the HSA, but the data are discontinuous.

74 *The Hospital*, 26 (1930), p. 159.

75 M. Powell, 'An expanding service: municipal acute medicine in the 1930s', *Twentieth Century British History*, 8 (1997), pp. 334–57.

76 Harris, *Origins*, p. 231.

77 *The Hospital*, 33 (1937), p. 260.

78 MRO, M610 MED 4/1, MHC, annual reports, 1930, 1936; WHSA, SHC, annual reports, 1929, 1938; Leeds Local and Family History Library, Leeds Central Library, Leeds Hospital Fund, annual report, 1933; BLSL, BHCA, annual reports, *passim*.

79   *Forward*, 7 January 1892.
80   WHSA, SHC, annual reports, 1937, 1945; BLSL, BHCA, annual report, 1928.
81   MRO, M610 MED 4/1, MHC, annual report, 1932.
82   *The Contributor*, January 1930, p. 708.
83   *The Contributor*, January 1934, p. 721.
84   *The Contributor*, January 1932, p. 12.
85   *The Hospital*, 26 (1930), p. 151.
86   *The Hospital*, 32 (1936), pp. 202–3.
87   'Free' legacies were donations which the hospital could use as it wished, as opposed to those earmarked for a particular purpose.
88   MRO, M610 MED 2/3/3/1, MHC, Distribution committee, 20 January 1929.
89   *Ibid.*, 17 October 1930.
90   BLSL, BHCA, annual report, 1928, 1931.
91   MRO, M610 MED 2/3/3/1, MHC, Distribution committee, 27 April 1933.
92   *Ibid.*, special meeting, 5 November 1934.
93   LMA, A/KE/11a/1, Contributory schemes committee, 1 August 1941, 30 October 1941, 11 June 1942.
94   Ministry of Health, *Hospital surveys* (10 vols) (London, 1945–46).
95   *The Hospital*, 30 (1934), pp. 334–5.
96   LMA, A/KE/11/1b, CSC, 11 June 1942.
97   Ministry of Health, *The hospital services of the north eastern area* (London, 1946), p. 89.
98   TNA: PRO, MH 66/721, Dr Lethem, 'Liverpool survey report' (1932), pp. 147–9.
99   *The Contributor*, February 1927, p. 93.
100 *The Contributor*, December 1928, p. 446, and January 1929, p. 35.
101 *The Hospital*, 31 (1935), p. 12.
102 *The Hospital*, 33 (1937), report of speech by F. B. Elliott, p. 65.
103 *The Hospital*, 35 (1939), pp. 299–300, and 37 (1941), p. 207.
104 For example: BCA, MS 1576/1, BHCS, MMC, 3 May 1929, 6 November 1929, 4 December 1929; MS 1576/3, BHCA, MMC, 19 December 1931; MS 1576/4, BHCA, MMC, 9 March 1932, 13 April 1932, 14 June 1932; MS 1576/5, BHCA, MMC, 13 September 1933, 8 November 1933; *The Liverpolitan*, June 1936, pp. 1–2.
105 BCA, MS 1576/3, BHCA, MMC, 19 December 1931; MS 1576/4, BHCA, MMC, 13 April 1932; Lethem, 'Survey report', pp. 149, 150; MRO, MHC, annual report, 1936.
106 Patients' Aid Association Archive (PAAA), Wolverhampton and Staffordshire Hospital, Hospital Saturday committee minute book, 3 July 1940.
107 BCA, MS 1576/5, BHCA, MMC, 12 July 1933; *The Samaritan*, March 1936, p. 14; for similar sentiment in Glasgow and Sunderland see ML, HB14/1/34, Glasgow Royal Infirmary minutes, 11 January 1919, and TWAS, HO/SRI/3/6, 19 January, 19 October 1946.
108 A. Atkinson, 'Municipal hospitals in relation to contributory schemes', *The Hospital*, 31 (1935), p. 12.
109 S. Cherry, 'Before the NHS: financing the voluntary hospitals, 1900–1939', *Economic History Review*, 50 (1997), pp. 305–26.
110 Chisholm, *Marketing survey*, pp. 111–17.
111 It is possible that some of these figures reflect reciprocal payments for patients treated elsewhere but we cannot determine this from this source of data.
112 Thompson, 'To relieve the sufferings of humanity', p. 254.
113 B. Doyle, 'The politics of voluntary health care in Middlesbrough, 1900–1948', in A. Borsay and P. Shapely (eds), *Medicine, charity and mutual aid: the consumption of health and welfare, c. 1550–1950* (Aldershot, forthcoming, 2006).
114 An extreme case makes the point: if a hospital derived an income of, say, £1 per bed from contributory schemes in 1926, and an income of £100 per bed in 1936, then this in percentage terms is a 9,900 per cent increase. The range of values is potentially extreme and violates assumptions of conventional statistical tests. The values can be transformed if we subtract the 1926 from the 1936 value, and divide this by the sum of the values. The

consequence is that all the values for change are constrained in the range zero to one: in this case, $(100 - 1)/(100 + 1) = 0.98$.

115 *HSA Contributor*, January 1939, p. 3.

116 BLSI., BHCA, annual report, various dates.

117 TNA: PRO, MH 99/18, Statistical memorandum.

118 J. Mohan, 'Voluntarism, municipalism and welfare: the geography of hospital utilisation in England in 1938', *Transactions, Institute of British Geographers*, 28 (1), 2003, pp. 56–74.

119 *The Hospital*, 31 (1934), p. 254.

120 *The Contributor, passim.*

121 A. M. Gray, 'A mixed economy of health care: Britain's health service in the inter-war period', in A. McGuire, P. Fenn and K. Mayhew (eds), *Providing health care: the economics of alternative systems of finance and delivery* (Oxford, 1991), pp. 233–60, at pp. 248, 250.

Chapter 4

The geography of hospital contributory schemes: membership, reciprocity and integration

If mass contribution was to save the voluntary system, as its advocates had hoped, then a key question was whether it could do so everywhere, or whether it would simply reinforce variations in the resources available to the hospitals. And in an era when the populace was becoming accustomed to the 'hospital habit', to what extent did membership of a scheme ensure that contributors could obtain treatment without having to undergo enquiries as to their means at all hospitals and not just the one with which their scheme was associated? To explore these questions, this chapter considers geographical variations in scheme membership and the associated issue of variations in the resources generated by the schemes.

The discussion is related to arguments concerning the strengths and limitations of voluntarism. First, there is the extent to which a voluntary system can steer resources to where they are most needed. Second, a question which was central to the development of the schemes was whether the inherent localism of voluntary activity could be overcome. There were clear tensions here, between the local loyalties and rootedness in community of many single-hospital schemes, and the broader view of multi-hospital funds, which recruited members over substantial territories. It might also be suggested that there was a tension between raising funds for a local cause, given concrete expression by a local hospital, and the abstract ideal of contributing to a collective fund. And could these problems be overcome through voluntary cooperation?

Comments on geographical variations in mass contribution can be traced back for over a century, when the hospital reformer Henry Burdett criticised the 'artisan classes' of London, who did 'not contribute to hospitals through the Hospital Saturday Fund in anything like the same proportion' as was the case in the provinces. He published league tables of per capita contributions to various Hospital Saturday funds and particularly praised the 'remarkable' success of the Birmingham fund.[1] The Cave committee (see chapter 2) began to assemble a more comprehensive picture and commented on the high level of membership in places such as Merthyr Tydfil, where 'practically every organised worker in the borough' was contributing a penny a week. In contrast, some witnesses to the committee referred to the difficulties of overcoming the 'lethargy of the country' − a comment, presumably, on the difficulties of organising mass contributory schemes in rural areas, though attention was drawn to successful rural initiatives in Oxfordshire, Hampshire and Wiltshire. The Cave committee attributed the problems of developing mass contributions in London to the 'absence of local patriotism'; hospitals were not so closely identified with their local community and it was 'difficult for a particular hospital to guarantee treatment'. There is also evidence that the committee regarded some locations – such as Manchester – as being relatively backward in scheme development.[2] However, there was no systematic analysis of variations in scheme membership. Academic work on contributory schemes has provided some regional comparisons of the proportions of hospital income generated by the schemes and of contribution rates.[3] As yet, however, there is no national picture of spatial variations in participation in, or the financial contribution of, the contributory schemes in the 1930s and 1940s. This chapter builds on previous research in three respects.

First, there is an assessment of variability in membership of contributory schemes between English counties. The catchment areas of the contributory schemes did not map neatly onto administrative boundaries, and some reassignment of scheme membership is undertaken, in proportion to the pattern of patient flows to individual hospitals. Estimates of the resources generated by the schemes are then produced by combining data on membership and average rates of contribution.

Second, there is a discussion of imbalances in the distribution of contributors, and of the problem of patients seeking access to hospitals which were not associated with the scheme of which they were members. The former problem arises from the classic 'free-rider' dilemma: individuals in need could not be excluded from hospital treatment but nor could they be compelled to join a contributory scheme. This problem was exacerbated by the logistic difficulties of collecting contributions in rural areas. The latter difficulty arose because most schemes were tied to a particular hospital and those seeking admission to other institutions risked incurring charges for maintenance. More generally, schemes did not operate over defined territories and there were several boundary disputes concerning whether large, multi-hospital funds had the right to encroach on what local schemes saw as their catchment area.

Third, the role of the schemes in the integration of hospital services is explored. Historians have argued that, in the first half of the twentieth century, there emerged general agreement on the desirability of regional organisation of hospital services, to ensure that medical expertise could be made available to all those in need of it. In the case of contributory schemes integration took several forms. The most common response was the development of reciprocal arrangements, whereby the fact that patients had been regular contributors elsewhere would be acknowledged if they were admitted to another institution, in the form of a payment to the hospital by the scheme to which the patient belonged. We discuss the development of such arrangements. We also examine the development of agreements between the schemes and municipal authorities, as well as the role of the BHCSA, the national representative organisation, in stimulating the formation of regional groupings of schemes.

Geographical distribution of contributory scheme membership

The *Hospitals yearbooks* give details of membership and the total value of contributions made for large numbers of individual schemes. Of 334 schemes
reporting to the *Hospitals yearbook* for 1938 in England, 213 supplied data on
both membership and income; for the other 121 schemes, which supplied data
on income but not membership, we estimated membership by applying national
average rates of contribution per head to the income data. Geographical variations in coverage can therefore be estimated by attributing the membership
of each scheme to the county in which it was based. However, this exaggerates
coverage in some counties while underestimating it in others, because large
funds had members in several counties. The HSA, for example, had 1,920,000
contributors in 1938, but while the scheme was based in London many of its
contributors resided in the surrounding counties. The membership of some
of the largest schemes has therefore been reassigned to geographical areas in
proportion to the pattern of patient origins as revealed by the wartime *Hospital
surveys*.[4] Thus, if 5 per cent of London's in-patients came from a given county,
then 5 per cent of the membership of the HSA and of the Hospital Saturday
Fund was reallocated there. This exercise was carried out for the twenty-four
largest schemes – those with over 75,000 subscribers; their 6 million members
accounted for over 60 per cent of the total for England. Smaller schemes were
usually linked to hospitals which treated few patients from outside the county
in which they were located, and reallocating their membership would have
involved disproportionate effort. Of course, there was not a perfect match
between the distribution of contributors and patients (the free-rider issue,
explored later in this chapter), but this method at least dampens down the
distortions which arise from attributing all contributors to the jurisdiction in
which the scheme to which they belonged was located. The main effects of this
adjustment are evident in major urban centres – for example, over a third of
the membership of the HSA was redistributed in this way. Information on the
pattern of patient flows, which is necessary for the estimation of county-level
membership rates, was not available for Scotland and Wales. For Scotland
we produced an initial estimate of 450,000 for members of contributory
schemes, but as the main Glasgow hospitals (whose schemes did not report a
membership figure) typically received some £60,000 per annum from workers'
contributions we should probably add at least 100,000 to that total. In Wales,
membership totalled 460,000, the largest schemes being in Swansea (114,000
members) and Cardiff (66,000).[5]

   The effect of our adjustment is to reduce the range of values for county-level
membership of schemes. The unadjusted values for membership ranged from
58 per cent of the local population to 1.6 per cent, but once adjusted the
range is from 44.8 per cent (Berkshire) to 7.9 per cent (Westmorland). When
the figures for England are mapped (figure 4.1) we can see that coverage was
greatest in East Anglia, Oxfordshire, Berkshire, Worcestershire and Leicester-
shire, as well as London. There is some consistency with the pattern of areas
with high levels of hospital utilisation (the latter show a strong north–south

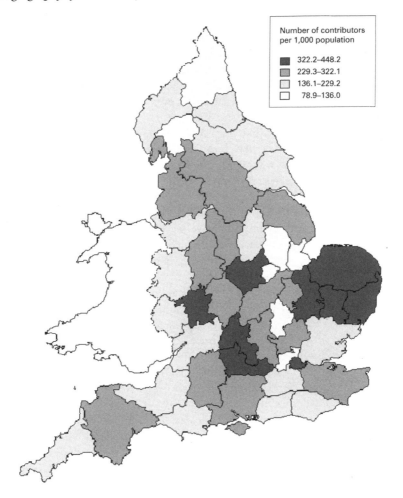

Figure 4.1. Ratio of contributors to total population in the English counties, 1938.

contrast, with a group of counties around London and extending westwards exhibiting high utilisation rates).[6] Most of the ten lowest-ranked counties were rural areas (Rutland, Lincolnshire, Shropshire, Herefordshire), perhaps reflecting the difficulties of organising collections in sparsely populated areas with few large urban centres, although East Anglia was clearly an exception. Although the principal schemes were all in large urban centres or conurbations (Birmingham, Liverpool, Manchester, Leeds, Sheffield) the counties of which these are a part did not feature in the highest-ranked areas, reflecting the difficulties of recruiting outside the main centres of population.

One caveat is that the schemes were not intended to cover the whole population; they were intended for those on low incomes (typically below £5–£6 per week), but there are no detailed data on the income distribution which would allow estimation of the proportion of households whose income was at this level. There are some estimates, for county boroughs (though not counties), of the number of households falling into four income bands, the lowest two of which (below £2 10s 0d per week; between £2 10s 0d and £5 per week) correspond to the income limits typically applied.[7] For English county boroughs covering roughly one-third of the country's population, on average 84 per cent of households were in these income brackets and the proportion exceeded 90 per cent in Warrington, Stoke and West Bromwich. In such places (and in the counties in which they were located) it seems reasonable to assume that nearly all the population was eligible for membership of contributory schemes, but this was not so elsewhere, such as in the eight boroughs where less than 75 per cent of households had weekly incomes of below £5. In such locations (e.g. Bournemouth, Coventry, Oxford) the estimated membership figures probably understate the comprehensiveness of coverage, though such towns may not be wholly representative of the income distribution in the counties of which they formed a part. In short, these data may underestimate the extent of coverage of the eligible population, though the margin of error is likely to be relatively small in the industrial Midlands and the North. There are just a few household surveys that allow direct corroboration of these estimates. These studies, undertaken in the late 1930s, suggested that 62 per cent of households in Bristol and 49 per cent in Blackburn subscribed to hospital funds. As the proportions of households within scheme income limits in those towns were 85 per cent and 81 per cent respectively, we may tentatively conclude that 73 per cent and 60 per cent of eligible households in Bristol and Blackburn were members of the schemes.[8]

Data on scheme income also allowed estimation of variations in the resources generated by the schemes. Averaging this out at the county level, figure 4.2 shows the income (in pennies per week) per contributor; only in Warwickshire did this figure exceed 3d. Income per contributor was typically in a relatively narrow band: 1.8d to 2.3d per week. Although some of the largest schemes asked for 3d per week as a typical contribution, the county-level averages do not approach this figure, reflecting cessation of contributions due to unemployment (one estimate, for Hull, was that at any one time 6.5 per cent of contributors were not paying their subscriptions) or short-time working,[9] and variations in weekly rates of contribution between schemes. For example, the average for London is brought down by the inclusion of the Hospital Saturday Fund – as it requested only 1d per week from contributors, which led to considerable friction with the HSA, with its standard rate of 3d per week. There is also evidence that contribution rates were the subject of contestation. Some schemes were unable to increase weekly contribution rates in the face of pressure from the trade unions (see chapter 6). At the level of individual schemes, the Sheffield 'penny in the pound' scheme was the most successful, generating around 4d per week per worker. This reflects the success of the fund in persuading employers to make matching contributions (see chapter 3). This is the principal reason why the West Riding of Yorkshire appears near the top of the rankings (fifth) on

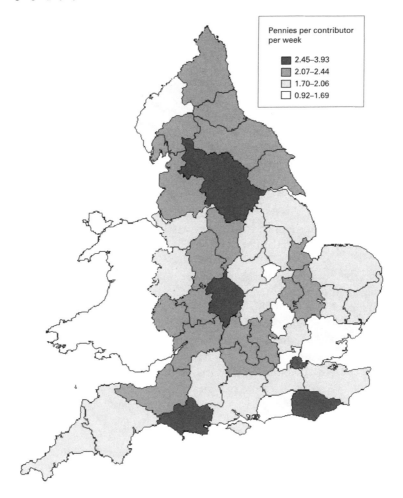

Figure 4.2. Income per contributor in the English counties, 1938.

income per contributor, when it is near the middle of the range on scheme membership.

At the onset of war, the schemes had experienced nearly twenty years of impressive growth (see chapter 3) and had a total membership of around half the population of England, but coverage was still highly variable. Again, it is not possible to be definitive because the proportion of the population above the income limits is unknown. But even if we assume two dependants per contributor (and schemes with which we are familiar assumed only one) this would still leave around 40 per cent of the eligible population outside the ambit of the schemes in most of the country, as shown by the lowest two categories on figure 4.1. The picture is further complicated by variations in the amounts received from each contributor (figure 4.2), which were primarily a function of the state of the labour market. Coverage and contribution interacted, as can be demonstrated if we combine membership and weekly contribution rates to produce an estimate of income generated by the schemes in each county. For those counties in which income per contributor was between 1.9*d* and 2.1*d* per week, income per bed ranged from £36 (Gloucestershire) to £119 (East Suffolk); this was largely a result of different levels of membership. When relatively high coverage combined with high weekly contributions, as in Yorkshire (West Riding) and Warwickshire, sums of up to £130 per bed could be generated. On this evidence the schemes had by no means redressed the substantial regional imbalances in funding which had been a feature of the voluntary system since the nineteenth century.[10]

Free-rider problems and boundary disputes: delimiting the territory of contributory schemes

Most of the contributory schemes were initiated to support a particular hospital. Identification with individual institutions was crucial because contributors would have tangible evidence of the improvements to local hospital services. However, tying benefits to specific hospitals became problematic for several reasons. In most areas scheme members were concentrated in urban areas so there were free-rider problems associated with people being admitted to hospital from surrounding districts, because the availability of specialist services in large cities attracted patients from afar. One effect of this was that contributors might be unable to obtain a bed in hospitals associated with their scheme. Other pressures resulted from social change. Thus, mobile workers, such as railway workers, could travel on a daily basis between regions and require treatment away from home if suddenly taken ill. Suburban growth meant that people were contributing, through their city-centre workplaces, to urban hospitals, but they might actually be treated at suburban hospitals which did not benefit from their contributions. Increased numbers of holidaymakers could also generate demands for treatment.

Contributors requiring hospitalisation might therefore find that they were admitted to a hospital other than the one with which their scheme was associated. In the absence of reciprocal recognition of their status as a contributor, they were then liable to be charged for the cost of hospital services. Moreover, adverse publicity resulting from denial of treatment to a contributor could undermine support for the schemes. These problems are briefly described here, followed by a discussion of attempts to resolve them.

The concern that the unsystematic growth of contributory schemes might distort, rather than stabilise, hospital income began to be articulated in 1923, even as the VHC was encouraging their spread. A meeting of a voluntary hospital committee representing institutions in Bristol, Somerset and Wiltshire pointed out that the hospitals in the urban centres of Bath and Bristol treated patients from surrounding rural areas yet derived no scheme income from them. In Frome, for instance, all contributory funds went in support of the town's 16-bed cottage hospital, which had neither resident medical staff nor visiting consultants.[11] And within Bristol itself the General Infirmary, which had markedly lower capacity and expenditure than the Royal Infirmary, received nearly the same amount from mass contribution. The Somerset committee duly called on the VHC to review the impact of the schemes.[12] H. N. Crouch, secretary of the VHC, argued that each scheme should extend over 'the whole area served by the hospital' and that all wage-earners therein should be made aware of the hospital's charges which their contributions would cover. If regional coordination of urban general hospitals and nearby cottage hospitals could be achieved, this would ensure that patients were referred to the appropriate institutions and that reimbursement from the schemes would follow accordingly.[13] This was an early and idealistic statement of the goal of regionalism, but putting it into practice was a different matter.

Similar concerns about imbalances in membership were expressed some years later by the MHC. Sydney Lamb, the Council's secretary, showed that over a four-year period it had cost Liverpool's hospitals some £102,000 to accommodate patients from outlying areas – yet these areas, it was estimated, had contributed only £51,000 from all sources to hospital funds. Lamb did acknowledge, however, that 'certain friends in these outlying areas remind us that they should be credited with many of the legacies received by Liverpool hospitals in the past'; this was perhaps an acknowledgement that, as Daunton has suggested, the charitable middle class had moved out of the city to suburban and rural areas.[14] Lamb's preferred solution was to strengthen recruitment efforts in order to bring 'outside' patients within the scope of the fund.

A response to such imbalances was the development of reciprocal arrangements whereby membership of one scheme was recognised if a patient was treated in an institution funded by another. The problem which then arose was variations in reimbursement rates; as Lamb pointed out, even where reciprocal arrangements were in existence, '50% of schemes pay adequately for services in outside hospitals, and 50% pay little or nothing'.[15] In public speeches Lamb made persistent reference to this problem and worked assiduously to solve it, but progress was not straightforward.

The tension between funds with different rates of contribution and remuneration, and between local and centralised funds, is clearly illustrated in the relationship between the HSA and various provincial schemes. The HSA had spread from its metropolitan base, partly through expansion in the South East and partly by recruiting in multi-site organisations such as railway companies and multiple stores. It had also struck agreements with a large number of provincial English voluntary hospitals (293 by 1937) to accept its 'green voucher' in lieu of payment.[16] While many hospitals seem to have welcomed HSA patients and accepted reimbursement from its fund for their treatment, others found the whole notion of an 'extra-regional' contributory scheme alarming.

Wolverhampton is one case in point. Problems arose first in 1932 over the treatment of the workforce of the Great Western Railway, of whom 2,000 were members of the Wolverhampton contributors' association, associated with the

Wolverhampton Royal Hospital, and some 400 were in the HSA.[17] The Royal had tried to bill the HSA for the treatment of its members at its standard maintenance rate of three guineas per week, but had received only two guineas, the HSA rate of reimbursement for London hospitals.[18] The hospital's board therefore informed the HSA that from January 1933 local HSA members would not be treated as in- or out-patients at the Royal.[19] The HSA took the matter to the Charity Commission, claiming that it was the right of workers to join whichever scheme they chose, but was rebuffed. The Wolverhampton Royal Hospital's board stood by its right to refuse treatment to those who were not contributors to the local scheme, and the Charity Commissioners concluded that they had no power to intervene.[20] The HSA was left with no further course but to pass a resolution condemning the hospital's board, to which the contributors' association responded with a message of support for the hospital, which it copied to both the BHA and the BMA.[21]

The dispute reflected the Royal's desire to retain a local membership base as well as concerns about the notional financial shortfall. The Royal claimed to be 'struggling for the principle' that local residents and workers 'should contribute to this Hospital and not to any London Collecting Society, that does not possess a single Hospital bed'. Note the dismissive terminology, which emphasises the importance attached to schemes associated with a specific hospital, in contrast to a city-wide fund. The board feared that the HSA 'apparently visualize a great contributory scheme for the country'. This would be 'fundamentally bad for provincial hospitals', as its own rates of contribution and low administrative expenses meant it could raise far more for the Royal than would the HSA's scheme. Indignantly, the board claimed that the HSA 'have in effect sold, without authority, the service of The Royal Hospital and its Honorary Staff for 3*d*. per week'.[22]

It may be that this defensive and insular stance arose from a previous negative experience. The Royal had had a dispute with the adjacent Birmingham contributors' association. In June 1932 the Royal's contributors' association had decided not to accept Birmingham vouchers from Wolverhampton-based workers employed by Birmingham and Midland Red Bus Company and Austin Motors. It had also refused to reimburse one of the Birmingham hospitals, St Chad's, for treating a member of the Wolverhampton scheme, resolving that 'Groups of men living in the Wolverhampton Hospital Area and working in Wolverhampton or elsewhere shall be expected to pay their contribution to the association'.[23] Thus the desire of individual hospitals to protect their income by putting geographical limits to eligibility and entitlement restricted the freedom of patients.

The Wolverhampton case was not the only example of an altercation involving the HSA. On Merseyside it was reported that the HSA had been 'unable to restrain their local honorary officers' from exceeding their brief of recruiting subscribers only from among railway workers employed by the London-based Great Western Railway.[24] *The Hospital* referred to negotiations regarding 'difficulties between the HSA and certain provincial hospitals'; these were institutions in the West Country, where the HSA had also initiated recruitment on the basis of its ties with the Great Western Railway.[25] However, it had subsequently used these ties as a bridgehead for the recruitment of other workers. Another dispute involving the HSA, with hospitals in Somerset, demonstrated the problems of differential rates of reimbursement. A reciprocal arrangement was concluded under which the HSA and the local scheme would each pay the same daily rate (6s), but the HSA wished to reduce this to 5s because its funds were being depleted by high levels of hospital utilisation. The local scheme criticised the HSA for failing to limit the growth of hospital use by its members and for offering a wide range of extra-hospital benefits rather than getting expenditure under control.[26]

The HSA–Wolverhampton dispute became the subject of mediation between the BHA and the HSA, and the BHA subsequently prepared a memorandum on the organisation of contributory schemes. Key propositions were that 'there should be no competitive organisations for the raising of money by contributory methods in the same area', that schemes should confine themselves to defined territories, and that reimbursement should follow the flow of patients to hospitals. The HSA responded with some rather bland and unexceptionable statements that it was its policy not to compete, but to cooperate, and that its general policy was to refer prospective contributors to their local schemes. It also declined to respond to the BHA's request that it confine its activities to the London area. What may really have riled the BHA, however, was the HSA's high-handed statement that, if provincial hospitals did not wish to cooperate with it, then contributors to the HSA in the relevant areas would be informed that they could expect almoners' enquiries if they were treated in non-cooperating hospitals. The clear implication was that the HSA was unwilling to negotiate with provincial schemes, and the BHA publicly stated that further negotiations were impossible owing to this stance. The matter was taken to the BHA's Joint Conference, in June 1933, at which the deeply felt local patriotisms of the movement were evident. According to Sir Harold Pink (Portsmouth), the chairman of the meeting, the BHA's preferred solution was for each scheme to have its own well defined area and the Association had been able to assist in defusing 'two or three' disputes (though details of these were not given). Pink thought that the HSA's attempt to 'spread their tentacles all over the country', on the pretext that companies with a head office in London 'really came under the HSA', would damage the movement as a whole. Other delegates criticised the HSA for failing to abide by undertakings it had given to 'refrain from canvassing' in their localities. Although one speaker claimed that the HSA had 'only come into those areas where there was not already a satisfactory scheme', he was quickly shouted down. The meeting concluded by endorsing the BHA's statement of principles.[27] The HSA claimed that its stance had the support of the executive of the BHCSA, but it transpired that the latter had either failed to convene appropriate meetings for discussion of the problem or had repeatedly postponed them on the basis of what one scheme secretary believed were spurious technicalities. This demonstrated the limited ability of the BHCSA to articulate the collective view of its members and develop an agreed policy.[28]

The problem of reciprocity was not confined to territorial disputes between schemes; there was a wider issue of the entitlements conferred by scheme membership. There were widely divergent views on this point. Concerns that patients were not obtaining admission to hospital through appropriate channels began to be expressed; as one scheme secretary expostulated, 'why should we give our contributors *carte blanche* to go anywhere for their treatment?' If this was allowed, contributors' 'imaginary preferences' for one hospital rather than another might mean that they would be treated in an expensive or inefficient hospital,[29] which would deprive their local hospital of resources. In contrast, it could also be argued that patients' choices were restricted, because they were largely compelled, perforce, to join the scheme associated with the hospital nearest to where they lived or worked. This led some administrators to deplore the isolationism of many schemes and the 'pettifogging and irritating restrictions' which they imposed. It was 'fundamentally unsound to force a patient to attend this or that particular hospital'.[30] Clearly, there was a need for a greater degree of integration and cooperation if the schemes were to maximise their impact.

Progress towards integration

The inter-war years witnessed discussions of, and some experiments in, the coordination of acute hospital services on regional lines. Indeed, as indicated in chapter 3, the foundation of some multi-hospital schemes was bound up with such proposals. The role of the schemes in coordinating hospital provision is the subject of this section, which considers the development of reciprocal arrangements between schemes, the role of the schemes in public–private partnerships after the 1929 Local Government Act, and the establishment of regional groupings of schemes under the auspices of the BHCSA.

Several multi-hospital schemes were established and they soon began to develop procedures for reimbursing hospitals (see chapter 3), as well as administrative structures, including local committees. There were also some amalgamations of schemes. Examples include the Cornwall Hospital contributors' association and the Bath region contributory scheme, which administered eight schemes in Somerset and Devon.[31] The unsystematic nature of this process is illustrated by the latter grouping, which covered an area between the Devon coast (Sidmouth) and Gloucestershire (Tetbury), overlapping with numerous other schemes on the way. This ran counter to a normative ideal of delimiting catchments within which the schemes could operate.

The most widespread response was the establishment of reciprocal arrangements. These were not universal and were not always possible; in some cases a scheme's constitution prevented it from entering into reciprocal arrangements which hinged on means testing of those admitted to hospital. This was the case with the Edinburgh Royal Infirmary, though it eventually amended its constitution in October 1942 and thereafter began to develop reciprocal arrangements with institutions as distant as Bristol and Coventry.[32] Here, we

summarise the evidence that we have concerning the extent of these arrangements and we point to some of the unresolved difficulties.

Following the lead given by officials such as Sydney Lamb, and the
endorsement by the BHCSA of the need for reciprocity,[33] the major urban
schemes began to develop reciprocal arrangements. Birmingham was an early
pioneer – the question of reciprocity had been one of the main reasons why
the leadership of the Birmingham scheme had argued for the establishment of
a national organisation in the first place (see chapter 2). Agreements had been
reached at an early date with smaller towns nearby, such as Lichfield, Worcester
and Hereford. Also, the nature of the West Midlands conurbation raised the
problem of employees who contributed through Birmingham workplaces but
lived in the city's hinterland, which necessitated agreements with hospitals in
such places as West Bromwich, Halesowen, Nuneaton and Walsall.[34]

The MHC was also actively developing such arrangements. It had invited
every contributory scheme in the country to agree to the principle of reciprocity,
and found a generally positive response – but most of its respondents were
schemes fifty miles or more from Liverpool, whereas the major problems of
cooperation were experienced in relation to schemes less than twenty-five miles
away.[35] In other words, it was easy to sign up to a reciprocal agreement if the
likelihood of having to honour it was small. By 1936 Merseyside had established
reciprocal arrangements with hospitals in 114 towns, rising to 150 in 1938,
entailing the recognition of each other's letters of introduction and reimbursement of costs incurred.[36] The Leeds Hospitals Fund began to record payments
to hospitals outside the city from 1932. However, this seems to have been a
rather *ad hoc* practice, because there is no mention in the annual reports of
formal procedures along the lines of the HSA's green voucher. A similar pattern
is evident for Sheffield, with greater evidence of progress towards cooperation
during the wartime years. In 1935 it was reported that reciprocal arrangements
were 'working very satisfactorily with a large number of other Contributory
Schemes affiliated to the National Association.'[37] During the war the scheme's
sphere of influence was extended, with full reciprocal arrangements with
hospitals in, for example, Barnsley and Rotherham, under the supervision of
regional committees of the Sheffield and District Hospitals Council.[38]

While the protection of voluntary hospital finances from free-riders, coupled
with the convenience of members, drove this process, it was also the case that
localist concerns impeded the equitable working of reciprocal agreements.
Subscription levels and benefits were far from uniform: single-hospital
funds, especially those in small communities, typically offered lower levels of
reimbursement than the great urban schemes. In Birmingham, for example,
three years of working the arrangements 'revealed that whereas "out-city"
hospitals were receiving the full cost of contributory patients' treatment, the
Birmingham hospitals were receiving barely 50% of the cost of the work done.'[39]
Smaller schemes worried that mutual agreements with a larger neighbour
would undermine local independence, by tending to regional standardisation,
and that they would cause contributors to desert, thus eroding the finances
of 'their' hospital. Gradually, however, such difficulties were resolved, partly

through the BHCSA-inspired development of regional groupings to hammer out compromise agreements of standard rates of reimbursement[40] (see below). Thus, in 1938 the Merseyside scheme agreed with the Manchester Hospitals Council that members of other schemes admitted to institutions in Liverpool or Manchester from outlying areas would be charged at 7s per day; in Birmingham, to maintain the 'goodwill' of neighbouring schemes, it was agreed that these would reimburse city hospitals at the same percentage of costs which they paid to their own institutions.[41]

Another aspect of reciprocity and regionalisation was the question of admitting the members of contributory schemes for treatment in local authority institutions (see chapter 3). While there had been concerns that any proposals to treat contributors in poor law infirmaries would be seen as an 'attempt to escape from an implied bargain',[42] some schemes were willing to contemplate this. For example, the once radical Birmingham Hospital Saturday Fund (BHSF) had initiated joint working with the corporation, arranging in 1924 that Dudley Road Poor Law Infirmary should treat fund contributors for a fixed annual fee, and then in 1926 handing over its tuberculosis sanatorium (after municipal authorities were given statutory power to treat patients with the condition).[43] The benefits of integrating public institutions into urban hospital systems were equally plain to others in the hospital world, particularly since the poor law and municipal hospitals were increasingly developing acute care facilities alongside their traditional remit of catering to the chronic sick. The Ministry of Health in the 1920s saw the virtue of using spare capacity in poor law infirmaries, as did some progressive local medical officers of health. Use of the public sector provided the opportunity to relieve voluntary hospital waiting lists of acute patients, and at the same time to remove patients requiring long-term care from voluntary beds. They also offered the possibility of broadening the cases and facilities available for teaching purposes.[44] For example, in Wolverhampton, New Cross Hospital was a poor law (public assistance, after 1929) infirmary which moved to extend its provision of acute services; by 1938, 294 of its 382 hospital beds were for acute medical, surgical or maternity patients, and it could draw on visiting consultants from local voluntary hospitals.[45] The Wolverhampton contributors' association reached an agreement with Staffordshire County Council public assistance officials in 1934 over the amount that the scheme would pay in respect of any members and dependants who were admitted.[46] The arrangement enabled the Royal Hospital to free up blocked beds by passing long-stay cases to New Cross, thus easing the pressure on its waiting list.[47]

Similar cooperation was evident in Birmingham, where the city's public health committee actively sought to build up municipal acute care, especially at Dudley Road Hospital; up to 14 per cent of the income of the contributory scheme went on treatment in municipal hospitals.[48] Local agreements for the admission of subscribers to the SHC into public hospitals antedated the 1929 Act,[49] and from 1931 arrangements were concluded with the corporation to reserve a number of beds at Sheffield's public hospital, the City General, in order to relieve pressure on the SHC's waiting list.[50] Admission was on

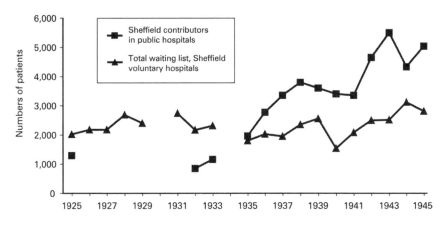

Figure 4.3. Contributors in Sheffield treated in municipal hospitals, and total numbers on the waiting lists of the Sheffield voluntary hospitals, 1925–45.

application to the medical superintendent, and assessment was carried out by the hospital almoner, thereby avoiding the stigma of being seen by the poor law relieving officer.[51] Coordination developed further from 1935; facilities at the City General were to be used 'for the treatment of accidents and home casualties within a defined area'.[52] In subsequent years, although the reports referred to an upper limit of 500 patients from the voluntaries' waiting lists going to the municipal hospitals, the overall number of patients whose care was reimbursed was greater, which suggests that some must have gone straight to the public institution.[53] The numbers of contributors availing themselves of municipal treatment in Sheffield rose between 1932 and 1939 from 850 to 3,500 (figure 4.3), though even then the money involved was only some 3 per cent of the sums going to the voluntary hospitals. None the less, the arrangement appears to have at least restrained the growth in numbers on the waiting list of the city's voluntary hospitals, which varied between 1,500 and 2,500, without any signs of increasing beyond this level (with the exception of 1944).[54] Finally, in Leeds, from 1931 the Leeds Hospital Fund made an arrangement with the local Public Assistance Committee of the Leeds Corporation that members and dependants should have access, free of charge, to two public sector hospitals, St James's and St Mary's, and 1,458 patients attended in 1933 for example. By the end of the sequence the sums going to the public hospitals were not insubstantial, though they remained far less than those directed to the voluntaries: in 1944, for example, £17,193 went to these two institutions, when the General Infirmary received £65,000.[55]

On the foregoing evidence we can see that the schemes played a growing role in the integration of hospital services. This could take the form of amalgamations, the establishment of multi-hospital schemes, negotiation of reciprocal agreements and the development of contractual arrangements with the public sector, the better to overcome capacity constraints in the voluntary hospitals.

These could be seen as pragmatic developments – recruitment would have been threatened if it was clear that scheme members were not getting treatment when needed – but there is also evidence that at least some figures in the contributory schemes movement had a broader vision of the problems and of how to resolve them.

The service of a hospital, or a hospital service?

The Cave committee (see chapter 2) had recommended the establishment of local voluntary hospital committees, the better to facilitate integration and coordination of hospital services and fundraising. This implied agreement on the areas to be served by hospitals, some conception of the role to be played by all the hospitals in a particular area, and the possibility of bringing public hospitals into association with the voluntary hospitals.[56] The need for integration was expressed succinctly by F. B. Elliott of the HSA, who argued that schemes were a 'fluid system of finance for modern conditions'; social change meant that 'the old watertight compartments within which hospitals worked … [were] breaking down'. Consequently, what the population required was not 'the service of a hospital, but a hospital service'.[57] Important figures in the movement, such as Sydney Lamb of the MHC and T. W. Place of the BHCA, made speeches at BHCSA conferences in 1932 and 1933. Place spoke of 'overlapping' being a symptom rather than the disease.[58] Lamb asked the 1933 conference to assist the BHA by 'determining … the recognised area in which each provincial contributory scheme should operate'. Such proposals for rationalisation had to confront the local patriotisms of the contributory scheme movement, which had inspired many scheme foundations, but by the mid-1930s there was a growing body of opinion deploring the 'narrowness of vision' in the movement. The inability of small, local schemes to extend membership, and their resistance to reciprocity, were clearly regarded as holding back the movement.[59] The HSA in fact tried to have its cake and eat it, in asserting that centralised funds were not incompatible with local patriotism.[60]

Conferences of the contributory schemes broadly agreed, then, on the goal of integration, but progress towards it proved slow. Eventually the voluntary hospital movement put its imprimatur on the regionalisation of the contributory movement in 1937. The occasion was the report of the Sankey commission, prepared for the BHA, which recommended that contributory schemes should henceforward be organised on a regional basis.[61] Its long-term financial goal was that each hospital region would organise its own 'conjoint collection', which would then be distributed equitably between the various institutions. Each scheme was to be regional with respect to organisation and benefits, though 'occasional exceptions' might be made for 'national workers' or patients requiring highly specialised treatment outside the area. The BMA's recommendation on the income limits of members was to be followed (a maximum of £200 per annum for single adults and £300 per annum for married couples with children) and there was to be no explicit 'insurance' element that would oblige the hospital to treat the contributor.[62] It was hoped that 'eventually' all schemes would follow 'the same model as regards contribution, benefit and administration' and that there would be reciprocal arrangements between contributory associations in each region.[63] Ironically, at least one member of the Sankey commission was unable to persuade his hospital to follow its recommendations. This was Alan Davies, chairman of the contributors' association at Wolverhampton Royal Hospital. Only during the war did Wolverhampton agree to reciprocal arrangements with most of the region's hospitals.

To what extent, then, did these calls from within the voluntary sector meet with a positive response? Much was left to the initiative of individual schemes, but the BHCSA's regional groupings also played a part. The formation of the BHCSA in 1931 was an attempt to overcome divisions and to achieve greater uniformity and cooperation among schemes (see chapter 3). One of its first challenges was to mediate between the HSA and Wolverhampton and, as we have seen, the BHCSA was perceived as ineffectual. Its first meeting resolved that local schemes should be free to operate in the areas served by their local hospitals, and that other schemes should not, with some exceptions such as railway workers, seek to recruit members from areas felt to be the territory of another scheme. There was broad agreement on this but the unresolved problem was that the BHCSA did not have the authority to define the areas to be covered by the schemes; such questions had to be resolved locally, through voluntary cooperation. The BHCSA hoped that each large scheme would convene a meeting of its neighbours, and some county-level groupings were formed, including a 'mid-southern' group and a Devon and Cornwall Association.[64] The desire to ward off external threats, like the HSA, underpinned the efforts of the Wessex Association of Hospital Leagues to define spheres of operation.[65] There are references in the papers of the BHCSA to nine regional groups; if survival of archival records is a guide, such groupings were largely absent from Yorkshire, the North West (apart from Manchester), the North East and the South West (apart from Devon and Cornwall).[66]

The Midland Group of Contributory Schemes was formed in 1938, though sceptical schemes such as Wolverhampton were assured that it was 'for purely consultative purposes'.[67] The report on its first meeting warily noted the discussion of the difficulties of 'dealing with vouchers from schemes without income limits'.[68] The Association was also happy to send Davies, along with W. Harper, secretary of the Royal Hospital, as delegates to meetings of the BHCSA.[69] The schemes in Shropshire, Staffordshire and Worcestershire were members of this grouping and during 1939 they discussed reciprocal arrangements with the BHCA. Reimbursement on the basis of a percentage of the cost of treatment, as initially requested by Birmingham, was inherently problematic for smaller and less well resourced schemes, which were concerned about how to limit their liabilities. It was agreed, apparently without much friction or negotiation, that reimbursement would be made at a standard rate per in-patient day.[70] This may of course have been pragmatism on the part of Birmingham; it would have made more sense to compromise on the amount to be reimbursed than to antagonise potential patients and supporters by holding out for a percentage cost reimbursement, especially when one recalls that the patient numbers involved were small.[71] Further discussions during the war resulted in standardisation of the rates of reciprocal payment to hospitals made by the region's schemes.[72]

The few surviving papers from other regional groupings reveal harmonious cooperation in East Anglia, where all the schemes in the constituent counties were members of the regional committee; apart from occasional comments about the encroachment of the HSA in wartime (partly due to evacuation of London-based firms) there is little sign of dissension.[73] Elsewhere, however, there was evidence of rivalry and competition at a very late stage in the schemes' existence. In Devon, during 1944, efforts to agree reciprocal payments of 7s per day were concluded without the participation of the Torbay scheme, which was demanding 10s per day. It was argued, however, that this would threaten the viability of the smaller rural schemes, and that this was Torbay's intention. Indeed, one scheme recounted that it had spent sixteen fruitless years attempting to develop a reciprocal arrangement with Torbay, but to no avail. Torbay was further criticised for attempting to negotiate with individual schemes rather than through the regional group.[74] And early in 1946 the BHCSA executive committee noted reports of disputes over reimbursement rates and catchment areas in the East Midlands and Kent, respectively.[75]

There is no national overview of the extent of these various forms of regional integration, but a sense of the slow progress towards this goal was conveyed in an address by Sydney Lamb, printed in the MHC's 1940 annual report, which urged the schemes to liaise with the voluntary hospitals and the BHA to ensure that their territorial groupings were 'in harmony with the new system of regional planning' promoted by the Nuffield Provincial Hospitals Trust (NPHT). This read as a normative goal rather than as a description of what was happening.[76] Yet again, in the 1943 annual report, under the heading 'More uniformity desired', there was a discussion of efforts to establish reciprocity which conveys the impression that the scheme was conscious of the slow progress being made nationally. By this time the MHC had agreements with 600 voluntary hospitals beyond Merseyside and 'many hospitals' controlled by local authorities, and it urged that 'now, more than at any previous period, it is of supreme importance that Letters of Introduction should have that universal validity which the Council has never failed to advocate'.[77]

Figure 4.4 juxtaposes two indicators of the progress of regional integration, with reference to Merseyside. The bars illustrate the scale of the MHC's grants to the municipal hospital, relative to the sums going to the voluntaries. Following the renegotiation of 1936, these payments increased in two steps to reach about one-third of the voluntary grants in the 1940s, although they fell back early in the war, perhaps reflecting the MHC's adjustment to the disruptions of the Emergency Hospital Service (EHS). Only after the NHS Act was passed, in 1946, did a really substantial sum go to the public hospitals. Thus, for most of this period, both sectors were interested in compartmentalising their sources of hospital finance, unless it was clearly in their interest to pool resources. The line in figure 4.4 shows the amounts received from other contributory schemes through reciprocal agreements. With the increasing number

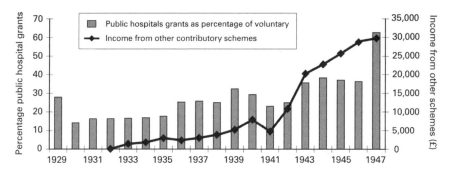

Figure 4.4. Merseyside Hospitals Council: the growth of regional arrangements, 1929–47.

of mutual arrangements made, it is not surprising that this sum increased rapidly, but it is doubtful whether the sums recouped covered the costs of treating patients from beyond Merseyside; at less than £5,000 per annum before the war, these reciprocal payments were around 10 per cent of the cost of treating non-Merseyside in-patients.[78] The rapid rate of increase from 1941 must partly reflect the greater mobility of the wartime labour market, but the growth of reciprocal payments continued after 1945. This suggests that, despite the numbers of reciprocal agreements struck in the 1930s and 1940s, the MHC did not succeed, until perhaps the very end, in organising a system which genuinely recouped the costs of treatment of contributors to other schemes.

Overall, there were conflicting assessments of the extent and success of reciprocity. In 1941 Sydney Lamb restated the principles of reciprocity and regional organisation which guided BHCSA policy but he also referred to 'delinquent' schemes which did not conform to BHCSA principles.[79] On the other hand, a Ministry of Health paper in May 1942 praised the BHCSA for its role in achieving 'almost complete' coverage of reciprocal agreements.[80] The BHCSA's response to the 1944 White Paper[81] included a reiteration of its acceptance of the need for strict demarcation of the areas to be served by the schemes. This declaration of intent was soon overtaken by events, in the form of the nationalisation of the hospitals. But even after that decision was taken, there was still evidence of territorial disputes between schemes (for example in Kent) and, in what might almost be seen as a verdict on the BHCSA's efficacy, the executive committee felt that neither the national association nor the regional groups had 'the power to insist on the fusion of schemes' when small contributing schemes were 'officially recognized and admitted to the BHCSA'.[82]

Conclusion

The growth of the contributory schemes was uneven; this, combined with variations in wages and labour-market conditions, meant that the resources generated varied substantially. Areas where membership was highest were not necessarily those which produced the most funds for hospitals. However, these variations received less consideration, and debate, than questions of inter-scheme rivalry and reciprocity. There were discussions about free-riders, reciprocal arrangements, the entitlements of patients and the extent to which they could be permitted to obtain treatment as and where they desired. The schemes played their part in regionalisation initiatives, and reciprocal arrangements were developed to facilitate the availability of services, but the process was not without dissension.

The inherent tensions had been well captured in a speech by Sydney Lamb to the conference of contributory schemes held in Harrogate in 1933. Lamb insisted that 'individuality, local patriotism and freedom to experiment were priceless features, which need not be jeopardised because you are asked to work in harmonious unity'.[83] In contrast the HSA, and others, saw the necessity of large-scale organisation. Regionalism was thus presented as an inevitable, and progressive, development. The dilemma was 'how to preserve all that is requisite of the autonomy of the unit and to secure all the strength and efficiency to be derived from a central unified policy'.[84] However, the fact that over 60 per cent of scheme membership was in large, often multi-hospital schemes might imply that 'local patriotism' – in the sense of an attachment to an individual hospital – was less important to contributors than Lamb suggested.

Problems of collective action were not resolved through voluntary co-operation. It does seem that extensive networks of reciprocal arrangements developed, and some regional groupings appear to have operated in a reasonably harmonious manner and to have resolved disagreements amicably. What is uncertain is whether there were failed efforts to promote regional groupings. The BHCSA endorsed the ideals of regional organisation at its annual conferences, but it had no effective levers which could be pulled to ensure that schemes settled their differences. Indeed, the history of the BHCSA records that it was supportive of regional groupings only where they had emerged spontaneously.[85] If this was so, the non-confrontational character of discussions within regional groupings is hardly surprising. Moreover, as the schemes were voluntary it was not clear how a national and comprehensive hospital service could be founded upon them; as a Ministry official argued in 1942, making membership of a scheme compulsory (and therefore universal) would destroy their voluntary character, but it was not clear that universal membership was possible without compulsion.[86] Thus, the localism on which many schemes were founded was both a source of strength and an obstacle to progress: their small size and voluntary character meant that many schemes simply lacked the organisational structure necessary to expand recruitment. The schemes therefore never attained comprehensive coverage, and a key factor in this was the question of attachments to individual hospitals. This was recognised as a potential threat to the movement – the secretary of the Eastern Group of the BHCSA argued that 'we will be bypassed if we do not burst out of watertight compartments and leap years ahead',[87] and ultimately this is what transpired.

Notes

1   H. C. Burdett, *Hospitals and charities* (hereafter *Burdett's*) (London, 1894), pp. cclxxv–cclxxvii ('London shows so badly [in the rankings] that comment is unnecessary'); *Burdett's* (1899), pp. 180–6; *Burdett's* (1914), p. 136 (Birmingham).

2   Ministry of Health, Voluntary Hospitals Committee, *Final report*, Cmd 1335 (London, 1921), pp. 19–24.

3   S. Cherry, 'Before the NHS: financing the voluntary hospitals, 1900–1939', *Economic History Review*, 50 (1997), pp. 305–26; S. Cherry, 'Regional comparators in the funding and organisation of the voluntary hospital system, c. 1860–1939', in M. Gorsky and S. Sheard (eds), *Financing medicine: the British experience since 1750* (London, forthcoming, 2006); B. Doyle, 'The politics of voluntary health care in Middlesbrough, 1900–1948', in A. Borsay and P. Shapely (eds), *Medicine, charity and mutual aid: the consumption of health and welfare, c. 1550–1950* (Aldershot, 2006).

4   Ministry of Health, *Hospital surveys* (10 vols) (London, 1945–46).

5   *Hospitals yearbook* (London, 1940), pp. 289–300.

6   J. Mohan. 'Voluntarism, municipalism and welfare: the geography of hospital utilisation in England in 1938', *Transactions, Institute of British Geographers*, 28 (1) (2003), pp. 56–74, figure 1.

7   C. Chisholm, *Marketing survey of the United Kingdom* (London, 1938), pp. 111–17.

8   C. Madge, 'The propensity to save in Bristol and Blackburn', *Economic Journal*, 200 (1940), pp. 410–48.

9   A. Atkinson, 'Municipal hospitals in relation to contributory schemes', *The Hospital*, 31 (1935), p. 12.

10 For a fuller discussion of these variations see J. Mohan, 'The caprice of charity: regional variations in finances of British voluntary hospitals, c. 1891–1944', in M. Gorsky and S. Sheard (eds), *Financing medicine: the British experience* (Routledge, forthcoming, 2006).

11 *Burdett's* (1922–23), p. 16.

12 TNA: PRO, MH 58/177, Crouch to Brock, 20 November 1923. In 1923 the Bristol General had 268 beds, against the Infirmary's 350.

13 TNA: PRO, MH 58/177, H. N. Crouch, 'Note on contributory schemes for provincial general hospitals', May 1923.

14 M. Daunton, 'Payment and participation: welfare and state formation in Britain, 1900–1951', *Past and Present*, 150 (1996), pp. 169–216, at pp. 188–9.

15 *The Hospital*, 29 (1933), p. 324.

16 *The Contributor*, January 1937, pp. 29–31, where readers were informed, cryptically, that the lists of hospitals accepting vouchers 'include some that are not fully co-operating'.

17 PAAA, Wolverhampton and Staffordshire Hospital, Hospital Saturday committee minute book, 10 August 1932.

18 This paragraph and the next are based on a loose-leaf memo inset in the cover of the Wolverhampton and Staffordshire Hospital, Hospital Saturday committee minute book (*ibid.*).

19 The Royal would, however, treat HSA subscribers who were 'itinerant' and suffered an accident or emergency while in Wolverhampton.

20 PAAA, Wolverhampton and Staffordshire Hospital, Hospital Saturday committee minute book, 4 January 1933.

21 *Ibid.*, 25 February 1933.

22 *The Hospital*, 29 (1933), p. 96.

23 PAAA, Wolverhampton and Staffordshire Hospital, Hospital Saturday committee minute book, 8 June 1932.

24 MRO, L610 MED 2–4, Merseyside Association of Hospital Contributors, Executive committee, 11 December 1928.

25 *The Hospital*, 29 (1933), pp. 205–7; examples were given from Exeter, Bath and elsewhere in the West Country.

26 BLPES, BHCSA 8/2, *Report of the 5th annual conference* (1935), p. 21.

27 The BHA's resolution, and the HSA's response, appear in *The Hospital*, 29, (1933), pp. 209–11; the report of the BHA's Joint Conference, from which these quotes are drawn, is at pp. 205–8.

28 *The Hospital*, 29 (1933), pp. 214–15, letter from W. H. Flear, secretary of the Mid-Southern Group of the BHCSA.

29 *The Hospital*, 30 (1934), p. 334, letter from the secretary of the Northampton and District Hospital Fund.

30 W. Parkes, 'Contributory schemes and their relations with voluntary hospitals', *The Hospital*, 30 (1934), pp. 290–3.

31 Bath: Chippenham, Clevedon, Devizes, Hambrook, Malmesbury, Ottery St Mary, Sidmouth and Tetbury; Cornwall: Hayle, Helston, Isles of Scilly, Newquay, Redruth, St Austell, Stratton, Truro. *Hospitals yearbook* (London, 1942), pp. 204–16.

32 LHSA, LHB 1/18/3, Edinburgh Royal Infirmary League of Subscribers, Executive committee, 9 October 1942, 17 February 1943, 23 January 1944.

33 BLPES, BHCSA, 7/1, *Report of the 3rd annual conference*, 1933, pp. 10–18.

34 BLSL, BHCA, annual report, 1934; BHCA, MMC, 17 June 1930, 14 January 1931, 8 March 1933.

35 *The Hospital*, 32 (1936), pp. 144–6.

36 MRO, M610 MED 4/1, MHC, annual reports, 1936, 1938.

37 WHSA, SHC, annual report, 1935.

38 WHSA, SHC, annual reports, 1941, 1943.

39 *The Samaritan*, 4 (December 1937), p. 26.

40 BLPES, BHCSA, 6/9, Wolverhampton group minutes, 4 January 1939, 6 September 1939, 3 January 1940.

41 MRO, M610, MED 4/1, MHC, annual report, 1938; BCA, BHCA, MMC, 8 March 1933, 10 May 1933.

42 Ministry of Health, Voluntary Hospitals Committee, *Final report*, p. 7.

43 BCA, MS 1576/4, BHCA, MMC, 13 April 1932; G. Hearn, *Dudley Road Hospital, 1887–1987* (Birmingham, 1987), pp. 43, 45; BHSF, *65 years history of the Birmingham Hospital Saturday Fund 1873–1938* (Birmingham, 1938), pp. 31–2, 38: the corporation also took over the substantial debt on the sanatorium.

44 TNA: PRO, MH/58/172, Hospital accommodation enquiry 1923–25, L. G. Brock to Onslow, 20 February 1924; M. Gorsky, '"Threshold of a new era": the development of an integrated hospital system in north-east Scotland, 1900–39', *Social History of Medicine*, 17 (2004), pp. 247–67.

45 Ministry of Health, *Hospital survey: the hospital services of the West Midlands area* (London, 1945), p. 44; TNA: PRO, MH/66/1079, C. J. Donelan, Wolverhampton CB: survey of health services, 1931, p. 70.

46 PAAA, Wolverhampton and Staffordshire Hospital, Hospital Saturday committee minute book, 27 January 1934, 7 February 1934, 7 March 1934, 6 June 1934, 18 June 1934. The union which New Cross had served before 1929 included parts of both Wolverhampton county borough and Staffordshire county council; it subsequently became the borough's hospital, with the county patients withdrawing in 1935 (see Ministry of Health, *Hospital survey*, p. 44).

47 PAAA, Wolverhampton and Staffordshire Hospital, Hospital Saturday committee minute book, 3 July 1940.

48 Hearn, *Dudley Road Hospital*, pp. 54, 57.

49 WHSA, SHC, annual report, 1926.

50 WHSA, SHC, annual report, 1931.

51 *Ibid.*

52 WHSA, SHC, annual report, 1935.

53 WHSA, SHC, annual report, 1936.

54 WHSA, SHC, annual report, 1932, 1939.

55 Leeds Central Library, Leeds and District Workpeople's Hospital Fund, annual reports, 1934, 1945.

56 The theme of hospital regionalisation is given much fuller treatment in Fox's work: see D. Fox, *Health policies, health politics* (Princeton, NJ, 1986).

57 *The Hospital*, 33 (1937), pp. 65–7.

58 T. W. Place, speech to BHCSA conference, Torquay, 1932, reported in *The Hospital*, 28 (1932), p. 279.

59 *The Hospital*, 32 (1936), pp. 144–6.

60 *The Hospital*, 33 (1937), pp. 65–7.

61 B. Abel-Smith, *The hospitals 1800–1948: a study in social administration in England and Wales* (London, 1964), pp. 414–15; C. Webster, *The health services since the war, vol. I* (London, 1988), pp. 263–7. The regions were intended to coincide with those of the BHA. The BHA subsequently proposed fourteen regional councils for England and Wales, made up of over sixty divisional councils, so the scale on which regional contributory arrangements were to operate was never clearly stated.

62 BHA, *Report of the voluntary hospitals commission* (London, 1937), pp. 32–3.

63 *Ibid.*, p. 34.

64 BLPES, BHCSA 7/1, Report of executive committee, 1932–33.

65 *The Hospital*, 30 (1934), p. 282.

66 The listing of BHCSA papers in the BLPES records groups in: Devon and Cornwall; eastern England; Kent; London; Shropshire, Worcestershire and Staffordshire; Warwickshire; and Manchester.

67 PAAA, Wolverhampton and Staffordshire Hospital, Hospital Saturday committee minute book, 12 January 1938.

68 *Ibid.*, 6 April 1938.

69 PAAA, Royal Hospital Wolverhampton Contributory Association, Minute book, 7 June 1942.

70 BLPES, BHCSA 6/9, Wolverhampton group minutes, 4 January 1939, 6 September 1939, 3 January 1940.

71 According to the hospital survey, in 1938 there were 33 patients from Wolverhampton, 188 from West Bromwich and 102 from Shropshire, though there were 1,507 from Staffordshire. Ministry of Health and NPHT, *The hospital services of the West Midlands area* (London, 1945), pp. 71–3.

72 PAAA, Royal Hospital Wolverhampton Contributory Association, Minute book, 7 July 1943.

73 BLPES, BHCSA 6/2, *passim.*

74 BLPES, BHCSA 6/1, Devon and Cornwall regional committee, 7 December 1944, 8 March 1945, 16 September 1946.

75 BLPES, BHCSA 2/6, Executive committee, 7 February 1946.

76 MRO, M610 MED 4/1, MHC, annual report, 1940.

77 MRO, M610 MED 4/1, MHC, annual report, 1943.

78 Estimate derived by calculating the proportion of in-patients at Liverpool hospitals who were not from Liverpool, Cheshire or the principal county boroughs on Merseyside, and applying this to the expenditure of Liverpool hospitals for 1938.

79 S. Lamb, 'The future policy of voluntary hospital contributory schemes', *The Hospital*, 37 (1941), pp. 131–2.

80 TNA: PRO, MH 80/34, Memorandum on contributory schemes development, 21 May 1942.

81 Ministry of Health, *A national health service*, Cmd 6502 (London, 1944).

82 BLPES, BHCSA 2/6, Executive committee, 7 February 1946.

83 *The Contributor*, October 1933, p. 625.

84 *The Contributor*, December 1935, p. 550.

85 A. T. Page, *Pennies for health: the story of the British Hospitals Contributory Schemes Association* (Birmingham, 1949), pp. 13–14.

86 TNA: PRO, MH 80/34, Memorandum…, 21 May 1942.

87 BLPES, BHCSA 6/2, note by E. Watkin, 8 August 1942.

Chapter 5

Hospital contribution and civil society: humanity not democracy?

This chapter turns to the contributory schemes' role as mediators of popular participation in health provision. Part of their self-image was as vehicles for patient involvement in hospital affairs, and they were subsequently admired as 'democratic in origin and in self-government ... a splendid way of showing how democracy can become an aristocracy of public service'.[1] As such they offer a hitherto unexplored resource for learning about the nature of active citizenship, augmenting the work of scholars such as Finlayson on voluntary involvement in social welfare.[2] More generally, they provide a case study of how institutions of civil society generate social capital. As noted in chapter 1, recent literature stresses the broader importance to political life of a vigorous voluntary sector. Following a Tocquevillian model, the argument is that active local citizenship achieves a broader social good by stimulating ties of trust and promoting political engagement in wider society. Moreover, proponents of greater mutualism and localism in the welfare state have suggested that past practice demonstrates the vitality of local governance: subscriber democracy was once genuine and effective, and so can be again.[3]

This chapter (and that which follows) will interrogate these ideas through the contributory schemes. First, it presents empirical evidence on the scope for grassroots or local involvement in decision-making, and explores the structures and procedures of representation. It illustrates the mechanisms available for popular participation and the channels by which the views of the small contributors were conveyed to hospital management boards. The next section asks how 'active' contributors were in the movement, in terms both of attendances in democratic forums and of the nature of the leadership which the movement selected to represent it. The ethos of the contributory schemes is then surveyed: were they perceived principally as sites of voluntary action, or simply as a practical necessity – as *public* interest or *self* interest? And, given the role of the labour movement in the gestation of the schemes, what does the relationship between the two reveal of notions of social citizenship held by trades unions and the Labour Party?

Representative structures

Multi-hospital schemes

The pan-city funds in Sheffield, Birmingham and Liverpool illustrate the representative arrangements of multi-hospital schemes with very large numbers of subscribers. Such schemes were closely affiliated to their local 'hospital councils', city-wide planning bodies (whose emergence was described in chapter 3) on which hospital managers sat alongside doctors, industrialists and academics. These sought to rationalise fundraising by developing existing Saturday funds into more extensive contributory schemes, and the process of constituting these raised the issue of contributors' representation.

The influential case of Sheffield demonstrates the creation of elaborate structures linking grassroots contributors to decision-making bodies. Initially the SHC consisted of thirty-six people, including five lay and medical members from each hospital, five university members and five employers or workpeople.[4] It quickly decided that direct representation of works contributors on both the Council and individual hospital boards was 'essential for the success of the voluntary scheme'.[5] The Sheffield trades and labour council assisted by convening a meeting of delegates from 264 contributing firms and in November 1921 the Association of Hospital Contributors was inaugurated.[6] In addition to fundraising for hospital and convalescence care, its constitution stipulated that it should articulate the views of members and dependants, ensure 'adequate and prompt treatment', represent contributors on the SHC and hospital boards, and meet the needs for treatment of the poor and unemployed. The Association had a pyramid structure. At its base were the committees in the city's workplaces, wards and outlying districts which organised income gathering, through either payroll deduction or collection, and also ran fêtes and bazaars to generate additional funds.[7] For every 500 subscribers it had, each committee could send one delegate to the Association's quarterly meetings and AGM, at which five contributor nominees were elected to serve a term of three years on the SHC. This number was increased to ten in 1922 and nineteen by 1926, though this did not imply a larger voice on the Council as it also grew, to sixty-two by 1923 and eighty-one by 1926. By this time it included representatives of general practitioners, the press, the trades council, clergy, the corporation, the Cutlers' Company and the poor law guardians.[8] The elected members on the Council also provided the pool from which were drawn the contributors' representatives on the board of each of the voluntary hospitals.[9] Finally, the mass meetings elected representatives to the Association's seventeen-strong executive committee, which was typically dominated by people from collieries, metalwork and engineering companies, the utilities, the Post Office and the railway.[10]

In Birmingham contributor representation was more diluted. The BHCA was managed by a committee established by the Birmingham Hospitals Council; it was chaired by a local businessman, Bertram Ford, and, as in Sheffield, had the mayor as president, signifying the Association's role as a high-profile civic initiative. There were initially two contributors' representatives on this committee, rising to six by 1936, from either large manufacturing concerns or district branches; a further seven, rising to ten by the mid-1930s, came from the Saturday Fund, now renamed the 'Industrial Section'.[11] Others came from the voluntary hospitals (in 1936, fourteen members), the Hospitals Council (four), the Chamber of Commerce (two), the national insurance panel committee (two) and the Hospital Officers Association (two).[12] There was no attempt to weight membership according to the proportion of income raised – some 75 per cent of which came from the Industrial Section. Thus, although workplace representatives dominated the Industrial Section's executive, the BHCA was led by voluntary and medical leadership and was, anyway, distinct from the Hospitals Council.[13] Ford rebuffed attempts by the Birmingham trades council to obtain direct representation, and in general Birmingham's labour organisations were kept at arm's length.[14]

In Liverpool, working-class patients had rather better representation on the MHC. Here the contributors' association was formed to provide 'a machinery for the expression of views'.[15] Any workplace could nominate a delegate to its AGM, with additional representation for firms with more than 500 members.[16] Elections were held for the fifteen members of an executive committee and for the ten members who represented the association on the 129-strong MHC; these members could serve for two years, with five retiring each year.[17] Four more representatives to the Council came from the 'area committees' in Liverpool and its hinterland, which raised funds from the self-employed and others.[18] The remaining MHC seats were allocated to 'organised labour' (thirty), local government health committees (fourteen), hospital subscribers and staff, local general practitioners, university, press and employers; workers were therefore in the minority.[19] Meetings of the contributors' association focused to a considerable extent on fundraising, although the executive committee's brief extended to the consideration of contributors' complaints and representing these to the Council.[20]

Direct representation was weaker in the HSA, the largest multi-hospital scheme, which provided no mechanism for grassroots contributors to sit on individual hospital boards. Following its inception in 1922, its membership climbed to some 2 million, organised around 'branches', in which volunteers canvassed local firms. Contributor 'groups' were formed within participating businesses; there were ultimately some 14,000 local groups, which often relied on the commitment of an individual secretary to recruit new members and obtain weekly contributions.[21] Examples of large concerns where early groups were formed included the Great Western Railway, the South Metropolitan Gas Company, W. H. Smith and Son, Hovis, Cadbury's, Brooke Bond, Truman, Hanbury, Buxton, LCC tramways, Harland and Wolff, Vickers, United Glass Bottle manufacturers, the Woolwich Arsenal, the Post Office and the metropolitan borough councils.[22] Initially, HSA branch secretaries were to arrange local meetings of group representatives, rather than large central meetings. Each group could nominate one 'member' for every 1,000 contributors (up to five per group) to attend the AGM, which in practice was a meeting of group secretaries.[23] Held in the Kingsway Hall, central London, they were the high point of the year for HSA activists and were attended by up to 2,000 people, who would be addressed by prominent politicians, religious figures, trade unionists and, occasionally, the Prince of Wales.[24] Groups were also entitled to nominate four members to the HSA's executive council.[25]

With this structure in place, the HSA deemed itself 'constitutional in the fullest sense'; it claimed that the group system offered each individual contributor a means of 'keeping in touch with the hospital problem' and that 'full facilities are provided for all to work together and to understand each other's views', from the 'contributor right up to the Chairman of Council'.[26] However, the only opportunity for group secretaries to raise questions about policy was at the AGM; even there, while the chairman of the executive council would respond to them, there was no opportunity for debate. In practice, power devolved to the small executive committee, on which the four contributor members were in the minority, the remainder being four 'hospital' and four 'general' members.

Single-hospital schemes

Where a scheme supported a single hospital, a variety of different arrangements for contributor governance existed. Typically a voluntary hospital called an AGM of all its subscribers to ratify any rule changes and elect a board of management, and, in large institutions, sub-committees to deal with such issues as finance, staffing, buildings and medical policy. The issue for contributors was therefore the extent of their representation at the AGM and on the board of management. Where a separate organisation – a contributory scheme or Saturday fund – oversaw fundraising, the questions arose of how ordinary contributors should be represented on the scheme's management body and of how the scheme should nominate representatives to hospital management boards.[27] In schemes administered directly by the hospitals, matters were simpler, with representation usually granted by reserving for contributors a set number of seats on the hospital's governing body.[28]

A few examples will illustrate local variations of hospital board membership. In Nottingham, a Saturday fund started and managed by hospital officers had reconstituted itself as an independent body in 1873, with any firm providing at least two guineas per annum entitled to have a delegate become one of the General Hospital's governors. By the Second World War the fund had six representatives on the hospital's monthly board and membership of the committee which selected honorary consultants.[29] Gloucestershire Royal Infirmary was less generous: it permitted workers three representatives on its general committee and only one on the weekly committee, which was responsible for day-to-day management of the hospital.[30] In the early 1920s Oxford's Radcliffe Infirmary proposed to allot seven of its twenty-eight committee seats to contributors.[31] In the same period Merthyr Tydfil's Joint Working Men's Hospital Committee had fifteen members, who also constituted one-third of the executive board.[32] Labour's position was better in Barrow-in-Furness, where contributors made up half the council of North Lonsdale Hospital, which attributed the scheme's success to this generous representation.[33]

The picture is therefore similar to the multi-hospital schemes, with large, lively contributors' associations, which had a significant, albeit minority, voice on hospital boards. For instance, Bolton Royal Infirmary's scheme was administered by a Hospital Saturday committee founded in 1877 by local trade union and friendly society activists, and in the inter-war period operated a contributory scheme that provided hospital and nursing benefits to members and dependants for 2*d* per week.[34] The committee was large, with 134 members in 1934–35, including representatives from the 'out-districts' and co-opted members from the trades council, the National Union of Teachers and the district nursing association.[35] It met each February to elect its officers and eight members (rising to twelve by the 1930s) to serve on the management committee of Bolton Royal Infirmary. There were two formal channels for grassroots input: complaints about the service were formally recorded and investigated by the committee; and members were entitled to submit a motion for discussion.[36] Within the hospital, however, the contributors' voice was smaller. The Infirmary retained a subscriber recommendation system and reserved twenty-four seats on its management committee for philanthropic subscribers, who, along with the medical staff, easily outnumbered the Saturday fund representatives. This arrangement did not reflect relative financial weight: in 1935, for instance, the scheme yielded over £24,000 against about £3,000 from subscription.[37] Bolton's trades council deplored this situation and the committee pressed for the Saturday fund to have 50 per cent representation on all Infirmary committees, for all fund members to be allowed to vote at AGMs, and for evening board meetings, to permit working-class attendance. By 1947, however, they still provided only twelve of the fifty-strong Infirmary management board.[38]

A similar situation obtained in the case of the Wolverhampton hospital, where frustration with under-representation surfaced only in 1944 (see chapter 8). Firms contributing at least three guineas annually could send two members to the contributors' association AGM, which was always well attended.[39] That association's purpose was to further 'projects for the good of the Hospital, especially … the adoption by all workers, of the weekly system of contributing'. This limited remit, which excluded the advancement of contributors' interests or views, was reflected in representative arrangements. The executive committee included the hospital's chairman, vice chairman and one member of its board of management, thirteen elected Wolverhampton fund members and the officials of outlying district committees. The duties of these local committees were restricted to the organisation of fundraising events, and only three members of the scheme had seats on the hospital board. However, the AGM also elected five house visitors, whose duty was to report to the association on the state of the hospital, and this potentially offered a conduit for the expression of users' views.

An example of an association with an even more restricted remit was the Winchester and District Contributory Scheme. Known initially as the

'Insurance Scheme', this was established by officials of the Royal Hampshire County Hospital, had 26,600 members and 284 branches by 1925, and was managed by the hospital's almoner, who carried out the assessments.[40] The Royal had little scope for expansion based on traditional charity, as it lacked either industrial wealth or an aristocratic presence; by the late 1930s two-thirds of its income came from payments by patients, the majority through the Scheme.[41] The Scheme's committee had originally been a hospital sub-committee, and its fundraising had been more through area collections than through payroll deductions, augmented by social activities such as whist drives.[42] Records of AGMs give little sense of open discussion; instead, the dominant feature was a speech from the chair of the Royal's court of governors, followed by a prize-giving to successful secretaries and collectors: in 1943 National Savings certificates for six people and certificates of merit for forty-three, the vast majority of whom were women.[43]

What was the situation in hospitals where no means test applied and where the scheme supported an 'open door' policy? In Edinburgh the absence of an insurance element appears to have lessened contributors' influence. Here the League of Subscribers set no flat rate for contribution; membership was conditional on payment of 1*d* from adults or ½*d* for juniors and although membership cards were issued these did not serve as a voucher for treatment.[44] The Infirmary's finance committee provided the League's accommodation and it was run by a small executive consisting of its president, vice-president, honorary secretary and organising secretary (who was also the Infirmary's secretary), along with three other members.[45] For its first ten years it had no seats on the Royal Infirmary's board, although this body did contain three representatives of local miners' associations and two from the trades council.[46] Subsequently AGMs saw the election of two League representatives to the board, on which they were in the minority. In 1938 there were twenty-eight members in total, with seven from the League and labour organisations, the remainder being from local government (two), the Royal College of Surgeons and Physicians (four), the university (two), commercial and professional associations (five), philanthropic subscribers (six) and Infirmary management (two).[47] This was not disproportionate to the relative income shares of philanthropy and contribution, though with over 100,000 supporters the League might legitimately have claimed a larger voice.[48]

However, where the shift away from philanthropy had begun early and the hospital's proportion of contributory income was high, 'open door' schemes were well represented and grassroots democracy was energetic. Two final cases, from the North East, will demonstrate this, and here it is likely that scheme activism was coloured by participants' experience of trade unionism, particularly in the collieries.

Sunderland Royal Infirmary's early extension of participatory rights occurred in 1881, when mass contribution first exceeded charity, and by 1900 the excess had grown (in 1900 contributions totalled £6,287 and subscriptions £1,994).[49] Elected representatives sat on a 'workmen's governors committee', which met regularly and elected delegates to the Infirmary board of management. Printed minutes of the committee's meetings and relevant sections of the Infirmary's rules were sometimes disseminated for consideration by workplace members.[50] By the inter-war period, these governors held a third of the seats on the Infirmary's board of management, the remainder being divided between subscriber representatives and medical staff. This tradition of transparency and participation set the stage for various conflicts, discussed in chapter 6.

Newcastle's Royal Victoria Infirmary allowed contributing firms in 1923 to nominate one governor for each £10 subscribed, and thirty-two of these sat on its seventy-six-strong governing board.[51] Their selection was made at meetings of six district committees of 'workmen' governors, of which Durham, North Tyne and Newcastle districts were the largest. Numbers of representatives rose over the period as the workmen lobbied for increases.[52] Procedures were scrupulously followed, with regular scrutiny of attendance records and concern with electoral mechanisms.[53] Efforts were made to disseminate information on hospital committee business to the mass of contributor governors, and some districts went to great lengths to ensure that the nomination process for the Infirmary's house committee (the hospital's executive) was not just delegated to governors but was also subject to workplace ratification.[54] Sometimes discussions became heated, as in the Durham district when a majority proposal to re-elect the current members *en bloc* led to such noisy opposition that the meeting had to be abandoned.[55] Indeed, Durham meetings were often spirited, perhaps because they were a forum in which other coalfield political tensions were expressed.[56]

Our survey therefore confirms the existence of representative procedures for contributors, but raises questions about their scope for real influence. Based on the evidence of the large urban schemes surveyed here, the usual arrangement was for a contributors' association to be formed, whose corporate identities ranged from active, democratic bodies dealing both with fundraising and patients' concerns to gatherings of voluntary collectors meeting infrequently at the hospital's behest. These associations typically provided the forum for the selection of a small number of representatives to the governing boards of joint hospitals councils or to individual institutions. In most cases, however, the numbers were small. Indeed, a minority position was recommended by the secretary of the VHC, H. N. Crouch, who advised in 1923 that a scheme should furnish no more than one-third of the management committee, and that 'its right of representation should not be such as to imperil the independence of the hospital'.[57] In the event, the VHC's published advice made no mention of this, concluding that it was unnecessary to warn explicitly of the 'dangers of over-representation', on the grounds that local committees 'can see that well enough for themselves'.[58] Evidence from the early days of the schemes suggests that hospital elites were diffident about such participation. A witness to the Cave committee from Newcastle commented that 'little was done' at the mass meetings, which he thought were 'not to the advantage of the hospital', while the chairman of Glasgow Royal Infirmary confided that 'one has to watch them [workmen governors] and humour them a bit'.[59] An even more telling illustration of this conceptual gulf came at the first meeting of Sheffield's contributor delegates, when the Royal Infirmary's senior surgeon, having expressed his delight at their 'valuable co-operation', went on to urge 'that they would think of the work of the hospitals more as Humanity than of Democracy'.[60]

Activism

Any conclusion about the capacity of the contributory schemes to foster social citizenship must hinge on the nature and extent of active participation of volunteers. This section asks whether involvement in the various organisational structures was extensive among the ordinary contributors and identifies the types of people who became activists in the associations.

Attendance

Attendance figures for mass meetings of workplace members paint a contradictory picture, in that while turnouts were usually large, representation seems to have been far from universal. In Sheffield 600 people attended the Association's fourth quarterly delegates' meeting in 1922, while 350 came to the 1924 AGM. Numbers had dropped by the early 1940s, with quarterly meetings attracting about 100 and AGMs about 50, though 300 delegates attended the hundredth quarterly meeting in 1946.[61] Even so, by 1926 there were around 2,500 firms contributing, and ninety-three separate wards and districts.[62] The picture in Glasgow is rather similar. The AGMs at which elections took place were well attended, with an average of 167 delegates over the inter-war period, and a peak in the late 1920s of about 200 people. Interest appears to have fallen off somewhat in the war years, when the average was 138 members, dropping to only 112 in 1948.[63] Here, in 1930 for example, out of 790 firms whose subscriptions entitled them to nominate delegates, only 300 did so, and of these only 187 attended the Saturday afternoon AGM.[64]

Much the same pattern is discernible elsewhere. The Edinburgh League's AGMs were well supported, even if, for example, the 270 people at the 1930 AGM were a small fraction of the 100,000 members.[65] Newcastle upon Tyne's busy AGMs also testify to popular engagement: in 1926, for instance, Newcastle district had 200 governors; Gateshead, 120; Durham, 350; North Tyne, 90; and South Tyne, 95. By 1939 levels had fallen somewhat in Newcastle and Durham (130 and 200, respectively) but had increased in North and South Tyne (140 and 150). So here significant public activism was still evident.[66]

Surviving sources for the HSA give little sense of participation in the constituent bodies. With some 2 million members and around 14,000 groups the average group size would have been about 150 members, though many would have been much smaller given the large scale of some workplaces. In such groups it is doubtful whether elaborate democratic procedures were necessary, and it is probable that everything devolved to the secretary. There are, for example, occasional letters from such officials in the HSA's magazine, *The Contributor*, complaining that most members were too lazy or unconcerned, interested only when they wanted a benefit, and dilatory in payment.[67] Conversely, the same source sometimes articulated complaints that procedures for involving individual contributors were either lacking or totally ineffective in many groups, though there appears to have been no formal response, such as central guidance as to standard practice.[68] Insofar as there are descriptions of the activities of groups, they usually relate to fundraising, apparently led by small numbers of committee members.

A further piece of evidence comes from data collected in Beveridge's study, *Voluntary action*, which provide participation rates for a wide range of 'third sector' associations.[69] Based on a 1947 survey of 3,000 people, mostly urban dwellers in England, Scotland and Wales, this found that 66 per cent were members of voluntary organisations. Of these, 93 per cent belonged to a hospital contributory scheme, which far exceeded the popularity of other voluntary groups (the nearest runner-up was the British Legion, with 12 per cent).[70] The vast majority of contributors, 97.1 per cent, took no part in the scheme other than subscribing; of the remainder, 2.4 per cent actually attended meetings and only 1 per cent (about eighteen people) attended meetings quarterly or more frequently.[71]

None of this is to underplay the commitment and, presumably, the altruism of the movement's volunteers. Surveying the 1934 AGM of the BHCA, its president observed that its success was attributable to over 9,000 volunteer workers, consisting of 7,100 works delegates, 700 nurses and ambulance staff, and 1,650 branch officials and district collectors, often retired people who canvassed street by street.[72] It should also be emphasised that devotion to the hospital cause encompassed charitable work as well. Leeds members, for example, carried out pub collections, put on an annual gala in a local park and organised through ward and district committees a series of carnivals and Sunday concerts.[73] In Sheffield the SHC, aided by the Rotary Club, made an annual distribution of Christmas presents to all patients and nurses.[74] The Glasgow scheme successfully garnered the support of 'Wireless enthusiasts' to install radios in the Infirmary's wards in 1928, and so on.[75]

Thus, while activism was tiny in percentage terms, the schemes typically fostered significant groups of volunteers, who led the fundraising initiatives and participated in electoral and social activities. The numbers of delegates attending the full AGMs were impressive, though in some places they declined over the inter-war period. None the less, it was still the case that many participating groups and contributors had no mouthpiece and therefore, probably, no real interest beyond the instrumental purpose of gaining cover for treatment. Gauging popular attitudes of contributors is difficult, but some corroboration of this last point is provided by the Nuffield Social Reconstruction Survey's investigation of health insurance. This found that people had 'little but praise' for the schemes, because of the entitlement to care they offered, and because payroll deduction involved minimal effort on the part of the contributor (though weekly collections were a nuisance). At the same time, respondents found it irritating that they had to contribute to multiple providers of health insurance, including a range of sick clubs and friendly societies as well as contributory schemes.[76] Overall, theirs was not a positive endorsement of voluntary contribution, more a measure of the perceived failure of NHI, and the surveyors reported that 'a great many people' felt that 'medical services ought not to be on a contributory basis'.[77]

The nature of scheme leadership

Who were the scheme activists? According to the Bolton Hospital Saturday committee its members were 'your relatives, your personal friends, your fellow workmen and women. They probably live on your street'.[78] Sadly the identities and motivations of such ordinary members are now impossible to retrieve, so assessment of those at the helm of local schemes must be limited to a few prominent individuals, either those who are notable from other spheres of activity or those whose biographical details were recorded in scheme literature because of long and dedicated service. The Beveridge survey noted above observed that about 25 per cent of hospital contributors were also members of other voluntary organisations, so it is not surprising that the movement's leaders were influential figures in other areas.[79] Specifically, they tended either to be drawn from local or even national elites, or to have entered public life through the labour movement.

The HSA's executive council provides an untypical example, in that it was dominated by the metropolitan elite. Early 'hospital' members included Viscount Hambleden (one of the partners in W. H. Smith and Son and a member of the King's Fund general council), Viscount Knutsford (chair of the London Hospital, with directorships in banking, railways and life assurance), Sir Arthur Stanley (treasurer of St Thomas's Hospital, member of the King's Fund general council, chair of the Royal College of Nursing and of the Joint Council of the British Red Cross and the Order of St John, and later president of the BHA) and Francis Whitbread (managing director of the brewing company, a governor of Guy's Hospital and vice-chairman of the National Society for the Prevention of Cruelty to Children).[80] 'General' members included General Sir Herbert Lawrence (chair of the private bank Glyn, Mills and Co.), Sir Edward Penton (member of the King's Fund general council), Stanley Duff (secretary of the Ancient Order of Foresters friendly society and of the National Conference of Friendly Societies, and chair of the Unemployment Insurance Board) and Sir Alan Anderson (son of 'England's first woman physician', Elizabeth Garrett Anderson, vice-chairman and later president of the HSA, honorary secretary of the King's Fund, deputy governor of the Bank of England, director of the Suez Canal Company and Conservative MP for the City of London, 1935–40).[81] The contributor members, meanwhile, were group secretaries from substantial businesses such as the General Post Office, the Great Western Railway and Siemens Bros, and one stalwart, Henry Lesser, of the South Metropolitan Gas Company, was president of the National Federation of Employees Approved Societies.[82]

A mix of industrialists and labour movement leaders was evident elsewhere. The MHC was chaired by Lord Cozens-Hardy, a director of local glassmakers Pilkington, a justice of the peace, deputy lieutenant for Lancashire and president of the National Association of National Insurance Committees.[83] Contributor representatives came from the major labour institutions: the trades councils of Liverpool, Birkenhead, Bootle and Wallasey, unions representing dockers, transport, municipal and general workers, and large employee groups such as the police, utilities and shipbuilders.[84] The Contributors' Association was led in the 1930s by A. N. Denaro of the Carters' and Motormen's Association, and in the 1940s by city councillor John Braddock of the Co-operative Insurance Society.[85] In Birmingham the chair of the BHCS was ex-army man Colonel Bertram Ford, general manager of three Birmingham newspapers, governor of the University of Birmingham, and board member and chair of the Birmingham Hospitals for Women. Ford later became president of the BHCSA, no doubt because of the key role of the Birmingham scheme in inaugurating the Association, and was knighted in 1936 for his hospital work.[86]

Labour men were more to the fore in other towns. In Sheffield the president of the scheme from 1922 to 1939 was Councillor Moses Humberstone, assistant secretary of the Sheffield trades and labour council. Humberstone typifies the dedicated working-class voluntarist, describing himself as 'in love with the movement'. When he retired as president aged seventy-eight he had a long record of local public service: a justice of the peace from 1912, city councillor and member of the Royal Infirmary's board from 1919, alderman from 1926, and later chair of the ambulance section of the SHC; he proudly recorded his attendance at 'upwards of 2000 meetings for the Movement'.[87] John Hardman, chair of the Bolton Hospital Saturday Committee, was cut from a similar cloth. Employed all his life at a local cotton mill, he had begun Saturday fund work as a representative of the Operative Spinners Association and spent forty-four years in the movement, including twenty on the committee of the Infirmary, of which he was made vice-president in 1933; the source of his commitment was apparently his shame on learning, as a child with a broken wrist, that charity would pay for his treatment.[88] With tragic irony he died in the Infirmary while still in office, having been struck by a lorry-load of timber in a street accident.[89] The friendly society movement also provided contributor leaders, such as J. S. Tudor, founder member and honorary secretary of the Bristol Medical Institutions Contributory Scheme, who also held high office in the Ancient Order of Foresters.[90]

The schemes in Scotland and the North East offer many similar examples of working-class activism rooted in trade union activity. Andrew Eunson, honorary secretary of the Edinburgh League of Subscribers from 1930 to 1947, was a skilled cabinetmaker who became president of the Edinburgh trades council and executive member of Edinburgh's Insurance Committee.[91] Newcastle upon Tyne's committee members were drawn from the region's heavy industries and from the labour movement; in 1913–14, for example, members worked for the Co-operative Society and the corporation, the Durham collieries, Jarrow shipyard, Swan Hunter and gas and railway companies.[92] Executives in the Glasgow fund included Thomas McGhie, manager of Burnbank Co-operative Society, James McDermid, secretary of the Scottish Union of Bakers and Confectioners, and William Cross, general secretary of the Amalgamated Slaters' Society of Scotland (who was once absent from a contributors' meeting owing to 'an adjourned conference on wages negotiations').[93] Locally and nationally the Co-operative Wholesale Society was active in the fund, alongside other charitable work, including its own convalescent homes, unemployment relief and the local 'Police Bootless Bairns Fund'.[94] Participation in hospital governance, then, was part of the broader social mission of the organised working class.

Finally, there were also members from white-collar backgrounds who became either scheme administrators or leaders. In Sheffield, Humberstone was succeeded as president by Oswald Steward, solicitor of the Derwent Water Board and vice-president of the BHCSA from 1942 to 1947.[95] The linchpin of the Edinburgh League of Subscribers was Russell Paton, the salaried organising secretary of the Infirmary and also secretary to the League. Sydney Lamb came to the Sheffield scheme from a wartime career selling War Savings Certificates. He had received an MBE in 1923 for his hospital work and had gone in 1926 from his post at the SHC to become appeals secretary at University College Hospital, London, before he moved to the MHC, where he was based when he became secretary of the BHCSA (1942–43).[96] His successor (1943–47) was William Newstead, general secretary of the BHCA. John Dodd started his career as assistant secretary to the MHC, working under Lamb, then in 1939 moved to the Bristol Hospitals Fund, before becoming secretary of the BHCSA (1947–48); he was later a leading figure in the survival and development of the schemes under the NHS.[97]

In sum, activists among the leadership were a combination of philanthropists from industry and the professions, professional scheme bureaucrats, and local trade unionists and Co-operative Society members. This mix provides some grounds for supposing that hospital voluntarism nurtured networks of trust between representatives of different social and occupational groups, jointly engaged in a civic project. However, it is argued below that this collaboration was not founded on an unproblematic consensus, and it is doubtful that it suffused other areas of public life.

Continuity of leadership

Given the make-up of scheme activists, what can be said about changes to leadership over time? The point of this question is to consider how the elaborate selection procedures operated in practice. Were elections hotly contested, thus indicating a vigorous democratic culture, or was the personnel of executives and board representatives generally stable?

Although electoral procedures were faithfully followed, there is a good deal of evidence for stability of leadership. Humberstone's long service was not untypical in Sheffield. Of the fifteen executive members in 1929, eight remained in 1935, while two others had become hospital board representatives, and of the fifteen board representatives in 1929, seven remained in place in 1935, despite the three-year term of service.[98] In Wolverhampton, where hospital control of the scheme was more pronounced, the chair and board representatives were regularly unanimously re-elected.[99] Self-perpetuation was furthered during the war, when the executive adopted the power to co-opt three new members 'to replace those who had not attended meetings'.[100] The chair was Alan Davies, alderman and member (later vice-president) of the Royal Hospital's board of management; its secretary was William Harper, who was also the Royal's secretary, having started as a canvasser in 1898, finally retiring in 1942, when he was made the scheme's honorary secretary.[101]

In Glasgow, too, continuity of leadership was the key note, with the aforementioned Cross and McDermid regularly re-elected to the executive committee.[102] Cross began as a representative in 1904, was re-elected up to 1931, and later resumed the role until 1948. McDermid served until his death in 1939.[103] Seats on the board were occasionally contested, as in 1920, when a member was unseated by a Co-operative Society representative.[104] Often delegates were simply renominated *en bloc*, and occasional attempts to replace this with individual nominations were defeated by 'a large majority'.[105] The London, Midland and Scottish Railway delegates were the keenest opponents of this status quo, at one point unsuccessfully seeking an agreement that two representatives should stand down each year.[106] The justification for rejecting this was that 'it took many years to get thoroughly acquainted with all the details of such a large Hospital', and therefore stable leadership was desirable.[107] Conversely, in the Chesterfield and North Derbyshire scheme, six worker representatives stood down each year to be replaced by six more, which, according to the hospital's chairman, meant 'continuity in administration is secure and the old members calm down the reform zeal of their newly elected colleagues'. Moreover, it was normal for some who stood down to be re-elected immediately.[108]

Power, then, devolved to those with the expertise and the commitment, and not to the victors of keenly fought electoral battles. This was because the work of the executive committees was mainly routine (see chapter 6). The Glasgow body coordinated the efforts of the district councils, attempted to raise a uniform weekly rate of contribution and received reports of the financial support given to the town's various hospitals.[109] Members would also work on other committees of the hospital: for instance, a Mr Kerr, an employee of the Co-operative Society's accounts department, was involved with the purchase of supplies, while Cross sat on the fabric and equipment committee, and ultimately became the Infirmary's vice-chairman.[110] Indeed, this aspect of voluntary service was a long-standing tradition for worker contributors: in 1897 Glasgow Victoria Infirmary was fortunate to have as a governor Robert Mason, a skilled mechanic who maintained the Infirmary machinery in his free time.[111]

Despite the vigour of grassroots participation in Newcastle upon Tyne, continuous service on the district committees was also typical. In 1930, for instance, a Newburn governor, Mr Redhead, was forced to retire after thirty-seven years when the steelworks he represented shut; Newcastle district representatives Robson, Walton and Gibson served throughout the inter-war period (the former two were Co-operative Society men); and in Gateshead Messrs Shipley and Walker both served between 1915 and 1939 (when Shipley died).[112] An effort in 1926 by some Durham miners to limit service in their district to only three years was narrowly defeated and it remained the case that power resided with a stable core of activists.[113]

Continuity also characterised the leadership of the Edinburgh League, with elections mostly uncontested and unanimous.[114] Peter Herd, of the Edinburgh and District Trades Council, had joined the committee in 1926 and became president in 1942; he succeeded J. W. Thompson, who had joined in 1925 was president in 1930; David Penman was a committee member from 1922 to 1948 (excluding the war years); Andrew Eunson, who joined in 1922 and became honorary secretary in 1930, remained in post until death in 1947.[115] Even though the constitution of the board of management specified a five-year term, Eunson and Herd simply carried on as representatives of a different organisation.[116] Continuity is partly explained by the key role which labour organisations played in the nomination process.[117] Another issue was that while meetings of the League executive took place in the evenings, those of the Infirmary board were held in the daytime, thus narrowing the field of possible representatives to 'those who could attend without incurring loss'.[118]

The evidence therefore suggests that the existence of democratic procedures did not produce fiercely contested elections with large numbers eager to take office. Instead, control and policy direction remained with a small number of motivated individuals who were active elsewhere in labour and medical politics or in local government. Continuity was assured because expertise in the humdrum business of fundraising and administration was acknowledged and because representation was dominated either by hospital insiders or by major labour organisations. This conclusion endorses the observations of Pickstone in his discussion of the Preston fund. He contrasted the lack of interest on the part of the broad mass of subscribers, for whom scheme membership was simply 'useful insurance', with the small number of committed leaders, driven by moral impulses and civic pride, who 'thought Infirmary, talked Infirmary and lived Infirmary'.[119]

The ethos of the contributory schemes

All this raises questions about the motivation of activists and the nature of the social citizenship which contribution engendered. Were the schemes perceived as a philanthropic endeavour: a diffusion down the social gradient of the long tradition of voluntary hospital charity, inspired by community responsibility and duty to others? Alternatively, were they understood within the framework of existing workers' mutualism, as an extension of the friendly society and co-operative movements, in which collective risk-pooling was coupled with a fraternal ethic and workplace democracy? Or were they seen as essentially a form of personal insurance and thus similar to participation in a commercial plan or the statutory NHI? This section focuses first on the schemes' public representations, as evidenced in their journals, annual reports and other publicity material, to explore the movement's identity and ethos. It then considers how this was shaped by its close affiliation with the labour movement and what this indicates about the nature of social citizenship which participation signified.

Charity or insurance?

From the early days of the Saturday funds a tension existed between an appeal to the self-interest of workers and a wish to identify with the existing milieu of hospital charity. In the 1880s the Birmingham fund produced a striking series of leaflets whose panels depicted the act of subscription, a gruesome industrial accident and recovery in hospital (figure 5.1). The message was clear – hospital contribution was an act of enlightened self-interest. However, beneath the graphics a verse typically appeared which reminded the reader of the altruistic aspects of the collections:

> 'Now don't turn away, but remember to-day
> Is the day of all days in the year,
> When the true working man says "I'll do all I can
> The sorrowing sick ones to cheer."
> Then don't turn aside, with a false sort of pride,
> Since you cannot give dollars or crowns!
> But *do what you can*, like a brave-hearted man,
> And give us a handful of "browns"'

One reason for maintaining this charitable ethos was no doubt because the hospitals could not risk alienating their philanthropic supporters by presenting mass contribution as a form of pre-payment. This idiom also resonated with notions of brotherly love recognisable from the friendly society movement.[120]

The post-war contributory schemes maintained this dual identity. In 1922 the King's Fund had agonised over whether the HSA would be a 'prudential scheme appealing to self-regarding motives rather than the altruistic motives … on which the Fund has hitherto worked'. Moreover, contributors 'would not understand that this is not a contract', so that extra demands for treatment were sure to follow.[121] Only when it had been confirmed that contributors would have no legal right of admission was the scheme launched.[122] Clearly, hospital leaders were under no illusions that mass contribution was a manifestation of popular philanthropy. Francis Colchester-Wemyss, a leading light of the Gloucestershire Royal Infirmary and the Red Cross, put it like this: 'A workman who pays a fixed sum each week to his hospital expects, and is

HOSPITAL SATURDAY,

22ND MAY, 1886.

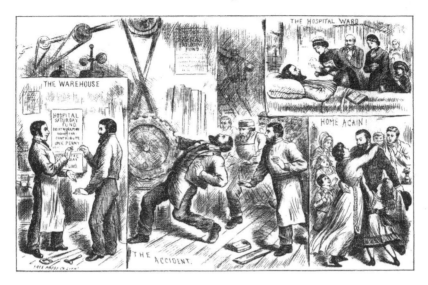

HOSPITAL SATURDAY,

MAY 12, 1888.

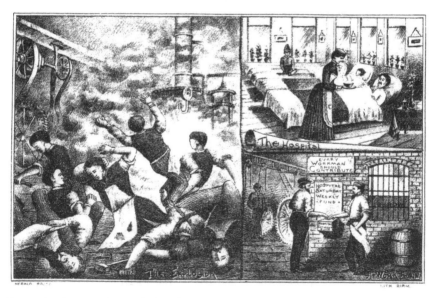

Figure 5.1. 'Hospital Saturday' leaflets, Hospital Saturday Fund, Birmingham (BLSL, LF.4663), collection of newspaper cuttings, etc., 1873–91. Reproduced by courtesy of Birmingham Library Services.

entitled to, a *quid pro quo*.... His subscription, in fact, amounts to an insurance premium.'[123] The professional journal of hospital administrators, the *Hospital Gazette*, editorialised more bluntly that it was 'self-evident' that 'the members themselves regard their periodical contributions as ensuring for them free hospital treatment if and when they require it'.[124] Finally, a 1930 survey of scheme administrators discovered that the basis of appeals to contributors was divided almost equally between 'a form of insurance' and the 'spirit of self-help and help to others'; it went on to note that while contributors had no legal right to treatment, they did 'possess a strong moral right'.[125]

Indeed, there were good reasons why the schemes comported themselves as charities rather than insurance funds. First, although income from the 'old form of subscriber' was now much less significant, it remained important for many hospitals which retained the ticketing system.[126] There was therefore a risk that philanthropy would be deterred if the bulk of hospital funding came from direct insurance. This would 'dry up the well of human sympathy' because treating the sick poor would become a 'secondary principle' as the hospitals became devoted to 'meeting the needs of contributors'.[127] Second, consultants who worked on an honorary basis did so on the understanding that they gave a service for the poor; if they now claimed payment, costs would be driven up. Third, a hospital's income tax exemption and a scheme's favourable assessment for local rates depended on charitable status.[128] Fourth, a contractual obligation to provide treatment could put pressure on resources, challenge medical authority over admissions and lay the hospital open to liabilities.[129] The hospitals must never become a 'members' club' according to Sir Robert Bolam of Newcastle's Royal Victoria Infirmary; they had to be able to select the most urgent cases on the basis of need.[130]

The public persona of the inter-war schemes therefore continued to manifest this dualism. For example, the 1937 annual report of the Bristol scheme admonished readers that 'The PRIMARY DUTY of every good citizen is the maintenance and support of our VOLUNTARY HOSPITALS', while the facing page proclaimed: 'A First-Class Investment for a Rainy Day! ... by contributing ... you will be assisting the beneficent work of Bristol's Voluntary Medical Institutions, and ensuring for yourself certain benefits, which, if the need arises, makes your investment a very profitable one.'[131] Bolton's scheme also advertised itself as an 'Investment.... If you do not need us today you MAY tomorrow'; its president simultaneously described it as 'the premier charity in the town'.[132] Similarly, the Merseyside scheme was depicted by its organisers as an example of 'that sturdy spirit of self-help which has had so much to do with the formation of British character', a contrast to the tendency of state welfare to 'sap individual enterprise and independence'. However, they also acknowledged that providence and a desire to avoid means testing were the contributors' prime motivation.[133]

The HSA exemplifies a scheme which actively promulgated an ethos of contribution, founded upon a compound of Victorian self-help and more contemporary notions of voluntary engagement. Unlike provincial urban schemes, with supportive newspapers and limited numbers of hospitals, it was more difficult to muster local patriotism in London, where a dispersed population utilised a plethora of institutions.[134] Efforts were therefore made to cultivate 'a fraternal spirit', for example through the development of an HSA sports league, in which groups engaged in 'bowls tournaments, darts contests, football, cycling and country rambles'.[135] The HSA also instituted a members' journal, *The Contributor*, in 1925 and this soon developed from a rather austere publication dedicated to fundraising and membership into a family magazine which included serialised fiction, reports of HSA sporting activities and, by the late 1930s, lifestyle features on DIY, recipes and gardening hints.[136] These changes, of course, could be interpreted as a sign that the membership required more than descriptions of the Association's core activities to sustain their interest. Another strategy was to convene mass gatherings to build 'mutual understanding' and 'closer association', such as the garden party in 1928 at Alexandra Palace, or the 1929 rally at Crystal Palace which provided the culmination to 'Green Voucher Week'.[137] Competitive solidarity between group secretaries was fostered by the HSA's 'corker club', whose members, identified by their group secretary lapel badges, would carry around with them a cork fixed with metal studs, one for each contributor they had recruited. When challenged by another group secretary with the word 'Corker!' the two would compare numbers of studs, with the loser paying the other a small forfeit (a drink, stamp or bus fare).[138] Partnership with other organisations also helped promulgate the image of the HSA as a social movement; this included Boy Scouts and Girl Guides undertaking mass leaflet drops, friendly societies helping to access large workplaces, religious organisations like the Brotherhood Movement assisting with appeals, and local councils providing contribution facilities at rent offices on housing estates.[139] The HSA felt it played a wider social role in the community; one writer claimed that many group secretaries acted 'almost as Advice Centres for their own districts' with regard to health services and spoke of the 'immeasurable value of this friendly cooperation'.[140] In terms redolent of concepts of social capital, it was suggested that the HSA cut across socioeconomic divides. It had demonstrated its capacity to 'vitalise entire neighbourhoods' and claimed that its 'watchword' was 'fraternal cooperation towards a common end', in an organisation where 'class distinction had been completely blotted out'.[141] It is of course true that the HSA brought substantial numbers of people together for its rallies and fundraising events but it is less clear that these activities negated social divisions. The schemes were aimed at a particular economic stratum, whose main interest lay in gaining low-cost insurance, while the voluntary hospitals' use of income limits and means testing reinforced class distinction rather than eliminating it.[142] Nor were the schemes really examples of spontaneous associational activity because, even if their public face was altruistic, individuals joined them with a very specific purpose in mind.

This dual thread of self-interest and humanitarianism was evident in the way the HSA message was dramatised. 'You can help your hospital and yourself today', announced a tableau at an HSA carnival in Mitcham, featuring the climactic scene from Dickens' *A tale of two cities* with Sidney Carton on the

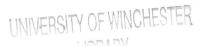

scaffold (a rather odd way to inspire confidence in the efficacy of health care!) and the inevitable slogan: 'It is a far, far better thing to do than you have ever done'.[143] *The Contributor* reconciled the two impulses by stressing the broader virtue of self-help: 'it is true charity to stand secure from the risk of becoming a source of drain upon other people's gifts'.[144] More positively, notions of the HSA as a collectivist venture were regularly iterated through the motif of individual members as 'single links in a great chain'; indeed, AGMs would occasionally begin with a song (to the tune of 'John Peel'):

> D'ye ken the links of the endless chain,
> That we forge with heart, and hand, and brain,
> D'ye ken how it binds and grows amain... [etc.][145]

However, HSA collectivism was firmly anti-statist, championing the virtues of voluntary action. *The Contributor's* editorial line was that 'officialism crushes individualism', whereas voluntary action was conducive to 'freedom and sympathy'.[146] Keynote speakers at AGMs regularly echoed this: 'The state can run my army, navy and postal service, but it cannot cure my sick child ... disease has to be fought by two things, sympathy as well as science'.[147]

The idealised HSA member was represented by the figure of 'Mr Bowcher' (the man with the voucher), hero of a cartoon strip in *The Contributor* (figure 5.2). Bowcher is depicted as a petit-bourgeois figure, perhaps to appeal to the aspirational nature of manual labourers, but also because London's economy necessitated a pitch to white-collar and service-sector workers. His process of joining the HSA is narrated as a transition from a light-hearted, jack-the-lad character to a responsible citizen, aware of his duties to family and society. Bowcher's rejection of the earlier *ad hoc* charity of flag days and boxes nicely illustrates the HSA's self-conception as the modernisation of traditional benevolence: it disparaged old-style collections as the 'efforts of amateur beggars out for a spree' and instead urged the public to embrace its 'business-like methods' and in a 'thoroughly modern spirit ... save systematically'.[148] Modernity signified not only an efficient, transparent approach in financial matters, but also a new model of 'good hospital citizenship', represented here by Bowcher's realisation of his domestic and social obligations.[149] Responsibility was the watchword: no more should 'honest and otherwise self-respecting people' expect to arrive at hospital and 'plead unpreparedness and poverty'.[150] In some respects such admonitions, which emphasised the socially demeaning aspects of accepting charity, echoed Victorian ideals of working-class respectability.[151] Yet, in the context of a nascent welfare state, they also posited a model of autonomous citizenship in contrast to the spectre of welfare dependency, wherein the country risked 'becoming a glorified almshouse ... in which men are seeking something for nothing and claiming their rights rather than performing their duties'.[152]

This was also a gendered conception of citizenship, as illustrated by Bowcher's portrayal as dutiful patriarch. Indeed, it was a recurrent tactic of appeals to play on notions of masculine responsibility for care of the self and the family, as in this *faux*-Cockney verse from *The Contributor*:

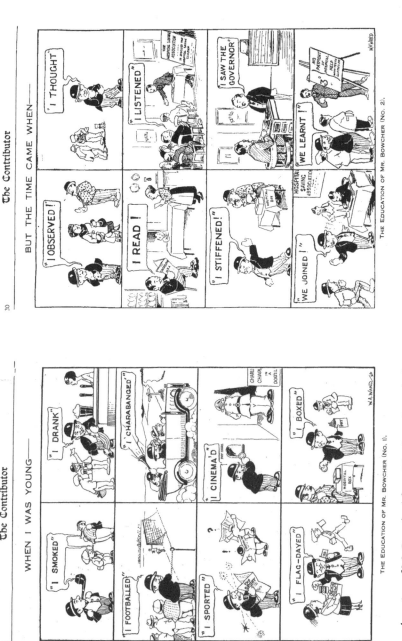

Figure 5.2 .'The education of Mr Bowcher', from *The Contributor* (February and March 1926). Reproduced by courtesy of the HSA.

'And when in "Orspital" yer goes,
Yer can "cut out" all yer woes ...
They'll fit yer up as quickly as they can.
When yer shows yer "Varcher Green".
They say, "right-o", all serene,
And then the feeling is "no kiddin" – you're a man.'[153]

Moreover, it was the 'duty of the head of every household to ... satisfy himself'
that the family had hospital coverage, and a 1936 advertising leaflet pointedly
asked: 'where is the man who can satisfy his wife on these points unless he
is in the HSA?'[154] These tropes were rooted in Victorian constructs of the
skilled male worker, for whom 'manly' providence was a norm, and they had a
continued salience in the inter-war years, as female labour market participation
declined and housewifery rose.[155]

Two further examples illustrate the tension between charitable and
mutualist elements. The BHCA, in which the balance of control was weighted
against the labour movement, produced a magazine (figure 5.3) which signified through its title, *The Samaritan*, its location within the framework of

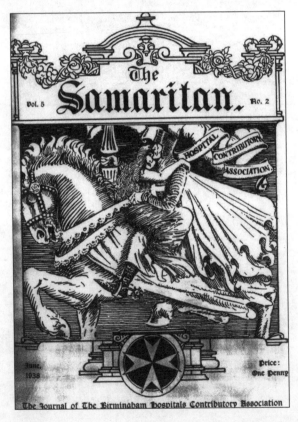

Figure 5.3. *The Samaritan*, 5 (2) (1938). Reproduced by courtesy of Birmingham
Library Services.

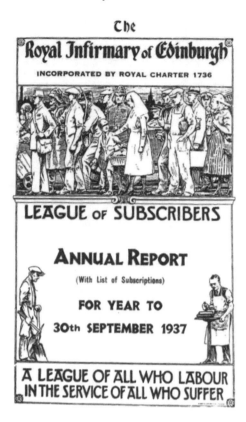

The
Royal Infirmary of Edinburgh
INCORPORATED BY ROYAL CHARTER 1736

LEAGUE of SUBSCRIBERS

ANNUAL REPORT

(With List of Subscriptions)

FOR YEAR TO

30th SEPTEMBER 1937

A LEAGUE OF ALL WHO LABOUR IN THE SERVICE OF ALL WHO SUFFER

Figure 5.4. Edinburgh League of Subscribers, annual report, 1937. Reproduced by courtesy of Lothian Health Services Archive, Collections Division, University of Edinburgh Library.

traditional charity. Its cover, resonant of the popular chivalric romances of the novelist G. A. Henty, depicts the Association as a crusade, in which contribution is an act of masculine gallantry. The tone of discussion in the journal's pages was primarily factual, although reports of public meetings regularly characterised the scheme as charitable, epitomising 'the wonderful spirit of giving, without necessarily expecting to get'.[156] As in the HSA, such rhetoric occasionally took on a more political tone: contributors were evidence of the 'initiative and independence and effort' of the voluntary sector, with its capacity 'to experiment in ways that statutory authorities can never do'. Indeed, this was a stark contrast to the European dictatorships, where totalitarianism had crushed voluntary activity.[157]

In contrast, the Edinburgh League of Subscribers chose a style of socialist realism for the cover graphic of its annual reports (figure 5.4). A band of working people, whose varied attire indicates the mix of local occupations, parades past in unison. The eye is drawn to the central character of the nurse, whose lowly status in the pecking order of the medical profession emphasises the democratic rather than hierarchical provision which mass contribution enables. The figures of the miner and printer below this tableau, archetypes of manual labour and artisan skill, are represented as resolute and high-minded, epitomising the sober respectability of working-class consciousness. The message is clear: participation in the League is an aspect of the forward march of labour, in which collective effort sustains the hospital service. As ever, though, the caption introduces notions of charitable service, rather under-cutting the intent of the illustration.

Relations with the labour movement

The ambiguous identity apparent in the artefacts of the contributory schemes reflected a deeper uncertainty at the heart of the movement. We have seen that the funds were typically the creations of hospital managers, who quickly realised they were dependent on the goodwill of organised labour if they were to make headway. Thus there was from the outset an uneasy coalition between two distinct voluntary traditions, on the one hand the urban philanthropy so central to middle-class culture, and on the other the trade union and labour movement.[158] How did these strange bed-fellows relate in practice, and to what extent was this form of social citizenship seen as an element of labour activism?

Even before 1914, efforts to develop contributory arrangements had met with resistance from workers who advocated public control and financing of hospitals. In Reading, for example, trade unionists and local members of the Social Democratic Foundation unsuccessfully challenged the establishment of the Reading Workpeople's Hospital Fund.[159] Similarly, in 1912 a resolution by the Sheffield trades and labour council denounced the lack of workers' control over contributory funds and declared support for municipal ownership of hospitals.[160] Others, however, had reconciled hospital schemes with the aims of labour politics. In the 1890s, the BHSF's journal, *Forward*, argued that the contributory system had ushered in the 'co-operative hospital', paid for by those who used it and quite distinct from traditional charity. The ideological bent of *Forward's* editors was underlined by such features as 'Thoughts on co-operation', which contained *aperçus* of thinkers such as Ferdinand Lasalle, Giuseppe Mazzini and John Ruskin.[161] In the same vein, the establishment of the BHSF's new convalescent home in Llandudno was an example of 'Constructive Socialism' in action, manifesting the capacity of 'the labouring classes to reorganise society by their own efforts without regard to the wealthier classes'; the latter were deemed too preoccupied by 'Self-interest whetted with an insatiable appetite for riches' to concern themselves with the poor. Hospital contribution was therefore framed within the politics of the progressive left: 'Have we in Birmingham happened to tumble quite accidentally upon a method by which the regeneration of society may be achieved?'[162]

However, by the time of the expansion of contributory schemes during the Cave era, the Labour Party was moving towards a new policy. In 1918 its advisory committee on public health envisaged a health service free at the point of use, funded largely by exchequer grants, and delivered through a network of public hospitals and health centres, which would incorporate the existing voluntary institutions.[163] Although these proposals were never formally adopted by the party, they indicate the sentiment of activists and the challenge faced by contributory funds. Scheme secretaries seeking support responded by appealing to pragmatism. Canvassing the Lothian coalfields in the early 1920s, the secretary of the Edinburgh League of Subscribers, Paton, found that 'it was usually presented [i.e. by the miners] as to the desirability of having State organised and subsidised hospital services'; his stock response was to agree, but to counter that in the meanwhile it would be necessary to 'keep an open door in the Scottish Capital for the sick and injured'.[164] Such counsel prevailed and the League was launched with a large public meeting at which representatives of the trades council, the engineering union and the shale miners addressed the crowd.[165] Such support was ongoing, with, for example, a 1938 'Trades Pageant' run by the trades council to raise money for the Infirmary's building fund.[166]

The incipient Merseyside scheme faced similar difficulties when the local trades council requested that members boycott the scheme.[167] In 1928, Luke Hogan, chair of Liverpool trades council and Labour Party, argued that a tax-based national health service was 'the only ultimate practical solution'. However, expediency persuaded him to support the scheme as an interim measure, not least because members of the National Union of General and Municipal Workers had begun to enrol.[168] Trade unionists, Hogan urged, should regard contribution 'not merely from the point of view of a political theory, but in the light of present day humanities and to think of the thousands of unemployed and poor people … dependant [*sic*] on these Medical Institutions'. Support, though, was clearly provisional: 'if the day comes to hand over our Voluntary System we shall be proud to hand over our … institutions in a prosperous and thriving condition'.[169] Cooperation also came at a price, in an extension of representation to workers and in the hospitals' open door to the unemployed.[170]

Labour also exacted concessions for its support in Sheffield, where the trades and labour council favoured municipal ownership and initially balked at the SHC's 'penny in the pound' proposals, with its plan for payroll deductions, employers' payments and contribution from trade unions, friendly societies and cooperatives at the annual rate of 2*d* per member.[171] Only at an advanced stage did the trades council meet with the SHC. At this meeting the labour deputation established its socialist credentials by arguing that hospitals should receive exchequer funding rather than relying on workers' subscriptions and that their own preference was 'for the hospitals to be Municipally controlled'.[172] Ultimately, however, pragmatism ruled and an accommodation was reached. The proposed employers' contribution of 3*s* per employee per annum was replaced by a system in which employers were to pay one-third of the amount raised by their employees, which had the advantage of enhancing the bosses' contributions at a time of rising wages in the Sheffield light and heavy trades.[173] The planned trade union contribution was dropped, on the grounds that individual workers would effectively be paying twice. Finally, representation was extended when the SHC's board was increased to forty-six members (increasing again in 1921 following lobbying by trades council man Moses Humberstone).[174] Thus placated, the names of the representatives of the trades council were duly added to a new circular that was sent to firms, and the scheme was launched successfully.[175] Support was henceforth widespread throughout the labour movement in Sheffield, and the trades council's annual report incorporated a yearly update on its progress, although the Amalgamated Engineering Union declined to recommend that its members join.[176]

To conclude, these examples demonstrate that labour movement engagement with the contributory schemes did not manifest a straightforward consensus in favour of voluntary social action. At the outset, the support of the organised working class was conditional, and though the schemes successfully modelled their procedures on existing mutualist associations, they had always to contend with a labour movement that was deeply ambivalent towards the voluntary hospitals. Thus, a speech by George Haynes, executive of the Birmingham scheme, to his local trades council argued for a 'state medical system' as the most fair and efficient system for ratepayers:

> As long as there remain 13 management committees attempting to do hospital work Birmingham will never get economy or a good service.… The only effective system is one hospital system in each town and in Birmingham this should be the Public Health Committee.[177]

Similarly, the one-time MHC chair, Lord Cozens-Hardy, told the 1935 BHCSA conference that he:

> entertained grave fears for the future of the British Voluntary Hospitals. He based his apprehensions on the fact that the main supporters of the Contributory system, on which the hospitals depend so largely today, are wage-earners and as such are likely to be Trade Unionists, and therefore to be identified with the organisations affiliated to the Labour Party. The Socialist party was bound to support the principle of a State Service, and therefore sooner or later, the voluntary hospitals of our country would come under State control.[178]

Clearly, then, any conclusions about networks of trust generated by voluntary work in this field must be tempered by an awareness of the political differences among scheme activists.

Conclusion

This chapter has sought to explore the role of contributory schemes as institutions of civil society. Their varied nature makes generalisation hazardous, and this analysis has been limited to several of the larger schemes; none the less, several conclusions emerge.

There is no doubt that, procedurally, the contributory schemes took their role as bastions of worker democracy very seriously. In most cases arrangements were in place for participating workplaces or districts to send representatives to mass meetings at which officials were elected to committees with a role in hospital management. The numbers involved were tiny as a proportion of all contributors, but attendance figures attest to a genuine popular participation. The remit of representatives varied, but certainly in some schemes the rationale went beyond fundraising, to include the articulation of patients' interests. Devoted civic spirit mobilised the voluntary effort of the scheme hierarchy, collectors and fundraisers, while trade union activism provided an *entrée* into hospital government for members of the organised working class.

That said, it is less clear that the contributory schemes were popular manifestations of social citizenship, in terms either of a commitment to the voluntary hospitals or of a genuinely democratic involvement. The confused identity of the schemes – part charity, part insurance – reflects the probability that the majority joined the movement with the pragmatic purpose of assuring free hospital treatment without a means test. Moreover, evidence from the 1920s, and the 1940s (see chapter 8), suggests that many contributors sub-scribed to Labour's goal of public control of hospitals; their participation was instrumental rather than signalling deep-rooted commitment. One indication of this may be the changing character of *The Contributor*, the HSA's maga-zine, which soon found that its members wanted a more lively, aspirational publication than one simply dedicated to organisational development. So while levels of membership were high, this did not translate into high levels of participation and nor were the schemes organisations which really cut across socioeconomic divides. Here, the argument is in accord with those social theorists who dispute the extent to which participation in civil society generates social capital.[179] It was also the case that, despite the vigour of democratic procedures, power devolved to a small number of enthusiasts with the time and experience to engage in hospital management, and typically rep-resentative of either local industry or major labour organisations. Ultimately, the minority position of worker governors on hospital boards meant that, numerically at least, control remained with the social and medical elites, as it had done in the nineteenth century.

These limits to direct democracy are aptly illustrated by occasional attempts of activists to enhance their position. For example, when one HSA group secretary suggested that the number of contributor members ought to be increased so that they were not outvoted on the executive council, Sir Alan Anderson replied that 'we have never had a party vote' of this kind.[180] Another request to increase the number of contributor members on the HSA council, in parallel with the growth in the number of contributors, was rebuffed on the grounds that the council was an executive body.[181] In a similar vein, com-plaints of under-representation were made at the 1941 AGM of the Leeds and District Workpeople's Hospital Fund:

> there is an old saying that 'he who pays the piper calls the tune'.... Yet they kindly give us a representation of only three out of a total representation on their Lay Board of 16 ... if a gesture of invitation was accorded to us to increase that representation it would be highly welcome.

Alderman Sir George Martin responded reassuringly:

> Don't worry about representation on the hospital boards ... they are not like
> a city council. They do not sit on each side of a table and vote according to
> numbers. Your representatives come to give us their best, and not only do they
> represent the Fund and its members, but also the suffering poor who come into
> the hospitals.[182]

This vignette illustrates to the central dichotomy. Were the contributory
schemes essentially voluntary charity, or a new forum of local democracy, or
simply a form of insurance which might equally well be delivered by statutory
means? This chapter suggests that, beyond the small layer of activists, for the
majority the latter is the most plausible construction. To complete this assessment of the schemes as conduits of active citizenship, their effectiveness as
patients' advocates is considered in the next chapter.

Notes

1   Lord Beveridge, 'The role of the individual in health service', speech to the Bristol confer-
    ence of the BHCSA, 1954.
2   G. Finlayson, *Citizen, state and social welfare in Britain, 1830–1990* (Oxford, 1994).
3   E. Mayo and H. Moore, *The mutual state* (London, 2002).
4   WHSA, Sheffield and District Association of Hospital Contributors, Delegates
    meetings, 3 July 1919; SHC, *Record of the penny in the pound scheme* (Sheffield, 1949),
    p. 7.
5   WHSA, Minutes of Sheffield Joint Hospitals Consultative and Advisory Council, n.d.
    but 1921.
6   Originally known as Sheffield and District Hospitals Contributors Council.
7   WHSA, SHC, annual report, 1926, pp. 27–8.
8   TNA: PRO, MH 58/200, Notes on responses to questionnaires; J. E. Stone, *Hospital
    organization and management (including planning and construction)* (London, 1927), p. 225;
    WHSA, SHC, annual report, 1926, pp. 1–3.
9   WHSA, SHC, annual report, 1935.
10 WHSA, SHC, annual report, 1936, p. 44.
11 BCA, Birmingham Hospitals Contributors Scheme (BHCS), *Report and statement of
    accounts*, 1928, p. ii, and 1936, pp. 4–5; one member represented the employers.
12 *Birmingham Post*, 4 March 1927.
13 BCA, BHCS, *Report and statement of accounts*, 1930.
14 BCA, MS 1576/4, BHCS, MMC, 10 February 1932.
15 MRO, M610 MED 4/1, MHC, annual report, 1970, Centenary of service, p. 24.
16 MRO, M610 MED 2/2, Liverpool Voluntary Hospitals Council, Minutes of all Council
    committees, note 'Contributors movement', 27 February 1928.
17 MRO, M610 MED 4/1, MHC, annual report, 1930, p. 27.
18 MRO, M610 MED 4/1, MHC, annual report, 1927/28, pp. 56–60.
19 MRO, M610 MED 4/1, MHC, annual report, 1930, p. 73.
20 MRO, M610 MED 2/4, Merseyside Association of Hospital Contributors: minutes of
    contributors meetings and the executive committee, 26 November 1928.
21 *The Contributor*, January 1938, p. 8.
22 HSA Archive, *Report of proceedings of the annual general meeting*, 1923. The five initial
    branches were St George's (Piccadilly), King's College Hospital area (Denmark Hill),
    Westminster, East London (Whitechapel) and St Pancras.

23 HSA Archive, HSA, annual report, 1924.
24 These meetings were typically reported in some detail in the January issue of *The Contributor*; for example, the fulsome discussion of the Prince of Wales's attendance at the December 1930 annual meeting appears in *The Contributor*, January 1931, pp. 10–11.
25 HSA Archive, HSA, annual report, 1924.
26 *The Contributor*, October 1926, p. 65, and September 1927, p. 199.
27 VHC, *Contributory schemes* (London, 1923), pp. 7–8.
28 *Ibid.*, p. 7.
29 A. Teebon, *The history of three Nottingham welfare schemes* (Nottingham, n.d., 1970s), pp. 3, 6–7, 28.
30 GRO, Gloucestershire Royal Infirmary, annual report, 1923.
31 TNA: PRO, MH 58/177, 'Summary of a number of contributory schemes': Oxford.
32 *Ibid.*: Merthyr.
33 *Ibid.*: Barrow.
34 Bolton Archive and Local Studies Library (BALSL), *Bolton Royal Infirmary, 1833–1933, Jubilee Carnival, Official Handbook* (Bolton, 1933), p. 7; BALSL, *Bolton and District Hospital Saturday Committee, rules, standing orders and contributory scheme* (Bolton, 1934), (henceforth *Bolton rules*), pp. 14–16.
35 BALSL, *Bolton rules*, pp. 3–4; BALSL, Bolton Hospital Saturday Committee, annual report, 1933, pp. 3–6.
36 BALSL, *Bolton rules*, pp. 7–10.
37 BALSL, Bolton Infirmary and Dispensary, *Rules adopted 1923* (Bolton, 1923), pp. 3–5; BALSL, Bolton Royal Infirmary, annual report, 1935, pp. 3, 30.
38 BALSL, Bolton and District Hospital Saturday Committee minute book, 13 June 1939, 'Local newspaper cuttings', and 'Bolton trades council', n.d. but 1948 or 1949.
39 PAAA, Wolverhampton and Staffordshire Hospital: Hospital Saturday Committee minute book, 15 December 1928, 25 July 1929.
40 HRO, Royal Hampshire County Hospital, annual reports, 1921, 1925.
41 *Hospitals yearbook* (London, 1938); B. Carpenter Turner, *A history of the Royal Hampshire County Hospital* (Chichester, 1986), p. 106.
42 HRO, 5M63/146, Contributory scheme sub-committee minute book; HRO, 5M63, Whist drive committee minute book.
43 HRO, 5M63/150, Royal Hampshire County Hospital, Contributory scheme minutes of annual meetings of hon. secretaries and collectors, cutting from *Hampshire Chronicle and General Advertiser*, 4 September 1943.
44 LHSA, LHB 1/1/56, Minute book, Royal Infirmary, 22 July 1918.
45 *Ibid.*
46 TNA: PRO, MH 58/200, Notes on responses; LHSA, Edinburgh Royal Infirmary, annual reports, 1918, 1919, 1927.
47 LHSA, Edinburgh Royal Infirmary, annual report, 1937.
48 In 1938, subscriptions plus donations totalled £30,183, while contributions from the League totalled £32,142; LHSA, Edinburgh Royal Infirmary, annual report, 1938, and *Hospitals yearbook* (1938).
49 TWAS, HO/SRI, Sunderland Royal Infirmary, annual reports, 1881, 1900.
50 TWAS, HO/SRI/1/7, General committee, 14 February 1884, 8 May 1884.
51 TNA: PRO, MH 58/200, Notes on responses; TWAS, Royal Victoria Infirmary, annual reports, 1921, 1923.
52 TWAS, HO/RVI/60, Royal Victoria Infirmary, Minute book: workmen governors' annual meetings, AGM 1921.
53 *Ibid.*, 4 February 1911, 18 March 1922, 10 March 1923, and see 10 March 1934.
54 *Ibid.*, 8 March 1919, 8 March 1924.
55 *Ibid.*, 14 March 1925.
56 TWAS, HO/RVI/34, Minutes, 8 March 1941.
57 TNA: PRO, MH58/177, Note on contributory schemes for provincial general hospitals, p. 7.

58 VHC, *Contributory schemes*, pp. 7–9; TNA: PRO, MH58/200, Minute sheet, Onslow to Brock, 22 July 1923.
59 TNA: PRO, MH58/204, Cave committee, evidence, day 15 (Newcastle), day 17 (Glasgow).
60 WHSA, Sheffield and District Association of Hospital Contributors, Delegates meetings, 16 November 1921.
61 *Ibid.*, 26 July 1922, 5 March 1924, 9 March 1940, 8 September 1942, 3 December 1946.
62 WHSA, SHC, annual report, 1926, pp. 30–72.
63 ML, HB 14/1, Glasgow Royal Infirmary minutes, *passim*.
64 ML, HB 14/1/40, Glasgow Royal Infirmary minutes, 1929–30, 11 January 1930.
65 LHSA, LHB 1/18/2, Minutes of meetings of the League of Subscribers to the Royal Infirmary of Edinburgh, November 1930.
66 TWAS, HO/RVI/60, Royal Victoria Infirmary, Minute book: workmen governors' annual meetings, 1926, 1939, *passim*.
67 *The Contributor*, July 1936, p. 203.
68 *The Contributor*, February 1932, p. 37.
69 The survey was conducted by Research Services Ltd: Lord Beveridge, *The evidence for voluntary action* (London, 1949), p. 69.
70 *Ibid.*, p. 78, table E.22.
71 *Ibid.*, pp. 81, 83, tables E.24, E.26; Beveridge also believed active participation had declined in the friendly societies: see B. Harris, *The origins of the British welfare state: society, state and social welfare in England and Wales, 1800–1945* (Basingstoke, 2004), pp. 192–3.
72 *The Samaritan*, 1 (2) (1934), pp. 10, 18.
73 Leeds Local and Family History Library, Leeds Workpeople's Hospital Fund, annual report, 1914, pp. 14–15.
74 WHSA, SHC, annual report, 1938, p. 26.
75 ML, HB14/1/39, Glasgow Royal Infirmary minutes 1927–28, 8 January 1927.
76 TNA: PRO, CAB 87/80, SIC (42) 64, Nuffield College Social Reconstruction Survey, 1942.
77 TNA: PRO, CAB 87/78, SIC (42), Twentieth meeting, 24 June 1942, Q5058–66.
78 Bolton Royal Infirmary, *Jubilee carnival*, p. 11.
79 Beveridge, *Evidence for voluntary action*, p. 79, table E.23.
80 *Who was who*: vol. *II, 1916–1928* (Hambleden); vol. *III, 1929–40* (Knutsford) vol. *IV 1941–1950* (Stanley, Whitbread); King Edward's Hospital Fund for London, annual report, 1923.
81 F. K. Prochaska, *Philanthropy and the hospitals of London: the King's Fund, 1897–1990* (Oxford, 1992), p. 288; *Who was who*: vol. *IV, 1941–1950* (Lawrence, Duff); vol. *VI, 1961–1970* (Penton); vol. *V, 1951–1960* (Anderson); King Edward's Hospital Fund for London, annual report, 1935; J. Manton, *Elizabeth Garret Anderson* (London, 1965, 1987 edn).
82 HSA Archive, HSA, annual reports, 1926, 1928; *The Contributor*, April 1926, p. 35.
83 T. C. Barker, *The Glassmakers: Pilkington 1826–1976* (London, 1977), p. 461.
84 MRO, M610 MED 4/1, MHC, annual report, 1936, pp. 33–4.
85 *Ibid.*, p. 34, annual report, 1945, p. 11; Braddock led Liverpool City Council from 1955 to 1961.
86 *The Samaritan*, 3 (1) (1936), p. 1.
87 WHSA, Sheffield and District Association of Hospital Contributors, Delegates meetings, 7 March 1939.
88 BALSL, Bolton and District Hospital Saturday Committee minute book, 1937–40, '44 years of service', news cutting, n.d. but November 1937.
89 *Ibid.*, 9 November 1937.
90 M. Wren, *Half a century of service 1935–1985* (Bristol, 1985), pp. 5–7, 13.
91 LHSA, LHB 1/18/4, Minutes of meetings of the League of Subscribers to the Royal Infirmary of Edinburgh, 4 September 1947.

92　TWAS, HO/RVI/60, Royal Victoria Infirmary, Minute book: workmen governors' annual meetings, 1913, 1914.

93　ML, HB 14/1/35, Glasgow Royal Infirmary minutes 1920, 10 January 1920; ML, HB 14/1/37, Glasgow Royal Infirmary minutes, 1923–24.

94　ML, HB 14/3/37, Memorandum regarding representation of the working classes, Request by Co-operative Societies, 1912; SCWS Employees' Amalgamated Charitable Funds; ML, HB 14/1/27, Glasgow Royal Infirmary minutes, 29 April 1912.

95　A. T. Page, *Pennies for health: the story of the British Hospitals Contributory Schemes Association* (Birmingham, 1949), pp. 6, 11.

96　*Hospital Gazette*, January 1926, p. 11; MRO, M610 MED 4/1, MHC, annual report, 1944, p. 10.

97　J. Dodd, 'The story of the Bristol Hospitals Fund I – 1939 to 1944', *Bristol Chamber of Commerce Monthly Journal*, 29 (12) (1954), pp. 29–35; MRO, M610 MED 4/1, MHC, annual report, 1930; Page, *Pennies for health*, p. 11.

98　WHSA, SHC, annual reports, 1928, pp. 26–7, 1934, pp. 38–9.

99　PAAA, Wolverhampton and Staffordshire Hospital: Hospital Saturday Committee minute book, 25 July 1929, 29 January 1930, 30 April 1932, 25 February 1933, 27 January 1934, 26 January 1935, 1 February 1936, 30 January 1937, 11 January 1939, 12 January 1941, 8 November 1942.

100　*Ibid.*, 14 February 1943.

101　*Ibid.*, 8 November 1942; WALS, L3621, N. Fox, *A history of the Royal Hospital*, pp. 38, 57.

102　ML, HB 14/1/38, Glasgow Royal Infirmary minutes 1925–26; ML, HB 14/1/40, Glasgow Royal Infirmary minutes 1929–30; ML, HB 14/1/46, Glasgow Royal Infirmary minutes, 14 January 1939.

103　ML, HB 14/1/38, Glasgow Royal Infirmary minutes, 10 January 1925.

104　ML, HB 14/1/33, Glasgow Royal Infirmary minutes, 12 January 1918; ML, HB 14/1/34, Glasgow Royal Infirmary minutes, 11 January 1919; ML, HB 14/1/35, Glasgow Royal Infirmary minutes, 10 January 1920; ML, HB 14/1/36, Glasgow Royal Infirmary minutes, 14 January 1922.

105　ML, HB 14/1/40, Glasgow Royal Infirmary minutes, 11 January 1930; ML, HB 14/1/44, Glasgow Royal Infirmary minutes, 9 January 1937.

106　ML, HB 14/1/41, Glasgow Royal Infirmary minutes, 9 January 1932.

107　ML, HB 14/1/42, Glasgow Royal Infirmary minutes, 14 January 1933; ML, HB 14/1/45, Glasgow Royal Infirmary minutes, 8 January 1938.

108　TNA: PRO, MH 58/200, Minute sheet, Brock, 8 May 1923.

109　ML, HB 14/1/39, Glasgow Royal Infirmary minutes, 8 January 1927.

110　ML, HB 14/1/40, Glasgow Royal Infirmary minutes, 12 January 1929; ML, HB 14/1/47, Glasgow Royal Infirmary minutes, 13 January 1940; ML, HB 14/1/48, Glasgow Royal Infirmary minutes, 11 January 1941.

111　S. D. Slater and D. Dow (ed.), *The Victoria Infirmary of Glasgow 1890–1900: a centenary history* (Glasgow, 1990), p. 35.

112　TWAS, HO/RVI/60, Royal Victoria Infirmary, Minute book: workmen governors' annual meetings, 7 March 1925, 22 March 1930 and *passim*.

113　*Ibid.*, 4 November 1926, 19 March 1927.

114　LHSA, LHB 1/18/2, Minutes of meetings of the League of Subscribers to the Royal Infirmary of Edinburgh, 29 November 1934, 28 November 1935; LHSA, LHB 1/18/3, 16 November 1938, 22 April 1942.

115　LHSA, LHB 1/18/2, LHB 1/18/3, LHB 1/18/4, Minutes of meetings of the League of Subscribers to the Royal Infirmary of Edinburgh, *passim*.

116　LHSA, LHB 1/18/4, Minutes of meetings of the League of Subscribers to the Royal Infirmary of Edinburgh, 17 July 1947.

117　LHSA, LHB 1/18/3, Minutes of meetings of the League of Subscribers to the Royal Infirmary of Edinburgh, 12 November 1942.

118　LHSA, LHB 1/18/2, Minutes of meetings of the League of Subscribers to the Royal

Infirmary of Edinburgh, 7 March 1934, 17 July 1934, 29 November 1934; from 1934 funds were voted to pay for attendance at board meetings.

119   J. V. Pickstone, *Medicine and industrial society* (Manchester, 1985), p. 254.
120   For example, *The lectures used by the Manchester Unity of the Independent Order of Odd Fellows* (London, 1846), p. 51.
121   LMA, A/KE/313, Meeting of president and general council, 1 January 1922.
122   LMA, A/KE/313, King's Fund, secretary – chairman, 27 February 1922.
123   F. Colchester-Wemyss, 'Contributory schemes', in F. Menzies (ed.), *The voluntary hospitals in Great Britain (excluding London): fifth annual report for the year 1923* (London, 1924), p. 102; *Hospital Gazette*, June 1925, p. 12.
124   *Hospital Gazette*, March 1929, pp. 39–40.
125   *The Hospital*, 27 (1931), p. 211.
126   A. Sanctuary, 'Contributory schemes', *Hospital Gazette*, June 1925, p. 12; S. Grew, 'The hospital ticket system', *Hospital Gazette*, March 1925, p. 8.
127   *Birmingham Post*, 13 January 1928, 6 March 1928.
128   Stone, *Hospital organization*, p. 539; MRO, M610, MED 7/5/3, Merseyside Association of Hospital Contributors, Delegates committee of enquiry into the council's operation and costs, Report by Councillor Braddock.
129   Stone, *Hospital organization*, pp. 218–19, 236–7.
130   *The Hospital*, 26 (1930), p. 149.
131   Bristol Contributory Welfare Association, annual report, 1937.
132   BALSL, Bolton Hospital Saturday Committee, annual report, 1939, p. 7, cover.
133   M610 MED 4/1, MHC, annual report, 1944, pp. 11, 13.
134   Sanctuary, 'Contributory schemes', pp. 12–13; Stone, *Hospital organization*, p. 218.
135   D. W. Orr and J. Walker Orr, *Health insurance with medical care: the British experience* (New York, 1938), p. 50.
136   See *The Contributor*, September 1926, p. 57, for an early statement of the journal's aims.
137   *The Contributor*, July 1928, pp. 364, 567, July 1929, p. 583, August 1929, p. 607.
138   *The Contributor*, August 1938, p. 238.
139   *The Contributor*, June 1929, p. 568, October 1930, p. 9, November 1931, p. 275.
140   *The Contributor*, June 1944, p. 22.
141   *The Hospital*, 32 (1936), p. 97 ('vitalising the neighbourhood'); *The Contributor*, September 1929, p. 645, August 1929, p. 607.
142   *The Contributor*, January 1938, p. 10.
143   *The Contributor*, August 1937, p. 235.
144   *The Contributor*, March 1926, p. 26.
145   *The Contributor*, July 1929, p. 584, December, 1930, p. 956.
146   *The Contributor*, February 1927, p. 93.
147   *The Contributor*, January 1926, pp. 13–14, February 1932, p. 40, January 1933, p. 339.
148   *The Contributor*, April 1927, p. 128, June 1932, p. 142, April 1935, p. 294.
149   *The Contributor*, June 1928, pp. 28–9.
150   *The Contributor*, May 1928, pp. 331.
151   *The Contributor*, October 1926, p. 59; S. Smiles, *Self-help, with illustrations of conduct and perseverance* (1859) (reprinted London, 1996), ch. 10.
152   *The Contributor*, January 1938, p. 16.
153   *The Contributor*, May 1926, p. 39.
154   *The Contributor*, April 1932, pp. 98–9, April 1936, p. 109.
155   K. McClelland, 'Masculinity and the "representative artisan" in Britain, 1850–80', in M. Roper and J. Tosh (eds), *Manful assertions: masculinities in Britain since 1800* (London, 1991), pp. 74–91.
156   *The Samaritan*, 4 (2) (1937), p. 13.
157   *The Samaritan*, 3 (2) (1936), and see *The Contributor*, January 1938, p. 12.
158   R. J. Morris, *Class, sect and party: the making of the British middle class, Leeds 1820–1850* (Manchester, 1990).
159   S. Yeo, *Religion and voluntary organisations in crisis* (London, 1976), p. 218.

160 S. Cherry, 'Regional comparators in the funding and organisation of the voluntary hospital system, *c.* 1860–1939', in M. Gorsky and S. Sheard (eds), *Financing medicine: the British experience since 1750* (London, forthcoming, 2006).

161 *Forward*, 1 (1) (1892), pp. 7–8, 31.

162 *Forward*, 4 (1) (1892), pp. 52–3, 54.

163 B. Abel-Smith, *The hospitals 1800–1948: a study in social administration in England and Wales* (London, 1964) pp. 286–7; A. Marwick, 'The Labour Party and the welfare state in Britain, 1900–1948', *American Historical Review*, 73 (1967–68), pp. 380–403, at pp. 388–9.

164 LHSA, Royal Infirmary of Edinburgh League of Subscribers, annual report, 1947, typescript appendix.

165 LHSA, LHB 1/18/14, Letter book, Edinburgh Royal Infirmary, League of Subscribers, 1920–21, Paton to Caldwell, 2 March 1920.

166 LHSA, LHB 1/18/3, Minutes of meetings of the League of Subscribers to the Royal Infirmary of Edinburgh, 16 November 1938.

167 MRO, M610 MED 2/2, Liverpool Voluntary Hospitals Council, Minutes of all Council committees 1927–1928, 15 June 1927.

168 *Ibid.*, 13 July 1927.

169 MRO, MHC, annual report, 1927/28, 'From Alderman Luke Hogan, J.P.'

170 MRO, M610 MED 2/2, Liverpool Voluntary Hospitals Council, Minutes of all Council committees 1927–28, 31 October 1927.

171 Sheffield Archives, LD 1368, Minutes of Sheffield trades and labour council executive committee meeting, 27 September 1920.

172 WHSA, Minutes of Sheffield Joint Hospitals Consultative and Advisory Council, 13 October 1920.

173 *Ibid.*, 20 December 1920; S. Pollard, *A history of labour in Sheffield* (Liverpool, 1959), pp. 208–9, 282–3, 302–3.

174 WHSA, Minutes of Sheffield Joint Hospitals Consultative and Advisory Council, 24 November 1920, 23 March 1921.

175 *Ibid.*, 20 December 1920.

176 *Ibid.*, 20 April 1921.

177 *Birmingham Post*, 8 June 1936.

178 *The Samaritan*, 2 (3) (September 1935), p. 2.

179 A. Portes, 'Social capital: its origins and applications in modern sociology', *American Review of Sociology*, 24 (1998); T. Skocpol, 'Unravelling from above', *American Prospect*, 25 (1996), pp. 20–25; D. Gaggio, 'Do social historians need social capital?', *Social History*, 29 (2004), pp. 499–513.

180 *The Contributor*, January 1938, p. 11.

181 *The Contributor*, January 1939, p. 5.

182 Leeds Central Library, Leeds and District Workpeople's Hospital Fund, annual report, 1941.

Chapter 6

Contributory schemes, working-class governors and local control of hospital policy

In contemporary political discourse about welfare provision, the active citizen is seen as preferable to the passive recipient. Direct participation, for example through stakeholding or mutual ownership, allows, it is thought, the wishes of users to drive service delivery, rather than the potentially flawed assessments of public sector bureaucracies. The inter-war contributory schemes offer a useful test of this premise. Clearly they were an idiosyncratic form of user group, in that involvement was rooted in the financial contribution rather than a more generalised sense of public spirit. None the less, they had a mass membership and strong representative procedures that allowed members a say in both fund management and hospital governance, and, as noted in chapter 5, some schemes specifically included the articulation of contributors' interests in their constitutions. Thus, while they do not offer a direct parallel with NHS bodies, they do provide useful evidence of citizen engagement with hospital policy.

This chapter seeks to determine whether contributor participation affected decision-making and signalled a genuine shift in control of institutions, making them more responsive to the needs of local users. The first section considers the routine work of scheme administrators, assessing whether they expressed patients' concerns about services. Next the implications of labour movement involvement are examined, to establish whether trade unionists were able to influence issues such as the pay and conditions of hospital staff. The third section details several episodes in which the wishes of contributor representatives clashed with the hospital establishment, and which demonstrate that ultimately power remained with providers rather than users. Finally, two areas are identified in which contributors successfully asserted their wishes: the retention of convalescence benefits and the rejection by schemes in Scotland and the North East of the hospital means test.

The contributors' role in scheme administration

The routine work of the schemes

An executive committee's work consisted for the most part of routine administration, as the characteristic example of the contributory scheme for the Wolverhampton Royal Hospital illustrates. The stable make-up of this

committee made for a comfortable relationship with the hospital.[1] Meetings heard regular reports on staffing, bed provision and accounts, as well
as broader hospital matters.[2] There was an annual round of nominations of
the officers and sub-committee members (house visitors, nurses home committee, women's hospital visitors).[3] Most meetings included an update on the
numbers of firms, district committees and individual members in the scheme.
Debate over contributors in arrears recurred regularly, as did the long-term
funding of chronically ill members.[4] Mutual support and solidarity flavoured
meetings, echoing the clubbable atmosphere of a friendly society. The achieve-
ments of hospital employees were honoured, and marriages or bereavements of
scheme representatives recognised.[5] Social activities included sporting events,
dinners and an annual excursion.[6] AGMs expressed consensual support for the
hospital's work, with invited lecturers speaking, for example, on the contributory scheme movement (Sydney Lamb and Bertram Ford), medical matters
or hospital politics (Ernest Brown MP).[7] Nominations for office were then
voted on, though throughout the 1930s nominees were always automatically
approved.[8] AGMs typically concluded with formal thanks to nursing and
medical staff, scheme officers and employers for arranging payroll deductions.[9]

Other schemes similarly used contributor meetings to stimulate public
involvement in hospital life rather than to provide a forum for debate. In
Glasgow contributors were encouraged to make Saturday afternoon visits
to the Royal Infirmary, while AGMs welcomed guest speakers on medical
themes: the hospital's work on diet and disease; histories of the Infirmary and
the 'voluntary principle'; a slide show on the history of X-rays, and so on.[10]
Contributors' meetings eschewed broader aspects of health politics: 'This was
not the place ... to discuss the Voluntary System, or the State-aided System'
the 1921 AGM was told by William Shaw, secretary of Glasgow trades and
labour council. Given that the national Labour Party was currently debating
just these issues, clearly in Glasgow hospital contribution functioned as a
sphere of consensual civic activism.[11]

For the large multi-hospital schemes, much of the work was similarly
routine and managerial, giving little scope for a distinctive contributors' role.
AGMs followed formal civic rites: set-piece reports on the fund's and the
hospitals' annual performance, followed by a speech from an invited dignitary,
then a public expression of gratitude by the chair to the voluntary workers and
hospital staff.[12] Popular engagement occasionally extended further, as when
the Merseyside contributors' association initiated a programme of health education lectures at its meetings.[13] For executive committees, fundraising matters
remained a key concern, and the larger schemes faced the additional problem
of how to distribute resources between institutions in a manner which fairly
rewarded work done and preserved incentives (see chapter 3). These were
essentially technical matters and not areas in which the ordinary worker governors had a distinctive stake. Similarly, as noted in chapter 4, the recurrent
question of public sector contracting in the big urban schemes arose not from
the expressed wishes of contributors but from the necessity of easing pressure
on the waiting lists of the voluntary hospitals at the cheapest price possible.

Nor was there a distinctive contributors' role in the framing of reciprocal agreements between the large urban funds and those in outlying areas. Again, the driving force was the logic of voluntary hospital finances rather than a response to grassroots needs. Indeed, institutional loyalties persuaded some worker governors actually to obstruct cooperation. In Sunderland the Royal Infirmary made overtures in 1923 to the Monkwearmouth and Southwick Hospital about joint working to ease pressure on beds.[14] However, contributors were hostile, despite Monkwearmouth's increased capacity after a new building opened in 1932; they regarded referrals to this neighbouring institution as a derogation of their rights.[15] Sunderland was consequently criticised for irrational duplication by Ministry of Health surveyors, who urged the two institutions to amalgamate so that the smaller hospital could specialise in orthopaedics and accidents.[16]

Patient advocacy

Amid this routine business there is sporadic evidence of contributor associations being used as a forum for members' concerns. For example, in 1930 Wolverhampton committee member E. J. Sherlock noted cases 'in which he considered more attention may have been devoted by the Staff'.[17] In 1938 a complaint was made against the almoner, though the executive committee expressed its confidence in him, and protests were made about increasing waiting times for tonsil and adenoid cases, though enquiries revealed these were unfounded.[18] During the war the question of whether to raise subscription rates from 3*d* to 4*d* to meet rising costs provoked localised protest; although the motion was easily carried, district committees received 'discretionary powers' to accommodate members unable to pay the new rate.[19] Wartime disturbance prompted marginally more patient advocacy, including a complaint regarding the casualty department in 1941, objections about the reduction of visiting hours, and a protest about the waiting area for the pathology department, which led to the construction of a temporary shelter from the rain.[20]

A similar menu of concerns appears elsewhere. At Glasgow Royal Infirmary complaints about treatment in 1919 were 'carefully scrutinised' and 'invariably satisfactorily explained'.[21] Unhappiness about waiting lists was aired at the 1922 AGM and delegates were reassured by the medical committee chair that the backlog of 900 patients 'should not … be invested with too much importance … as there was not now the same hesitation and disinclination to go to Hospitals that was prevalent, say, twenty years ago'; this, too, was a 'satisfactory explanation'.[22] Support for management was maintained in a dispute about proposals to demolish the old 'Lister ward', which some nurses, and the local press, felt should be preserved for posterity; the working-class representatives disapproved of 'sentimental affection for the dead'.[23] At Sunderland Royal Infirmary the worker governors were concerned, *inter alia*, with: excessive waiting times for admissions; neglect of a chronically ill patient; inferior treatment received by a person transferred from the Infirmary to a poor law institution;

the early discharge of a child tonsillectomy patient without notification of the parents; the discrepancy between ordinary visiting hours and those enjoyed by paying patients; the regulations over 'the age of kiddies being allowed to visit patients'; and the delays experienced by people awaiting non-urgent X-ray results.[24] Meetings of the Merseyside contributors' association also provided a mechanism for airing patients' concerns, such as the perennial problem of waiting lists and the quality of visiting facilities.[25]

It is rarely possible to establish the outcome of such grievances, though they certainly were communicated to doctors and governors. In 1928, for instance, the Sunderland contributors protested that a patient with a bad leg had been moved to the long-stay pavilion and had not seen a consultant for eight weeks; his doctor acknowledged the oversight and moved him back to the wards.[26] Other cases were less easy to resolve. In 1938 a vociferous workman governor locked horns with the board of management over a miner from Dawdon colliery who had suffered a hernia after an accident two years before, and had languished so long on the Infirmary waiting list that he had gone elsewhere for an operation that cost thirty guineas. The board's defence was that, given the time lapse, his was a non-urgent case and not liable for immediate admission.[27] In an atmosphere of resource constraint, contributor advocacy won no special treatment.

To summarise, these cases indicate cordial collaborative working between hospital managers and a small, stable group of contributors' representatives; indeed, they conform well to the hopes articulated in the early 1920s that scheme mechanisms would foster 'personal interest' and 'charitable instinct' among the workers.[28] The majority of the representatives' business was the routine work of raising and allocating income; major concerns like reciprocal agreements and public sector contracting arose not from contributor pressure but from a widely shared concern with the efficient use of resources. Evidence that representatives acted as advocates for patients and ordinary contributors is sporadic, not ubiquitous. Although undeniably manifesting 'local' needs, such complaints typically focused on issues which would concern any population of hospital users, such as waiting lists, infrastructure and the quality of doctors' care. Although outcomes are not always easy to discern, it seems that sometimes complaints were satisfactorily addressed and sometimes limited resources prevented this.

The influence of the labour movement

Scheme executives included significant representation from trade unions, friendly and cooperative societies and local Labour parties. Their participation was required to smooth the acceptance of workplace payroll deductions, to lead appeals and to popularise membership.[29] Were they also able to implant labour politics in hospital government?

Where inter-war unemployment was high and wages depressed, worker governors agitated to improve the pay and conditions of hospital staff. In

Sunderland, for example, miners' lodges were behind a 1935 resolution that nursing probationers' off-duty time should be augmented by a weekly half-day holiday.[30] The result was a partial victory: the board was sympathetic, though concerned about costs, and conceded a half-day off per fortnight.[31] In the 1940s representations were regularly made on behalf of the local nurses' guild that the hospital was opposed to trade union membership for nurses and that the Infirmary's nursing committee was not engaged in dialogue with staff.[32] The worker governors expressed the concerns of the local trades council, supported wage increases for porters and stokers, and ensured the unionisation of hospital painters.[33] In the 1940s a tussle over non-unionised labour occurred with a contractor responsible for the Children's Hospital gardens (wartime shortages apparently necessitating the employment of elderly workers paid below union rates).[34] The board of management finally acceded to proposals that all ancillary workers should be trade union members and publicly welcomed the facility this provided for negotiating wages and conditions with organised bodies.[35]

However, the ability and inclination of worker governors to champion employees' rights was compromised by their simultaneous concern, as contributors, with controlling costs. The tendency was therefore towards compromise. In Glasgow, for example, the claim of the National Amalgamated Workers' Union for standard wages for fire-fighters, labourers and porters in the three main voluntary hospitals was refused by the board on the grounds that the hours worked differed by institution, to which the worker governors raised no objection.[36] In 1937 Glasgow contributors also reluctantly supported management in rejecting the recommendations of a forty-eight-hour week by the committee on nurse training.[37] Only in the late 1930s, when the issue of nurses' pay and status was regularly raised at AGMs, did labour issues assume prominence.[38] Pressure for the forty-eight-hour week was maintained in 1939, along with calls for a superannuation scheme for skilled ancillary staff.[39] Contributors continued to seek assurances during the war that elected executives would fight for nurses' wage increases, keeping the issue of pay and conditions on the agenda.[40]

Newcastle upon Tyne's Royal Victoria Infirmary also presents a picture of compromise. Organised labour was well represented and worker representatives achieved positions on key committees (hospital policy, wages, buildings and properties), where they presumably exerted influence.[41] AGMs, however, were constrained by a constitutional ruling that prevented delegates passing resolutions on hospital policy.[42] Governors' meetings only rarely dealt with issues such as waiting times or complaints over admissions, and when these were raised they seem to have been brushed aside.[43] Labour concerns arose in 1933 when wage cuts for ancillary and maintenance staff were implemented without consultation: those earning over £100 per annum faced cuts of at least 4 per cent, and lower earners of 2.5 per cent.[44] Protests from some governors that most hospital managers were not 'acquainted with the conditions of their employment or the nature of the work they were called on to do' were to no avail.[45] With the National Union of General and Municipal Workers leading the campaign, the governors' annual meeting and some of the main works committees joined with local trade unions to 'press for the restoration of the wages cut until a negotiated settlement has been arrived at'.[46] Despite a promise to examine each case on its merits only the building workers had their wages restored.[47] Not until 1934 and recovery from the slump were the cuts rescinded, and this time the pressure came not from worker governors but from the National Union as well as engineering and electrical unions.[48] Again, then, contributor representatives kept the issue before management but were ultimately acquiescent.

In Liverpool the uneasy concordat with organised labour that launched the scheme meant that at the outset the MHC 'yielded to Trade Union pressure' in agreeing union rates for its own employees.[49] Then, against a backdrop of high local unemployment, in 1933 anxiety rose over the administrative costs of the scheme, which were nearly £15,000 in 1932, some 12 per cent of total expenditure on benefits.[50] A contributors committee of enquiry chaired by Labour activist John Braddock was set up and eventually reported that in fact costs were 'fair and reasonable', with salaries of clerical and ambulance workers at trade union rates (though it is notable that administrative expenses were henceforth more constrained as a proportion of expenditure).[51] Contributor ire was sparked again in 1944 by the issue of the retirement pension due to the MHC secretary, Sydney Lamb, which the outraged members of the local Labour Party and trades council deemed excessive.[52] There were calls for greater workers' representation on the MHC and criticism of the president's 'dictatorial' style; in 1945 a new executive committee was elected and Lamb's pension was cut.[53]

Worker governors with trade union links also mediated between the schemes' tendency to push for ever higher contributions and local workers' capacity to meet these. Rising utilisation rates and the costs of medical advance exerted constant pressure on expenditure, especially on the pay of nurses, ancillary workers and residents, while ambitious developments meant additional demands.[54] In Birmingham, for example, the building of a new hospitals centre commanded broad support.[55] Here there was much discussion of whether to raise contribution rates from 2d to 3d per week, with branch representatives uncertain whether all workers could afford this. Eventually the BHSF accepted the proposal, though the trades council 'strongly deprecated any coercion' to secure the extra penny and as a concession pensioners and blind persons escaped the increase.[56] Similar pressures operated on Merseyside, where the MHC sought sufficient income to reimburse hospitals for the actual costs of treatment and looked jealously at the higher rates levied in 'London, Birmingham or Sheffield'; however, given high local unemployment and casualisation of labour, it proposed instead that workers should increase subscriptions by a penny in the 'part of a pound'.[57] Little progress was made until wartime when, with a hospital deficit of £43,000, the trades council finally acceded to a minimum of 2d per week, though insisting that for those under eighteen and those on the lowest incomes the subscription remained at 1d; it was also agreed that 50 per cent of the additional revenue would support local war charities.[58]

These examples show that labour movement representatives on scheme executives sought to improve the pay and conditions of fund and hospital employees. Given their dual role as workers' spokespeople and guardians of the fund, such conflicts were resolved through compromise, with resource constraints sometimes militating against improvements. They also ensured that the level of contribution demanded by schemes did not exceed the capacity of local labour markets. For many, then, their activism was largely an extension of their role as trade unionists.

Conflict with the medical establishment

Thus far the discussion has concentrated on a broad set of concerns common to different contributory schemes. This section considers more specific cases of local grievance which pitted worker governors against the medical establishment – both doctors and hospital managers. Friction between contributors and practitioners had a long history, extending back to the nineteenth century: as with other forms of contract practice, doctors were concerned that their status should not be undermined and that they should not lose paying patients to contributory funds, while contributors were keen to assert entitlements.[59] Did the machinery for contributor participation in the schemes in the interwar period tilt the balance of power towards the ordinary patient? This section uses three specific examples to evaluate the matter.

The Gloucester smallpox epidemic

An unusual conflict between contributors and local medical leadership occurred in Gloucester in 1923. A popular contributory scheme had recently started, quickly doubling the sums raised hitherto from workplace collections, from £2,564 in 1921 to £4,989 in 1922 (21 per cent of total income).[60] Gloucestershire Royal Infirmary's management included Sir Francis Colchester-Wemyss, national advocate of mass contribution as the 'only alternative' for the voluntary hospital and a strong proponent of worker governors.[61] However, the Workpeople's Hospital Committee, which ran the scheme, was almost immediately 'in conflict with the Authorities of the Infirmary', over the temporary closure of three wards during a smallpox epidemic. The disease had appeared among the hospital patients, prompting the weekly committee (on which the workers had only one representative) to order the ward closures, against the wishes of the Infirmary's ordinary contributors.[62] Why should this apparently sensible precautionary move have set the scheme against the managers?

The answer lies in the local medical politics of smallpox, for Gloucester had long been a centre of opposition to compulsory vaccination. This stance dated back to the nineteenth century, when increasingly harsh statutory powers were adopted to enforce infant vaccination.[63] Anti-vaccinationism had developed in various towns (Leicester and Gloucester were notorious), supported largely by members of the respectable working class who resented the intrusiveness of the legislation and the association of vaccination with the despised poor law.[64] In 1896 Gloucester had been the centre of one of the last serious smallpox outbreaks, when 413 had died.[65] Since then the law had been progressively liberalised to allow parents to declare themselves 'conscientious objectors' and thus be excused the penalties for failing to have their children vaccinated.[66] Despite this, the tradition of anti-vaccinationism lingered, so Gloucester's response to the new epidemic was a highly sensitive issue. In 1923 the bulk of the medical profession and local government favoured rigorous application of the standard precautions of notification, isolation and vaccination. The situation was exacerbated by the local medical officer of health (MOH), who not only defied official advice but also claimed the cases were chickenpox; in fact it was a mild strain of variola, with a mortality rate of only three out of 507.[67]

This was the context in which anti-vaccinationism flared, as the local authority responded by sacking the MOH and bringing in an outside expert, who used magistrates' orders to remove infected persons to isolation hospitals.[68] For this he was threatened and insulted in the streets, while opponents inveighed against the 'bunkum of vaccination'.[69] The weekly committee claimed that its ward closures were necessary because unvaccinated persons had introduced the disease. Clearly, the committee identified with official policy, for in excluding smallpox patients it endorsed the sole alternative: removal to the public isolation hospital. Conversely, the workers' desire for the wards to remain open reflected the aspiration that 'their' hospital might offer an alternative response, in tune with the popular mood. The episode illustrates well the limits of the voluntary hospital's transformation into a 'community resource'. Power over essential decisions remained firmly with local and national medical and political leaders. Indeed, Colchester-Wemyss later drew on Gloucester's experience to advise administrators intent on setting up a contributory scheme that: 'Politics and discussions of controversial subjects, such as anti-Vaccination … be rigidly banned'.[70]

Sunderland – doctors and workers' compensation

Sunderland, as noted above, was characterised by a strong trade union presence among worker governors.[71] A recurrent sensitive issue was the role of the hospital with respect to workers' compensation. For instance, in 1931 representatives of Lumley Pit complained that a consultant had issued a medical report that prejudiced a compensation claim and asked Infirmary doctors not to undertake this work.[72] Three years later Houghton-le-Spring lodge protested about the private use of the Infirmary's X-ray apparatus by a doctor under contract to an employer in a compensation case. The Infirmary's standing committee tried to cool tempers, pointing out that consultants were at liberty to act for either the lodges or the employers in such cases.[73] Colliery activists were unconvinced that this was 'fair and equitable', asserting instead that since their funds had paid for the X-ray equipment they should have a say over its use for private work.[74]

This issue dramatised a paradox of workers' contribution. In towns such as Sunderland the hospital relied on mass funding – in 1934 workers provided 51 per cent of ordinary income, against only 11 per cent from charitable subscriptions and donations.[75] Why, when popular opinion was expressed through the appropriate representative networks, should the majority donors not have their way? The rancour of the compensation row generated further tensions, initially within the workers' committee itself, when Lumley Pit objected to the nomination procedures for its membership.[76]

In the mid-1930s worker governors challenged management policy more frequently, with J. Devlin of Dawdon Colliery, the chief spokesman, articulating complaints over waiting lists, non-unionisation and nurses' working hours. Opposition to private work hardened, with protests against some patients receiving 'preferential treatment by payment of a consulting fee' and objections that the Infirmary was 'for poor people who could not afford to pay fees'.[77] The compensation issue resurfaced in 1937, when the board of management bent the rules on retirement in favour of a doctor who was unpopular with the contributors because he worked for the employers. Why, Devlin wondered, should a consultant 'have full access in treating our people and then be able to give evidence against them'?[78] Devlin's view did not prevail in the hospital's court of governors, and he therefore attempted to extend workers' representation on this body. In 1938 worker governors raised the issue at the annual court, only to have the hospital's president, local MP Samuel Storey, inform them, in a statement which highlighted the tension between the charitable and insurance aspects of the schemes, that the current situation was 'quite fair' and that the board's function was 'not simply to represent a sectional interest'.[79] A formal resolution to ask the board for 'more equal representation' was then put, though the issue was postponed and ultimately dropped during the war.[80]

So, in sum, where medical politics and class politics intertwined, in this case over the rights of doctors to conduct private work, the minority representation of the worker governors ensured that the status quo was undisturbed.

Edinburgh – access to the municipal hospital

The failure of the Edinburgh League of Subscribers to secure its members' rights of access to the local municipal hospital provides another good example of the difficulties ordinary citizens experienced in influencing hospital governance. In common with other schemes, the League was an occasional advocate of contributors' concerns, on such issues as the quality of care in the eye and skin departments, visiting hours and the use of artificial stone in building works (which prompted a trades council delegation).[81] The dispute over the municipal hospital was more serious. It arose from members' long-running dissatisfaction with the Edinburgh Royal Infirmary's waiting list, which by 1930 ran to 2,400 people.[82] A potential solution presented itself in the development of the city council's hospitals, which in 1930 were taken over from the poor law institutions under the Local Government Act (Scotland). The council's aim was to improve the hospitals' standards, to develop acute care facilities, to introduce clinical teaching and to extend their clientele beyond the impoverished and infirm.[83] In common with municipal hospitals elsewhere, those in Edinburgh operated a system of means testing and charging; those too poor to pay were admitted as public assistance patients (just as they would have been under the poor law), while others were subject to charges. The result was that about half of all admissions made some payment, and the city assiduously pursued its debts.[84] The question therefore arose of whether League members unable to gain admission to the Infirmary should be required to pay if they entered the municipal hospital instead.

We have seen that in Sheffield, Birmingham and Merseyside the schemes responded by establishing contracting arrangements with the public sector, and the League's executive now came under similar pressure to act. Members were aggrieved to find that if admitted to the municipal hospital, thus relieving the waiting list of the Infirmary, they might be charged up to 25s per week. But had they not already subscribed for their hospital care?[85] This issue was 'always cropping up' during membership drives: if workers were expected to pay in public hospitals, what point was there in subscribing to the League as well?[86] Several possible solutions were discussed. One was to adopt the approach followed elsewhere, and for the League to make a payment from its funds to cover charges on members.[87] Another option was to press the council to abandon charging and make the municipal hospital free to all, as had been done, for example, in Aberdeen.[88] This had strong support from a range of labour organisations, including the National Union of Railwaymen, the Leith National Unemployed Workers Movement, and the local Co-operative Women's Guild.[89] Finally, the League might urge the Infirmary board to negotiate special terms for League members.[90]

The first two proposals were soon rejected. Edinburgh town council refused to allow free admission for League members, arguing that charging was a legal obligation.[91] The League studied SHC's approach, where *pro rata* grants were made by the scheme for members treated in the municipal hospital. However, this model was deemed unsuitable in Edinburgh, because it threatened two features of the League popular with contributors: the lack of standardised contribution rates and the 'open door' system of admission to the Royal Infirmary. If a systematic tariff of charges was introduced for members using the municipal hospital, then it would be necessary to impose a standard rate of contribution to maintain equity between members (many of whom currently subscribed less than the recommended 2*d* per week). Once standard rates and municipal charging were in place, this would strengthen the hand of those hospital managers who wanted to replace the Royal Infirmary's 'open door' with the English system, of user fees coupled with means testing (see below).[92] The Cardiff model, in which scheme members within the city paid a premium of an extra 1*d* to cover municipal charges, was also rejected, on the grounds of extra bureaucracy and the undesirability of discriminating between city and county members.[93] This left the option of the Infirmary, rather than the League itself, negotiating a payment from the hospital to the city council for

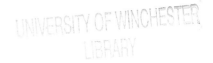

any patient taken off its waiting list.[94] Talks between the hospital and the town council then proceeded fruitlessly through the late 1930s and into the war, although the urgency was eased by the wartime EHS, which imposed a temporary solution by funding a ward at the municipal hospital to clear the waiting list.[95] Eventually broad agreement was reached that League members who subscribed at least 2*d* per week would receive a voucher which would entitle them to have the cost of treatment in the municipal hospital covered by the Infirmary.[96] Even then, the parties continued haggling over the size of the payment.[97] Only in September 1945 was the arrangement finally put into practice, some eleven years after members had first begun to voice their concern about this issue.[98]

Throughout the long deadlock the public interest was sacrificed because of the poor relationship between two sections of the medical establishment: the Infirmary doctors and the city's public health department. Municipal hospital reorganisation sought to rationalise the distribution of acute, 'sub-acute' and chronic cases. However, the efforts of the MOH, John Guy, to develop the Western General for acute and maternity cases, with teaching and nurse training facilities, were thwarted by the Royal Infirmary's determination to retain a local monopoly on acute cases.[99] This prevented the Western General offering its probationers operating theatre experience and thus also delayed it gaining the recognition of the General Nursing Council for its teaching.[100] The excess burden of chronic cases rankled; it made for 'somewhat monotonous' work and was unattractive to probationers.[101] Guy's objective was a common admission procedure for the municipal and voluntary sectors, with a reciprocal nurse training arrangement whereby voluntary hospital probationers learnt chronic care in the municipal sector.[102] The Infirmary took the opposite view. As a busy teaching hospital it required a variety of acute cases, and so did nothing to dispel the sense among local general practitioners that the poor law 'aura' still surrounded the municipal hospitals.[103] From its point of view, its long waiting list was due to patients blocking beds who required only nursing care: why should the municipal hospitals not take these chronic cases?[104]

The deadlock was broken not by contributor pressure but by the wartime EHS, under which both the Western General and the Eastern General Hospitals were opened to casualties and began to receive significant numbers of acute cases.[105] Staff shortages finally pushed the two sides into an agreement over nurse training in late 1939.[106] Moves were also made to agree payments for League members treated in the municipal hospitals.[107] Even then, the city council remained hostile to the League, and once planning for a national health service began in 1942 its own declared position was that the hospitals should be funded by an increase in NHI payments.[108] Thus the poor relations between different sections of Edinburgh's medical establishment greatly delayed a concordat which ordinary contributors desired.

These three cases represent the particular concerns of contributors in different locations. They demonstrate that where these were at odds with the position of the local hospital leadership, the wishes of contributors were ignored. In the Gloucester smallpox case, local doctors and the 'men in Whitehall' were assumed to 'know best'; in Sunderland, the freedom of practitioners to undertake compensation claim work was deemed sacrosanct; in Edinburgh, the rivalry and mutual suspicion between the municipal and voluntary sectors prevented a settlement in the contributors' interests. As the Sunderland case showed most graphically, the worker governors' minority position on management boards ensured that ultimate power resided with medical and managerial elites, just as it had previously.

Contributors ascendant: convalescent homes and the 'open door' policy

Birmingham and Merseyside – convalescent homes

Contributors proved more able to assert their views where doctors and lay governors accepted that concessions were necessary for the maintenance of income. One such example in the multi-hospital schemes was the workers' support for convalescent homes, which had been enthusiastically developed since the late-Victorian period. By 1939 the BHSF was running homes for men, women and children at Llandudno, Blackwell, Malvern, Weston-Super-Mare and Droitwich (where Highfield Hospital provided brine baths for the treatment of rheumatism).[109] On Merseyside the initial approach was to pay for patients to be sent to other homes, such as those in Woolton, Buxton and Southport: numbers rose from 499 in 1928 to nearly 3,000 by 1939. During the war, with many homes requisitioned for the EHS, the MHC purchased its own institutions in Windermere and Colwyn Bay.[110] Convalescent homes could represent a significant item of scheme expenditure, both on maintenance and on the transportation of patients: in Birmingham this averaged 11 per cent of all spending over the period 1928–46.[111]

Why were working-class subscribers so enthusiastic about these institutions? There was a clear perception that they were the product of cooperative endeavour, coupled with a sense of ownership by 'the workers' own great Movement'.[112] Thus, in 1930s Liverpool, the chair of the MHC's after-care committee was trade union organiser and Labour activist Mary Bamber.[113] Nominally the homes catered to patients whom a medical referee considered in need of convalescence after physical illness.[114] In addition, brine baths were held to benefit 'nervous ailments and … rheumatic and kindred disorders' and 'tone up your whole system' if you were 'run-down' or had been '"over-doing" it'.[115] This 'tonic' effect hints that convalescence was also considered worthwhile for the social and psychological benefits it offered manual labourers. Much play was made of the restorative power of 'romantic woodlands' and 'enchanting views'; the emphasis was on 'enjoyment', 'comfort' and 'sympathetic understanding'. So pleasurable were the stays for Birmingham contributors that 'Home Clubs' were organised for fellow patients to reunite on their return.[116] The homes therefore provided relief from 'the grinding days of continuous hard work' and in wartime offered 'rest breaks for those suffering strain from war conditions'.[117]

Doubts about the therapeutic value of the homes, coupled with concern about their costs, soon pitted fund leadership (determined to maximise resources for the hospital) against contributor representatives (who sought to extend the range of benefits offered) (see also chapter 3). The context was the financial strains of the 1930s. Birmingham hospital leaders were anxious to finance the building of their new hospitals centre, just as the slump depressed income; the BHSF, meanwhile, was planning a model convalescent home for women, at Kewstoke, in Weston-Super-Mare.[118] The accusation was made that these were no more than 'holiday homes' and that constraints should be placed on the BHSF's expenditure.[119] Liverpool's crisis came slightly later, following the failure to elicit the additional 'penny in the part of a pound' earned, with some voluntaries, such as the David Lewis Northern Hospital, facing deficits.[120] In Birmingham matters came to a head when the BHSF sought approval to increase its spending on convalescent homes and a divisive meeting saw the representatives of the voluntary hospitals all voting against the motion. However, it was carried, with Ford persuading the majority to make a gesture of goodwill, to which the BHSF would later reciprocate with an increase in subscription (it did, in 1931).[121] A similar split occurred in Liverpool, where elements within the MHC proposed the closure of the after-care department and called for the resignation of secretary Sydney Lamb when he refused to acquiesce. A local journal criticised the policy, not because it opposed the principle of recuperation but because of the consequent shortfall suffered by the hospitals: 'Trade unionists ... should be ashamed to "sweat" the doctors'.[122] Again though, the crisis passed, Lamb remained in place and convalescence benefit was retained.

Why were medical and managerial elites prepared to concede this point, despite professional doubts about convalescence? First, the homes did have a worthwhile auxiliary role for the voluntary hospitals in freeing 'blocked' beds.[123] Second, convalescence could be construed as socially beneficial because it hastened recovery and return to work.[124] Third, the existence of after-care departments permitted schemes legitimately to represent themselves as striving for 'a complete and ideal Health Service', and thus attuned to the movement for more integrated provision.[125] Above all, though, the perception that 'the workers ... will not give up that branch of the work' meant that convalescence benefit was integral to the consensus upon which the whole edifice of hospital contribution rested.[126]

Scotland and the North East: resistance to the means test

The 'English' model of contribution, with means testing of in-patients on admission and the waiver of hospital charges for scheme members, was never universally accepted. Major schemes in urban Scotland and the cities of the North East retained an 'open door' policy, which meant that voluntary hospitals were free to all comers, the only criterion being medical need. This was not simply a regional quirk but reflected the wishes of worker governors. Implicit in their rejection of an almoner's means test was the renunciation of formal maintenance charges for non-contributors, which in turn undermined the justification for a fixed rate of contribution. Resistance to the means test therefore represented both opposition to commercialisation of hospital services and a defence of the employees' right to contribute at a rate set in the workplace rather than decreed centrally.

In Glasgow, for example, trade unionist William Cross quickly nipped in the bud proposals to introduce an English-style system of charges, declaring his opposition was 'from his own convictions and as voicing the Working-Class Contributors'.[127] Here, although the executive recommended a standard, graduated weekly rate of contribution, many firms set their own flat rate or used the 'penny in the pound' approach.[128] This commitment to flexibility was popular with contributors, and remained sacrosanct, even during the depression of the early 1930s, when funding shortages prompted discussion of means testing to catch free-riders 'who were selfish enough to use the Infirmary without giving the slightest aid'.[129] However, rather than allowing themselves to be bounced towards assessment and charges, the Glasgow contributors made limited concessions on private beds, and eventually accepted the opening of paying accommodation, at the Victoria Infirmary in 1927 and the Royal in 1931.[130] An almoner's department was opened in 1935, but with a limited remit of weeding out middle-class free-riders and developing hospital social work.[131] Glasgow therefore went some way towards introducing assessment, but pulled back from organising a full-scale contributory scheme due to affection for the open door principle and dislike of standardised rates.

Edinburgh's League of Subscribers took a similar stance when a formal pre-payment scheme, with flat-rate contributions and means testing, was suggested in 1931.[132] The upshot was that Infirmary managers were unable to impose a general admission charge and were constrained to limit this to the new maternity block.[133] In 1936 pay-beds were mooted again for the cancer wards, on the grounds that middle-class patients had no other access to this treatment.[134] Matters came to a head following the publication of a Scottish Department of Health report which favoured charging in voluntary hospitals, and the Infirmary began taking legal advice on the necessary constitutional changes.[135] The League's AGM heard proposals to convert the scheme to the Birmingham model, with fixed payment and a 'joint hospital service' of voluntary and municipal institutions. However, when board member Lord Fleming attempted to sell the new plan he was met with hostility: 'If you say "free treatment for all" ... that would mean that a man with an income of £3,000 or £4,000 would be entitled to go into the Infirmary and not pay a penny. I would ask you all to consider whether you are in favour of that sort of thing. (Cries of "Yes" and "We are")'.[136] The League therefore firmly opposed any breach in the open door principle, even if (in contrast to Glasgow) the middle class were also beneficiaries.

In Newcastle upon Tyne, plans for patient assessment were also bound up with a drive towards regional integration. This followed the city council's efforts to develop Wingrove poor law institution as a municipal general hospital. In 1930 Sir Robert Bolam, physician and chair of the Royal Victoria Infirmary's honorary staff, championed joint working to facilitate the coordinated use of accommodation in both sectors. A contributory scheme spanning Newcastle, County Durham and Northumberland would ensure payment from all patients above a certain income level, whether in the state or voluntary sectors.[137] With the depression affecting hospital incomes, initial proposals were made for a pay-bed extension with a sliding scale of charges.[138] However, the system of free admissions was firmly entrenched among contributors, who even balked at accepting the HSA's green vouchers.[139] The staff suggested a compromise, with charges applicable only to patients from beyond Durham and Northumberland, but to no avail: the house committee was 'not prepared to entertain the institution of a Contributory Scheme'.[140] Here, too, the preference for flexible levels of contribution was a key issue, as evidenced by the failure of efforts in wartime to double income from workers through the imposition of a flat weekly rate of 1½*d.*[141] Even this fell well short of the true rate for maintenance coverage, which was estimated in 1930 to be 2*d.*[142]

Sunderland's workers also opposed Bolam's regionalisation proposal, though the board of the Sunderland Royal Infirmary favoured it, since in 1930–31 the hospital had reached its credit limit and faced ward closures.[143] None the less, the worker governors argued it would mean they 'would lose their association with particular Hospitals'.[144] Later debates about introducing a flat-rate contribution suggest that this was also a central impediment to acceptance.[145] Indeed, the best explanation of regional preference for the open door policy probably lies with wage differentials. In the inter-war period average earnings in the coalfields of the North East had fallen markedly behind those of other English mining areas, and for parts of the 1920s were 'even below adequate subsistence levels'. Also, in the 1930s miners in Northumberland and, more particularly, Durham experienced comparatively higher levels of full, as opposed to temporary, unemployment.[146] An ingrained reluctance to raise contribution rates is therefore understandable, and despite further discussion uniform deductions were never imposed.[147]

Thus, while contributor governors were only partially successful in improving pay and conditions in the hospitals, they did manage to assert their rights over convalescent homes and maintain the 'open door' policy. With respect to subscription rates and benefits, the involvement of trade unionists and worker representatives in the contributory funds ensured that the interests of the low-paid were protected.

Conclusion

The evidence presented here lends only limited support to the proposition that active citizenship in contributory schemes enhanced the responsiveness of the hospital system to the needs of users. As shown in chapter 5, worker representatives were small cliques of public-spirited volunteers, principally focused on administering the funds' routine business in a collegial relationship with hospital managers. The concerns of the broad mass of contributors did not intrude on this arrangement; probably most were entirely content with the operation of the schemes and saw no need for active participation. This should not surprise us: the late-twentieth-century conception of the patient as critical consumer of medical services was still a long way off.[148] Moreover, the notion that service delivery would improve if patients exercised more choice between competing institutions was absent. Instead, it was thought that efficiency gains would flow from a greater degree of regional planning and joint working, to match institutional capacity to patterns of need, a process which was not led by the contributors' associations and which some worker governors actually impeded.

The 'local' needs which the contributors' representatives advanced fell into three categories. First, there were the relatively minor complaints and concerns of users about the quality of medical care and institutional facilities; this form of advocacy was intermittent and not prominent in the sources. Second, there were the efforts of the labour movement to secure acceptable pay, conditions and union recognition for hospital employees. These were typically resolved by compromise within executive committees according to the constraints of available resources. Third, though, were a set of genuinely local issues which pitted contributors against hospital managers and doctors. In cases of conflict the minority representation of contributors on hospital boards meant that the status quo prevailed: the medical profession would not, ultimately, bend before the popular will. However, on the issues of convalescence benefit and the means test it did back down, because not to have done so would have threatened the reciprocal understanding on which mass contribution was based. Finally, it is striking to note that the most substantive area in which local wishes *did* triumph was the resistance to fixed charges and means testing in Scotland and the North East. Ironically enough, then, successful localism and active citizenship in the pre-war health system was in defence of the very principles which the NHS later perpetuated: free access at the point of use and an equitable burden of payment which did not penalise low-paid workers.

Notes

1 PAAA, Wolverhampton and Staffordshire Hospital, Hospital Saturday committee minute book, 30 May 1931.
2 *Ibid.*, 7 September 1929.
3 *Ibid.*, 3 May 1937.
4 *Ibid.*, 7 September 1932, 6 February 1935, 5 September 1935, 7 October 1935, 2 March 1938, 6 March 1935, 3 April 1935, 14 June 1933, 16 September 1933, 27 January 1934; 5 April 1939.
5 *Ibid.*, 25 February 1933, 5 October 1938; PAAA, Royal Hospital Wolverhampton Contributory Association, minute book, April 1942, 4 June 1947.

6   PAAA, Wolverhampton and Staffordshire Hospital, Hospital Saturday committee minute book, 5 April 1933, 5 September 1934, 25 May 1936.

7   *Ibid.*, 27 January 1934, 14 June 1941, 3 October 1942, 7 July 1943; PAAA, The Royal Hospital Wolverhampton Contributory Association, Minute book, 9 January 1944.

8   PAAA, Wolverhampton and Staffordshire Hospital, Hospital Saturday committee minute book, 8 March 1930, 7 March 1931, 30 April 1932, 25 February 1933, 27 January 1934, 30 January 1937, 5 February 1938, 4 February 1939.

9   *Ibid.*, 1 February 1936, 30 January 1937, 26 January 1941.

10 ML, HB 14/1/33, Glasgow Royal Infirmary minutes, 12 January 1918; ML, HB 14/1/38, Glasgow Royal Infirmary minutes, 10 January 1925, 9 January 1926; ML, HB 14/1/39, Glasgow Royal Infirmary minutes, 8 January 1927; ML, HB 14/1/43, Glasgow Royal Infirmary minutes, 12 January 1935.

11 ML, HB 14/1/36, Glasgow Royal Infirmary minutes, 8 January 1921; for a similar case in Newcastle, see TWAS, HO/RVI/60, Royal Victoria Infirmary, Minute book: workmen governors' annual meetings, 24 March 1928.

12 BCA, MS 1576/5, BHCS, MMC, 20 March 1933.

13 MRO, M610 MED 4/1, MHC, annual report, 1930, pp. 27–9.

14 J. Mohan, *Planning, markets and hospitals* (London, 2002), p. 53; TWAS, HO/SRI, Sunderland Royal Infirmary, annual report, 1925.

15 TWAS, HO/SRI/3/6, Sunderland Royal Infirmary, Workmen's governors minute book, 2 April 1938, 6 May 1939.

16 TNA: PRO, MH 66/917, Dr E. Donaldson, Sunderland CB: public health survey; TNA: PRO, MH 66/022, Sunderland: coordination of health services, 18 November 1938.

17 PAAA, Wolverhampton and Staffordshire Hospital, Hospital Saturday committee minute book, 29 January 1930.

18 *Ibid.*, 2 March 1938, 6 April 1938.

19 *Ibid.*, 6 April 1941, 7 May 1941, 14 June 1941, 2 July 1941, 12 July 1941; PAAA, Royal Hospital Wolverhampton Contributory Association, Minute book, 3 September 1941.

20 PAAA, Royal Hospital Wolverhampton Contributory Association, Minute book, 8 October 1941, April 1942, June 1943, 7 July 1943.

21 ML, HB 14/1/34, Glasgow Royal Infirmary minutes, 11 January 1919.

22 ML, HB 14/1/36, Glasgow Royal Infirmary minutes, 14 January 1922.

23 ML, HB 14/1/37, Glasgow Royal Infirmary minutes, 13 January 1923; J. Jenkinson, M. Moss and I. Russell, *The Royal: the history of Glasgow Royal Infirmary 1794–1994* (Glasgow, 1994), pp. 172–3.

24 TWAS, HO/SRI/3/6, Sunderland Royal Infirmary, Workmen's governors minute book, 12 May 1928, 5 April 1930, 5 July 1930, 6 October 1934, 5 October 1937.

25 MRO, M610 MED 4/1, MHC, annual report, 1930, pp. 27–9.

26 TWAS, HO/SRI/3/6, Sunderland Royal Infirmary, Workmen's governors minute book, 12 May 1928, 7 July 1928.

27 *Ibid.*, 5 March 1938, 2 April 1938, 14 May 1938, 11 June 1938.

28 J. E. Stone, *Hospital organization and management (including planning and construction)* (London, 1927), p. 241.

29 ML, HB 14/1/32, Glasgow Royal Infirmary minutes, 10, 13 and 22 January 1917.

30 TWAS, HO/SRI/3/6, Sunderland Royal Infirmary, Workmen's governors minute book, 19 January 1935, 9 March 1935.

31 *Ibid.*, 6 July 1935, 9 November 1935, 7 December 1935.

32 *Ibid.*, 11 May 1940, 26 April 1947, 10 January 1948.

33 *Ibid.*, 2 May 1936, 6 June 1936, 21 April 1945.

34 *Ibid.*, 20 January 1940, 16 March 1940, 11 May 1940.

35 *Ibid.*, 22 April 1944, 7 October 1944.

36 ML, HB 14/1/35, Glasgow Royal Infirmary minutes, 2 March 1920.

37 ML, HB 14/1/44, Glasgow Royal Infirmary minutes, 9 January 1937.

38 ML, HB 14/1/45, Glasgow Royal Infirmary minutes, 8 January 1938.

39 ML, HB 14/1/46, Glasgow Royal Infirmary minutes, 14 January 1939.

40 ML, HB 14/1/48, Glasgow Royal Infirmary minutes, 11 January 1941.
41 TWAS, HO/RVI/60, Royal Victoria Infirmary, Minute book: workmen governors' annual meetings, 27 March 1926.
42 TWAS, HO/RVI/34, Royal Victoria Infirmary, Minutes 1922–47, 10 March 1945, 9 March 1946.
43 TWAS, HO/RVI/60, Royal Victoria Infirmary, Minute book: workmen governors' annual meetings,15 March 1924, 14 March 1925, 21 March 1931.
44 TWAS, HO/RVI/2/54, Royal Victoria Infirmary, Minute book house com. no. 12.
45 TWAS, HO/RVI/58, Royal Victoria Infirmary, Wages committee minutes, 24 January 1933.
46 TWAS, HO/RVI/60, Royal Victoria Infirmary, Minute book: workmen governors' annual meetings, 4 and 11 March 1933; TWAS, HO/RVI/58, Royal Victoria Infirmary, Wages committee minutes, 14 March 1933.
47 TWAS, HO/RVI/58, Royal Victoria Infirmary, Wages committee minutes, 18 March 1933, 11 April 1933, 27 June 1933.
48 *Ibid.*, 20 March 1934.
49 MRO, M610, MED 7/5/3, Merseyside Association of Hospital Contributors, Delegates committee of enquiry into the council's operation and costs, Report.
50 *Ibid.*; MRO, M610 MED 4/1, MHC, annual report, 1932.
51 MRO, M610 MED 7/5/3, 7 July 1933; Merseyside Association of Hospital Contributors, Delegates committee of enquiry into the council's operation and costs, Report by Councillor Braddock, 19 July 1933; MRO, M610 MED 4/1, MHC, annual reports, *passim.*
52 *Liverpool Echo*, 24 November 1944; *The Liverpolitan*, April 1935 and June 1936; MRO, M610 MED 2/3/1/1, MHC, Minutes of council and annual meetings, 12 September 1939, 20 June 1939, 24 October 1944, 19 June 1945.
53 MRO, MHC, *News Bulletin*, 8 (July 1945); *Liverpool Echo*, 24 November 1944.
54 M. Gorsky, J. Mohan and M. Powell, 'The financial health of voluntary hospitals in interwar Britain', *Economic History Review*, 55 (3) (2002), pp. 533–57.
55 S. Barnes, *The Birmingham Hospitals Centre* (Birmingham, 1952).
56 BCA, MS 1576/5, BHSC, MMC, 6 May 1931, 9 September 1931, 10 February 1932.
57 MRO, M610 MED 4/1, MHC, annual report, 1936.
58 MRO, M610 MED 2/3/1/1, MHC, Minutes of council and annual meetings, 12 September 1939, 12 March 1940; MRO, M610 MED 4/1, MHC, annual report, 1939.
59 F. B. Smith, *The people's health 1830–1910* (London, 1979), pp. 282–3; *Forward*, 1 (1) (1892), pp. 5–6.
60 GRO, HO 19/8/6, Gloucestershire Royal Infirmary, annual reports, 1922, 1923.
61 F. Colchester-Wemyss, 'Contributory schemes', in F. Menzies (ed.), *The voluntary hospitals in Great Britain (excluding London): fifth annual report for the year 1923* (London, 1924), pp. 101, 103.
62 GRO, HO 19/8/6, Gloucestershire Royal Infirmary, annual report, 1923.
63 D. Porter and R. Porter, 'The politics of prevention: anti-vaccinationism and public health in nineteenth century England', *Medical History*, 32 (1988), pp. 231–52.
64 N. Durbach, '"They might as well brand us": working-class resistance to compulsory vaccination in Victorian England', *Social History of Medicine*, 13 (2000), pp. 45–62.
65 *British Medical Journal*, 4 August 1923, p. 208.
66 L. Barrow, 'In the beginning was the lymph: the hollowing of stational vaccination in England and Wales, 1840–98', in S. Sturdy (ed.), *Medicine, health and the public sphere in Britain, 1600–2000* (London, 2002), pp. 205–23, at pp. 219–20.
67 *Lancet*, 23 June 1923, pp. 1254–8, 22 September 1923, pp. 625–6; *British Medical Journal*, 23 June 1923, pp. 1109, 1072, 7 July 1923, p. 40, 28 July 1923, p. 157, 4 August 1923, pp. 207–8, 8 December 1923, pp. 1080–2.
68 *British Medical Journal*, 23 June 1923, p. 1071; *Lancet*, 22 September 1923, p. 625.
69 *British Medical Journal*, 30 June 1923, pp. 1110–11, and 7 July 1923, p. 40.
70 Colchester-Wemyss, 'Contributory schemes', p. 102.

71 TWAS, HO/SRI/3/6, Sunderland Royal Infirmary, Workmen's governors minute book, 5 October 1929.
72 *Ibid.*, 24 January 1931.
73 *Ibid.*, 3 March 1934, 5 May 1934, 11 May 1935.
74 *Ibid.*, 5 May 1934, 2 June 1934.
75 TWAS, HO/SRI/1381/111, Sunderland Royal Infirmary, annual report, 1934.
76 TWAS, HO/SRI/3/6, Sunderland Royal Infirmary, Workmen's governors minute book, 7 December 1935, 18 January 1936.
77 *Ibid.*, 6 July 1935; TWAS, HO/SRI, Sunderland Royal Infirmary, annual report, 1935.
78 *Ibid.*, 1936.
79 *Ibid.*, 1937.
80 TWAS, HO/SRI/3/6, Sunderland Royal Infirmary, Workmen's governors minute book, 2 April 1938, 5 November 1938, 1 April 1939, 8 July 1939.
81 LHSA, LHB 1/18/2, Minutes of meetings of the League of Subscribers to the Royal Infirmary of Edinburgh, 7 March 1934, 28 February 1935; LHSA, LHB 1/18/3, 10 October 1943, 5 November 1944.
82 LHSA, LHB 1/18/2, Minutes of meetings of the League of Subscribers to the Royal Infirmary of Edinburgh, 25 November 1930.
83 *Annual report of the Public Health Department for the year 1930* (Edinburgh, 1931), p. ix; *Annual report of the Public Health Department for the year 1932* (Edinburgh, 1933), p. vii; E. F. Catford, *The Royal Infirmary of Edinburgh, 1929–1979* (Edinburgh, 1984), pp. 22–4.
84 LHSA, LHB 1/18/2, Minutes of meetings of the League of Subscribers to the Royal Infirmary of Edinburgh, 28 February 1935, 25 June 1935, 22 November 1935, 24 September 1936; Catford, *Royal Infirmary of Edinburgh*, p. 25; Edinburgh City Library, Edinburgh Corporation committee minutes: public health committee, 1940–41, pp. 331, 356, 368.
85 LHSA, LHB 1/18/2, Minutes of meetings of the League of Subscribers to the Royal Infirmary of Edinburgh, 19 January 1934; LHSA, LHB 1/18/3, Minutes of meetings of the League of Subscribers to the Royal Infirmary of Edinburgh, 11 November 1938; LHSA, LHB 1/18/1, Royal Infirmary of Edinburgh League of Subscribers, annual report, 1935.
86 LHSA, LHB1/18/2, Minutes of meetings of the League of Subscribers to the Royal Infirmary of Edinburgh, 9 November 1937; LHSA, LHB 1/18/3, Minutes of meetings of the League of Subscribers to the Royal Infirmary of Edinburgh, 26 January 1938.
87 LHSA, LHB 1/18/2, Minutes of meetings of the League of Subscribers to the Royal Infirmary of Edinburgh, 16 April 1936, 9 June 1936.
88 *Ibid.*, 25 June 1935, 13 October 1936.
89 Edinburgh City Library, Edinburgh Corporation committee minutes, public health committee 1935–36, pp. 176, 235.
90 LHSA, LHB 1/18/2, Minutes of meetings of the League of Subscribers to the Royal Infirmary of Edinburgh, 13 October 1936.
91 *Ibid.*, 19 March 1935, 11 September 1936; LHSA, LHB 1/18/3, Minutes of meetings of the League of Subscribers to the Royal Infirmary of Edinburgh, 21 February 1939.
92 LHSA, LHB 1/18/2, Minutes of meetings of the League of Subscribers to the Royal Infirmary of Edinburgh, 22 June 1937, 7 July 1937, 24 November 1937; LHSA, LHB 1/18/1, Royal Infirmary of Edinburgh League of Subscribers, annual report, 1937.
93 LHSA, LHB 1/18/3, Minutes of meetings of the League of Subscribers to the Royal Infirmary of Edinburgh, 29 August 1940.
94 *Ibid.*, 12 November 1939.
95 *Ibid.*, 30 September 1941.
96 *Ibid.*, 23 October 1940, 17 November 1940.
97 *Ibid.*, 9 March 1941, 4 March 1945, 19 April 1945.
98 *Ibid.*, 9 September 1945, 23 January 1946, 17 July 1946; Edinburgh City Library, Edinburgh Corporation committee minutes: public health committee 1944–45, pp. 172, 264, 330.

99 *Annual report of the Public Health Department for the year 1932* (Edinburgh, 1933), p. vi.

100 *Ibid.*, p. vii.

101 *Annual report of the Public Health Department for the year 1933* (Edinburgh, 1934), pp. x–xi; *Annual report of the Public Health Department for the year 1935* (Edinburgh, 1936), pp. xi, 89; *Annual report of the Public Health Department for the year 1936* (Edinburgh, 1937), p. 96.

102 *Annual report of the Public Health Department for the year 1937* (Edinburgh, 1938), p. viii.

103 Catford, *Royal Infirmary of Edinburgh*, p. 24.

104 LHSA, LHB 1/18/3, Minutes of meetings of the League of Subscribers to the Royal Infirmary of Edinburgh, 16 November 1938.

105 *Annual report of the Public Health Department for the year 1939* (Edinburgh, 1940), p. 4; *Annual report of the Public Health Department for the year 1942* (Edinburgh, 1943), p. 43.

106 LHSA, LHB 1/18/3, Minutes of meetings of the League of Subscribers to the Royal Infirmary of Edinburgh, 12 November 1939.

107 *Ibid.*, 26 April 1939.

108 Edinburgh City Library, Edinburgh Corporation committee minutes: public health committee, 1941–42, p. 265.

109 BHSF, *65 years history of the Birmingham Hospital Saturday Fund 1873–1938* (Birmingham, 1938), *passim*.

110 MRO, M610 MED 4/1, MHC, annual report, 1928, p. 14, 1966, p. 5.

111 BLSL, BHCS, annual report, 1928, *passim*.

112 BHSF, *65 years*, pp. 22, 41.

113 'Ma' Bamber was the mother of 'Battling' Bessie Braddock, the socialist Liverpool MP: see J. Braddock and E. Braddock, *The Braddocks* (London, 1963); MRO, M610 MED 4/1, MHC, annual reports, 1936, 1938.

114 BCA, MS 1576/5, BHCS, MMC, 23 September 1930; MRO, H q 362 CUT, Hospitals: newspaper cuttings 1930–1974, Application Form Merseyside Hospitals Council, n.d. but 1943?, p. 67.

115 *The Samaritan*, 6 (1) (March 1939), p. 17.

116 BHSF, *65 years*, pp. 7, 9, 24, 39, 40.

117 *Ibid.*, p. 40; MRO, M610 MED 4/1, MHC, annual report, 1966, p. 5.

118 BHSF, *65 years*, pp. 19, 21.

119 BCA, MS 1576/5, BHCS, MMC, 23 September 1930, 5 November 1930.

120 MRO, M610 Med 2/3/3/1, MHC, Minutes of the distribution committee 1928–41, 20 September 1937.

121 BCA, MS 1576/5, BHCS, MMC, 5 November 1930, 9 September 1931.

122 'Penny in the pound friction', *The Liverpolitan*, April 1935.

123 BHCA, annual report, 1938, pp. 15–16.

124 *The Samaritan*, 3 (1) (March 1936), p. 14.

125 *The Samaritan*, 1 (2) (June 1934), p. 9.

126 'Penny in the pound friction'.

127 ML, HB 14/1/37, Glasgow Royal Infirmary minutes, 12 January 1924.

128 ML, HB 14/1/39, Glasgow Royal Infirmary minutes, 8 January 1927.

129 ML, HB 14/1/42, Glasgow Royal Infirmary minutes, 14 January 1933, 13 January 1934.

130 ML, HB 14/1/38, Glasgow Royal Infirmary minutes, 10 January 1925; S. D. Slater and D. Dow (eds), *The Victoria Infirmary of Glasgow 1890–1900: a centenary history* (Glasgow, 1990), p. 53; ML, HB 14/1/41, Glasgow Royal Infirmary minutes, 10 January 1931; ML, HB 14/1/41, Glasgow Royal Infirmary minutes, 9 January 1932.

131 ML, HB 14/1/43, Glasgow Royal Infirmary minutes, 12 January 1935, 11 January 1936; Jenkinson *et al.*, *The Royal*, pp. 183–4.

132 LHSA, LHB 1/18/2, Minutes of meetings of the League of Subscribers to the Royal Infirmary of Edinburgh, 3 September 1931, 26 and 29 November 1931, 17 December 1931.

133   *Ibid.*, 29 April 1931, 28 November 1931.
134   *Ibid.*, 11 September 1936.
135   Department of Health for Scotland, *Committee on Scottish Health Services report*, Cmd 5204 (Edinburgh, 1936); LHSA, LHB 1/18/2, Minutes of meetings of the League of Subscribers to the Royal Infirmary of Edinburgh, 25 November 1936.
136   LHSA, LHB 1/18/2, Minutes of meetings of the League of Subscribers to the Royal Infirmary of Edinburgh, 25 November 1936.
137   TWAS, HO/RVI/2/54, Royal Victoria Infirmary, Minute book house com. no. 12, 6 March, 27 March, 5 June 1930.
138   *Ibid.*, 5 March 1931.
139   TWAS, HO/RVI/60, Royal Victoria Infirmary, Minute book: workmen governors' annual meetings, 21 March 1931.
140   TWAS, HO/RVI/2/54, Royal Victoria Infirmary, Minute book house com. no. 12, 4 December 1930, 16 February 1932; TWAS, HO/RVI/60, Royal Victoria Infirmary, Minute book: workmen governors' annual meetings, 12 March 1932.
141   TWAS, HO/RVI/34, Royal Victoria Infirmary, Minute book: workmen governors' annual meetings, 7 and 14 March 1942, 6 March 1943.
142   TWAS, *Proceedings of the Newcastle Council*, 5 March 1930.
143   TWAS, HO/SRI/3/6, Sunderland Royal Infirmary, Workmen's governors minute book, 4 October 1930, 10 October 1931.
144   *Ibid.*, 11 April 1931.
145   *Ibid.*, 6 February 1943, 13 March 1943, 22 January 1944.
146   B. Supple, *The history of the British coal industry. Volume 4, 1913–1946: the political economy of decline* (Oxford, 1987), pp. 445–53, quote on p. 445.
147   TWAS, HO/SRI/3/6, Sunderland Royal Infirmary, Workmen's governors minute book, 22 January 1944, 22 April 1944, 21 July 1945, 20 October 1945, 19 January 1946.
148   J. Pickstone, 'Production, community and consumption: the political economy of twentieth-century medicine', in R. Cooter and J. Pickstone (eds), *Medicine in the twentieth century* (Amsterdam, 2000), pp. 1–19.

Chapter 7

The 'impending cataclysm': the state and hospital contribution, 1941–46

The National Health Service Acts of 1946 and 1947 were a watershed for the contributory schemes, as they were for the rest of the British health system.[1] They appeared to signal the end of the mixed economy of health care in Britain, which had combined private, voluntary and public financing. In its place they instituted a health service funded by direct taxation and nominally universal, comprehensive and free at the point of use.[2] The voluntary hospitals were nationalised and brought under the administrative aegis of appointed regional boards, alongside municipal institutions. Their assets were also taken over by the state, though teaching hospitals in England and Wales were permitted to retain control of their endowments.[3] Bereft of their financial *raison d'être*, many contributory schemes folded, while the remainder began to transform themselves into non-profit insurance associations, providing additional health benefits for subscribers who wished to continue.

Why was the policy option of retaining voluntary sector social insurance discarded in the planning of the new health service? Histories of the coming of the NHS have detailed the ministerial and bureaucratic deliberations, and the lobbying activities of the BMA and the voluntary hospitals' BHA. However, little is known of the contributory schemes' role in this policy process. Abel-Smith cursorily dismisses them by noting that:

> With the possible exception of the HSA, the pre-payment agencies ... were unbusinesslike, ineffectively co-ordinated and run by persons without power or influence. They were swept into the background without antagonising any important section of opinion.[4]

Webster alludes briefly to government consideration of the schemes' reten-tion, before suggesting that this option had been dropped by 1943, once the Scottish Hetherington committee firmly rejected voluntary contribution as a basis for hospital funding in Scotland (see below).[5] Honigsbaum charts the discussions between 1941 and 1943 in which the twin pressures of Treasury parsimony and voluntary sector lobbying kept alive the possibility of contribu-tory payment for hospital care; he detects a vein of hostility towards voluntary hospitals and the schemes among some civil servants.[6] However, these accounts neglect the responses of the schemes themselves to these developments and the lobbying efforts of the BHCSA. The memoir of the civil servant John Pater also overlooks their significance, summarily recording their representations as an occasional adjunct to those of the BHA.[7] Beyond this, accounts of pressure group influence have focused particularly on the BMA, and to a lesser extent the BHA and representatives of local government.[8]

Can Abel-Smith's stress on amateurism and lack of coordination adequately explain the schemes' failure to assert their position before the 'impending cataclysm' of a state health service?[9] After all, they had some 10 million members and provided a major channel for public involvement in hospital affairs.[10] Moreover, official willingness to consider contributory funding within a voluntary framework was expressed in several major policy initiatives between 1941 and 1944. To address this question, this chapter charts the development of the official policy towards the idea of voluntary contribution within the health service. The next chapter turns to the schemes' response.

Planning before 1941

Pressure for some form of health service reform had been growing through the 1930s, driven by two key problems.[11] The first was finance, for, notwithstanding the sums flowing into voluntary hospital coffers from the schemes, many institutions found it increasingly hard to balance their books.[12] Expenditure rose inexorably as a consequence of expansion of hospital capacity, technological advance and increases in staff costs.[13] Conversely, traditional charitable sources of income had ceased to grow in real terms, so that by the late 1930s many institutions were experiencing deficits in their annual maintenance accounts.[14] The second problem was the long-standing lack coordination between the different elements of the health service. The Dawson report of 1920 had suggested the hierarchical integration of primary, secondary and tertiary care,[15] while the Cave committee in 1921 had advocated formal cooperation between the voluntary hospitals (see chapter 2). However, real momentum for integration came only in 1929, when the Local Government Acts broke up the poor law and initiated the process of municipal 'appropriation' of public assistance institutions for use as general hospitals.[16] The legislation also called for joint consultative committees of local authority and voluntary hospital interests (on the model of the hospitals councils), although the establishment of these boards was patchy and not all were effective.[17]

Policy proposals to address these concerns emanated first from non-governmental organisations. The BHA-sponsored Sankey report made specific proposals for regional structures in which the voluntary sector dominated, with a central council to oversee the different hospital regions.[18] The aim was to develop joint working in areas such as the ambulance, almoner and blood transfusion services, to achieve administrative uniformity of patient and financial records, and to rationalise fundraising and the purchase of supplies.[19] Sankey envisaged contributory schemes reorganising themselves within this framework, with a scheme committee coordinating funds in each hospital region. National maximum income limits were to be adhered to, and reciprocal arrangements between schemes were to be attained through the standardisation of contribution and benefits.[20] This was broadly in line with the aims of the BHCSA leadership (see chapter 4), which also advocated reciprocal agreements and regional groupings, though only where 'this was the outcome of spontaneous local action'.[21]

Another influential voice was Political and Economic Planning (PEP), a right-of-centre group dedicated to 'capitalist planning'.[22] Its 1937 report on Britain's health services won a popular readership, with 25,000 copies in paperback, and is indicative of the broadening base of support for an organised system.[23] The sections on contributory schemes acknowledged their scope but cast doubt on their claims to represent a grassroots mobilisation in favour of voluntary provision. In comparison to NHI, with its state and employers' contributions, the schemes represented 'a regular drain on the weekly income of ... the lower income groups'.[24] Nor had they been 'thrust up from below by the spontaneous enthusiasm of a group', but rather were 'created by official initiative from above ... in order to fill a gap which government does not find it expedient to occupy'. The schemes were in fact 'service organisations for limited purposes ... it is not apparent that much interest is taken in their affairs, or much control exercised by any except the paid officials'.[25] Though not calling outright for the dissolution of the schemes, the report hinted strongly that hospital benefits should be consolidated within NHI, or provided through 'compulsory contributory schemes' with a flat-rate charge covering all workers and dependants.[26]

Further left on the political spectrum, the prospect of a full state medical service financed by taxation was more firmly advocated. Of particular significance was the Socialist Medical Association (SMA), which shaped the health programme on which the Labour Party fought the 1945 election.[27] The SMA was a pressure group dominated by radical doctors such as Somerville Hastings and David Stark Murray, and had exerted influence over the London County Council's health policies in the 1930s.[28] It conceived of health as a right of citizenship and consequently supported a free, unified health service funded by general taxation, in which doctors were salaried employees. Administration would be in the hands of local government and thus democratically accountable.[29] Contributory schemes were symptomatic of the makeshift, wasteful and fragmented nature of the existing system and a manifestation of popular aversion to means testing.[30] Dislike of the 'capricious and diminishing assistance' of the voluntary sector also pervaded SMA thinking, which held that 'cherished traditions' would have to be 'scrapped without pity' in the interests of 'equality of opportunity to the means of health'.[31] The Labour Party itself had first flirted with the idea of nationalising the voluntary hospitals in 1909. By the mid-1920s it was struggling for a consistent policy, with some members supporting the extension of NHI to cover institutional care (the option favoured by the trade union movement) and others advocating the voluntary hospitals' gradual merger into the municipal system.[32] Gradualism remained the keynote of the mid-1930s, when the party approved a staged progression towards a 'unified and comprehensive service' run by local government, in which the voluntaries would be taken over 'by agreement'.[33]

Brown's statement and policy discussions, 1941–42

The government formally signalled its intention to reform the post-war health service on 9 October 1941, in a parliamentary statement by the Minister of Health, Ernest Brown. A 'comprehensive hospital service ... available to every person in need of it' would be established, administered in partnership by local authorities and voluntary hospitals. It would not be free, however, and patients would be expected to meet the costs of their care, 'either through contributory schemes or otherwise'.[34] However, although this implied that the schemes would be integral to the reformed system, the announcement did not reflect a well considered policy position. Instead it was largely a response to proposals from a non-governmental body, the NPHT, for regionalisation organised around the catchment areas of the voluntary hospitals. This had antagonised the local authorities, which had pressed Brown to reassert his commitment to 'the democratic and local government element in hospital administration'.[35] Brown's limited consultations did not include representatives of the schemes, and the subsequent Commons debates revealed no consensus as to their role. Brown praised the 'welcome and increased' work of the schemes in his rebuttal of Aneurin Bevan's charge that voluntary fundraising offended 'civilised notions of organised society'.[36] The left railed against the 'snobbishness' of the teaching hospitals and asserted that 'indiscriminate charity' should now give way to community provision and state ownership, while moderate opinion endorsed the statement's implied support for the existing income mix.[37] Hector McNeil MP (Labour, Greenock) pointed out the wasteful transaction costs of hospital charges ('a method of keeping chartered accountants in business') and advocated the extension of NHI to cover institutional care. To him, the schemes' success indicated working-class willingness to pay, not an attachment to voluntarism.[38] Only Samuel Storey MP (Conservative, Sunderland) offered a clear defence of the contributory schemes, in arguing that they ensured efficiency and responsiveness on the part of hospital administrators and guaranteed democratic control through workers' representation.[39]

The lack of a firm policy line reflected uncertainty within the Ministry of Health. Furthermore, the Treasury was anxious that the burden of voluntary hospital finance should not fall on the state, but also entertained doubts about the sector's future. Early official discussions envisaged a post-war system based on some form of contributory insurance, but with admission to hospital based solely on medical need. Incorporation of hospital benefit into NHI was thought impractical, not least because, as one official put it, 'you can't compel people to insure for hospital treatment unless and until you can guarantee the beds'. Thus attention focused on creating a 'really effective system' of recovery of charges from the contributory schemes.[40] An early assessment of the schemes' role had been made before Brown's statement, by Sir John Maude, the Permanent

Secretary to the Minister of Health, and Sir Laurence Brock.[41] As the one-time secretary of the Cave committee, Brock was an authority on voluntary hospitals and doubted that they could now survive without public money. He was also sceptical of creating regional voluntary hospital authorities, since his experience as chairman of the Board of Control of mental health services persuaded him that a good local authority was more efficient.[42] Brock's advice, building on the whole thrust of inter-war policy, was therefore to extend still further the role of local government, and this posed awkward questions about the schemes:

> [If the Minister were to place] a duty on the local authority to provide a complete hospital system it is not clear on what ground a limited section of the community can reasonably be asked to tax themselves to meet the cost of a service which would otherwise fall on the rates and which would be more equitably distributed if it did so fall.[43]

These problems were developed further in a briefing paper on contributory schemes by Ministry of Health official John Pater, in which he detailed the movement's lack of uniformity.[44] Alert to the ongoing rift within the BHCSA, he pointed up the division between those schemes which emphasised members' benefits, on a quasi-insurance model, and those which maintained their primary purpose to be fundraising for designated hospitals. Beyond this he noted the diversity of benefits offered, such as convalescence services (to which 55 per cent of members had access), ambulances (35 per cent), ophthalmic treatment (45 per cent), nursing services (25 per cent) and dental care (35 per cent).[45] Pater also observed that only about 37 per cent of contributors were in schemes which observed the BMA's recommended income limits, which anyway were not seriously policed. Variations also obtained with respect to methods of collection, waiting periods for the receipt of benefits and rates of reimbursement to municipal hospitals. He concluded that, given their scale, policy-makers would have to take 'some account' of the schemes, but that major reforms were needed to achieve uniformity. Discussions held by Maude within the Ministry of Health arrived at a more relaxed view, that uniformity would be necessary in two areas only: inter-availability (scheme benefits should be payable at any hospital within a given region) and reciprocity (identical benefit rates should obtain for a region's voluntary and municipal institutions).[46]

Maude also received an upbeat assessment of the practicalities of retaining the schemes from representatives of the voluntary sector, including Ernest Pooley, honorary secretary of the King's Fund, William Hyde and William Goodenough of the NPHT, and T. W. Place, honorary secretary of the BHCSA. Hyde argued that contributory schemes were the optimum method of charging for hospital services: assessment by almoners was difficult and the sums elicited usually less than the real cost, while an extension of NHI would shift costs to employers and the Treasury.[47] Hyde proposed that schemes be required to obtain statutory 'approval' (as with friendly societies operating the NHI scheme), conditional upon standardising income limits, rates, coverage and hospitals reimbursements.[48] Place suggested that the schemes would accept such standardisation and statutory approval if they were made the main agents of voluntary hospital funding, through which Treasury subventions were channelled. He also appealed to sentiment: 'it would be an ungracious act to overlook the national value of the Voluntary Service of tens of thousands of men and women'.[49] Goodenough also favoured directing state grants through the schemes, so that money 'would "follow the patient"' and thus ensure hospital developments were responsive to demand.[50] Several problems were unresolved, however. Would state approval make scheme membership universal in the absence of compulsion?[51] Unless membership *was* compulsory, free-riders would remain in the system, either burdening hospital authorities with the need to chase payments or burdening insurers by taking out policies only when hospital treatment was imminent.[52] And should the state intervene to such a degree? Maude, who regarded the schemes as the 'sheet anchor' of the voluntary system, worried that excessive standardisation of these pluralist associations would be 'a straight-waistcoat' which 'might well squeeze the life out of them'.[53]

In sum, preliminary discussions inclined towards retaining the status quo, though civil servants realised the difficulty of incorporating the movement into a comprehensive national service. In late 1942 Ernest Brown made an appeal at a speech to the King's Fund for the 'better correlation' of the activities of the contributory schemes, signalling that this would ensure them a place in future plans.[54] However, by this time a new momentum for change had developed as a result of the Beveridge report.

The Beveridge report and the 'hotel charge' debate, 1942–44

Sir William Beveridge's *Social insurance and allied services* is widely regarded as the blueprint for the post-war welfare state.[55] Its principal concern was social insurance and it referred to health planning only briefly, in 'Assumption B', which envisaged a 'national health service for prevention and for cure of disease' as a concomitant of social security reform.[56] Though he believed this should include institutional care, Beveridge offered no firm proposals on the relative roles of voluntary and public hospitals, or on the continuation of contributory schemes. Instead, he set out a choice between funding the system by extending NHI contributions, which would undermine voluntary hospitals' finances, or maintaining the current approach, with the risk that citizens not covered by schemes might delay their hospital treatment.[57] He noted the schemes' recent growth, citing the widely accepted estimate that they covered 10 million people, and claimed that they raised some £6,500,000 per annum.[58] He was also optimistic about the trend towards standardisation, noting that 'contribution to a [*sic*] Hospital Saving Association' in London entitled members to enter both voluntary and public hospitals. However, he felt the scale of the movement indicated only a widespread willingness to make such contributions, not the inherent worth of this mechanism.[59] Significantly, the sections which discussed the continuing scope for voluntary insurance within the new social security system made no mention of the contributory schemes, and focused instead on trade unions, friendly societies and voluntary sector superannuation and life insurance schemes.[60]

Beveridge had left open a place for contributory schemes in the new health service but he was highly ambivalent about their value. What was the thinking that informed his position? His correspondence with Maude suggests he regarded the schemes' popularity as indicative of a general readiness to countenance an extension of compulsory contributions.[61] This perspective echoes the conclusion to the PEP report, in which the 'astonishing sums' raised by 'working class contributory power' were cited in support of consolidating other benefits within NHI.[62] In other words, the authors of both reports felt the growth of the movement indicated first and foremost a willingness to pay, not an attachment to voluntarism. Beveridge later made explicit his debt to PEP as a source of information and, as did its report, he depicted the contributory movement as having arisen to 'fill the gap in the provision for medical treatment under the National Insurance Act'.[63] As with the friendly societies, Beveridge heaped praise on the voluntary sector for pioneering new forms of social action, but at the same time he regarded the schemes as a temporary expedient in the forward march of social insurance.[64]

The movement itself failed to present Beveridge with an alternative view. A BHCSA deputation of Bertram Ford and Sydney Lamb had met with him in July 1942, though their evidence appears to have been considered marginal: it was not included in the published memoranda of the Beveridge report; nor does the BHCSA appear in the appendix listing individuals and organisations submitting evidence.[65] By contrast, several organisations which favoured the extension of NHI to include hospital benefit were given prominence. Thus the deputation from the Trades Union Congress derided the 'frantic endeavours' of 'money-raising schemes such as the Hospital Savings [*sic*] Association' to sustain expansion and modernisation of hospital care.[66] Similarly, the National Labour Organisation urged the integration into NHI of voluntary insurance schemes which 'supplement the State system', while the National Conference of Friendly Societies wanted NHI to cover medical attendance in hospital outpatient departments.[67] More pertinently, the Nuffield Social Reconstruction Surveyors, led by G. D. H. Cole, were questioned by Beveridge on popular attitudes towards the contributory principle; they argued that while people valued the entitlement which scheme membership conferred, there was little positive support for organising medical services on a contributory basis.[68]

With the Beveridge report launched to popular acclaim, the pressure was now on the Ministry of Health to bring forward concrete proposals and on the schemes to achieve uniformity in the areas Maude had identified.[69] Government statements in the Commons were encouraging. Sir John Anderson, the Chancellor of the Exchequer, envisaged a new health service in which voluntary and public organisations cooperated and where 'there would be no doctrinaire scrapping of good existing resources'.[70] Herbert Morrison also made emollient comments about the preservation of the voluntary hospitals, and noted the importance of voluntary public service to the health of British democracy.[71]

Behind the scenes, however, civil servants were starting to have serious doubts about the administrative and financial viability of voluntary contribution. Armed with Beveridge's alternative vision, of merging hospital insurance into a single social security contribution, Pater, along with Niven McNicholl of the Scottish Office, now argued forcefully in favour of abandoning the schemes.[72] They reiterated the importance of uniformity among the schemes, over and above Maude's prerequisites of inter-availability and reciprocity. If government wanted to preserve the current system, it had two choices. Either it could make the schemes uniform and compulsory, in which case there would be two parallel national insurance systems, an 'odd arrangement' which employers would not relish. Or it could introduce an organised system of charging and leave patients free to choose which of the schemes they wished to join; this undermined the principle of free access and added the risk that charging would deter early treatment. On balance they argued that reform of the schemes 'would be a troublesome process' and guessed that including hospital insurance within a single social security contribution would 'appeal to most people as the sensible course'. They then provided estimates showing that the sums hospitals could expect to receive as their share of the social insurance budget would be virtually identical to that raised by the schemes.[73] Crucially, Pater and McNicholl challenged the idea that the popularity of mass contribution meant that it had to be accommodated in the reform. Instead they claimed:

> there is little or no sentiment surrounding membership of most of the schemes, the workers regard them as a ready way of insuring against the contingency of having to go into hospital and of avoiding inquiry into means which non-membership would involve. Many workers speak of them as 'a bit of a nuisance' – but a tolerable nuisance in default of a better organisation of hospital service.[74]

Here was the first clear indication of Ministry scepticism that the schemes were a manifestation of active citizenship.

Detailed consultations on the future of hospital financing began in 1943, with the Ministry initially proposing to retain the schemes in a reconfigured funding mix that would combine charity, subventions from the rates and (following Beveridge) a unit grant from the national insurance fund to cover the costs of care. The schemes' role would be to insure against 'maintenance charges', effectively the 'hotel' costs of hospitalisation.[75] This notion of a hotel charge derived from the Beveridge report's observation that, since the social insurance scheme would pay a disability benefit to persons unable to work owing to illness, that benefit ought, in cases of hospitalisation, to go to the institution, notionally to cover costs of food and fuel.[76] Beveridge himself considered this a 'minor question' and there is no reason to suppose hotel expenses were suggested as a lifeline for the schemes. None the less, discussions were held in the first half of 1943 between Maude and the BHCSA on how they might cover contributors for the hotel charge. At a meeting in August Ernest Brown reassured BHCSA leaders that the schemes would have a place in the NHS, though he was careful to declare his remarks non-committal and unofficial.[77]

Events now moved out of Maude's hands, as the plans for the health service were debated by the Cabinet Reconstruction Priorities Committee.[78] Others have shown how the Committee came to reject the idea of hotel charges, and with them a continuing role for the contributory schemes.[79] Doubt had first been cast on Maude's plans by the Hetherington committee, which reported in August 1943 on the future of the hospital service in Scotland. Hetherington argued emphatically against the use of contributory schemes to collect patients' charges, on several grounds. First, Scottish voluntary hospitals did not apply means testing on admission.[80] Scottish contributory schemes therefore lacked the quasi-insurance character of their southern counterparts and had no experience of reciprocal payment to municipal hospitals. Hetherington's medical witnesses had argued that the abrupt introduction of hotel charges would have 'adverse psychological effects' and deter the poor from early hospitalisation.[81] Second, there were serious obstacles to using the schemes to collect insurance contributions. Membership was concentrated in the urban centres and even then was far from universal, and it would be difficult to collect in remote areas.[82] Strikingly, Hetherington's private papers suggest his guiding assumption was that 'an all-in contributory insurance system' was the way forward, and more positive evidence from the schemes and hospitals failed to influence his report.[83]

Thus persuaded of the case for free maintenance funded by the social insurance contribution, the Secretary of State for Scotland, Tom Johnston, stood out against the hotel charge when Brown put it before the Reconstruction Committee.[84] The two ministers were charged with preparing a paper on voluntary hospital finance, and this undermined Brown's position, as the paper confirmed the much smaller role of contributory scheme finance in Scotland.[85] Moreover, hospital administrators welcomed the Hetherington proposals because they had doubts about maintenance charges, seeing them as a device designed solely to force people into contributory schemes.[86] In January 1944 the Reconstruction Committee decided that the hotel charge was 'illogical' given the aspiration to provide a comprehensive service and, anyway, 'individual payments would become more and more an anachronism'. It duly restricted the hotel charge to the marginal role Beveridge had originally outlined, as applying only to those in receipt of disability benefit.[87] There were concerns about the likely reaction of the voluntary hospitals – Goodenough had previously made dire predictions of the demise of the voluntary hospitals without the democratic element which the schemes provided and further discussions took place with hospital representatives.[88] At these, the hospitals conceded the dropping of the maintenance charge, provided government made it clear that a funding gap remained to be filled from voluntary sources, though concern was expressed about those provincial hospitals that were without a significant charitable base.[89] The chairman of the Reconstruction Committee, Lord Woolton, was convinced that the voluntary hospitals were crying wolf, using fear to stimulate charitable donations, and that they should move their appeal for charity 'to a higher plane'. Accordingly, the subsequent White Paper, published in February 1944, made no mention of maintenance charges.[90]

Webster argues that party politics underpinned the divisions over this issue, with Johnston supported by his Labour colleague Ernest Bevin, who felt that 'the industrial contributory scheme caused a great deal of work and some friction'.[91] The left was particularly hostile to the means testing implicit in hospital charges, and presumably Labour members viewed the mix of social insurance and rate funding as more redistributive than voluntary schemes, in which employers' contributions were variable and unsystematic.[92] Some horse-trading may also have been involved over the final shape of the White Paper: Labour had already yielded ground on its plans for a full-time salaried general practitioner service, so the concession on voluntary hospitals was perhaps a *quid pro quo*.[93] Beyond this, two other, non-party figures were crucial, the Chancellor of the Exchequer, Anderson, who had supported Johnston and Bevin, and Lord Woolton. Probably cost containment and administrative tidiness were the determining influences on these men. The Treasury was concerned to avoid fee-for-service insurance in general practice, and endorsed a fully salaried service as the best means of ensuring costs were restrained and predictable.[94] In the hospitals, too, reliance on contributory scheme insurance would introduce a large element of unpredictability: the schemes were not universal and there was no immediate prospect of their achieving uniformity. And placing the duty of recovering hotel expenses onto the hospitals added a further transaction cost, which the hospitals themselves did not want, where the record of recovery from uninsured patients was already poor, and which in Scotland was likely to 'raise a storm of protest'.[95]

The NHS White Paper, 1944

Honigsbaum argues that the rejection of the hotel charge in January 1944 dealt a 'death-blow' to the schemes.[96] The 1944 White Paper made no specific mention of them and from then on the Ministry abandoned attempts to integrate them into the NHS.[97] Officials were also discouraging: 'we can't see any rosy prospects ... [and] don't want to mislead with promises'.[98] However, there is a certain amount of hindsight in the judgement that all was now lost. Policy remained in flux as the new Minister of Health, Henry Willink, undermined the White Paper's authority by emphasising its role as a provisional proposal rather than a statement of intent. A phase of 'infinite regress' ensued, in which different parties exacted various concessions.[99]

The White Paper's proposals for hospital finance left some room for the schemes to operate, but now solely as a channel for voluntary support.[100] Two main sources of voluntary hospital income were proposed. First, the voluntary hospitals would contract to provide services with the new joint authorities that were to oversee institutional care. These authorities were to be combinations of county and borough councils, and the funding to pay for hospital services would come from local rates supplemented by Exchequer grants. In addition, there would be a direct grant to the voluntary hospitals from the national insurance fund, and this was explicitly intended to replace the existing contributory scheme component. Crucially, the joint authority element 'was not to be assessed as a total reimbursement of costs incurred'.[101] This left an unspecified element of the hospital budget to be filled from voluntary sources, and it was here, by implication, that an attenuated role for the schemes would be found. It was emphasised strongly that government wanted voluntary hospitals to retain their autonomy and that this could be achieved only if they were able to draw on 'personal benefactions and the continuing support of those who believe in the … movement'. Effectively, government was challenging the voluntary sector to make good its claims to embody a genuine reservoir of public support. If the reality was that this support was based on pragmatism rather than benevolence, then the schemes, and with them the voluntary hospitals, would perish.[102]

Willink clarified all this to Parliament, stressing his own conviction that the schemes were certain to continue under the new arrangement, albeit in a different form. Since today's 'contributors were not merely paying an insurance premium but were paying to maintain a system in which they believed', then surely they would continue to make an additional voluntary contribution, even when the state met the cost of their hospital care?[103] The Ministry's parliamentary secretary, Florence Horsburgh (Conservative, Dundee), gave the proposals a different spin, justifying the demise of the schemes in terms of the administrative efficiency of unifying all social insurance contributions. However, this was not so much an 'end' to mass contribution as the government using taxation to make 'universal and compulsory' a system which the voluntary sector had begun.[104] As to why anyone should wish to continue contributing after the proposed reform, Horsburgh was evasive, particularly when challenged by Leslie Haden Guest (Labour, Islington North) to confirm that the government envisaged the future schemes offering provident insurance for private patients. However, she expected that both mass contribution and philanthropy would continue, that the voluntary hospitals' independence would be maintained and that the schemes would still provide an outlet for voluntary public service.[105] In the Lords debate Woolton took a similar line: he emphasised that 'we shall not pay out of public funds the whole cost of the services' and trusted that contributors' 'pleasure and pride' in 'beneficent work' would maintain voluntarism.[106]

The proposition that voluntary contribution could continue once state funding was in place met with incredulity from most MPs. Dr Frank Howitt (Unionist, Reading) frankly asserted that the 'contributory scheme is dead', while Sir Arnold Gridley (Unionist, Stockport) derided the government's claim that voluntary contributions would survive: the White Paper paid them only 'lip service' while sounding the hospitals' 'death knell'.[107] Others regretted the schemes' passing, believing that they represented public 'interest' in the hospital service and that there was a moral value in the 'pride' they instilled. However, such eulogies led only to unspecific pleas that the Minister 'preserve that spirit in some way or other'.[108] Beyond this, Parliament appeared to accept the dropping of the hotel charge, though two calls were made for the schemes' continuation as separate, earmarked funds within the national insurance arrangements.[109] Again, though, these were extremely vague and made in the context of general concern with the preservation of the voluntary hospitals' separate status. None of this prompted officials to reconsider their view of the hotel charge as 'impracticable as well as indefensible'.[110]

Indeed, MPs who spoke on hospital contribution did not make a positive appeal based on the virtues of non-profit insurance, but yoked the fate of the schemes to broader issues of finance and control. The Sunderland MP, Storey, suspected that the putative gap between the cost of services and income from contracting authorities was a ruse to ensure financial shortfalls, which would ultimately force voluntary institutions into state service. But rather than proposing the preservation of a separate insurance component, he advocated more substantial state reimbursement.[111] A Scottish MP voiced similar concern about the gap in revenue, before proposing a centrally distributed block grant that would provide all voluntary hospital income, modelled on that made by the University Grants Committee.[112] The other great concern was that voluntary hospitals should remain outside local authority control. For example, Howitt urged that, in recognition of the schemes' tradition of public service, the voluntary hospitals be allowed greater representation in the proposed Local Health Service Councils.[113] Percy Jewson (Liberal National, Great Yarmouth) also regretted the threat to the schemes' 'very valuable piece of social work' and warned that some members of voluntary hospital boards 'are not suited, temperamentally … to what we commonly call political life' and would therefore be lost to public service.[114]

Parliamentarians did not identify the schemes with the interests of the labour movement. Only John Craik Henderson (Conservative, Leeds North-East) gestured towards this when he extolled the efforts of 'workers' committees and … working men and women on the committees'. Again, the context was an appeal that regional hospital management should not be dominated by local authorities.[115] Labour MPs, meanwhile, welcomed the freeing of the hospitals from the 'undignified' business of fundraising.[116] They regarded the panegyrics for voluntary service as veiled attempts to preserve the 'pomp and circumstance' and 'sheer snobbery' of hospital governorship; there was, after all, plenty of opportunity for public service in trade unions or in local government.[117] More pointedly, Fred Messer (Labour, South Tottenham) welcomed the end of the 'humiliating … inquisition' by almoners and saluted the 'equal distribution of liability' which the new arrangements promised.[118]

The debates on the White Paper therefore saw the voluntary hospitals' supporters alluding to the schemes principally in the context of more general appeals for concessions and a similar approach was taken in the next round of Whitehall consultations with the representatives of voluntary hospitals. The NPHT accepted the demise of the hotel charges plan as a *fait accompli*, but argued that the u-turn on the schemes had implications for the scale of state aid which the hospitals would now require.[119] Once public funding began, voluntary income would 'eventually fail' to plug the financial gap and this had implications for the calculation of state subventions.[120]

Memoranda from organisations such as the NPHT, the BHA and the King's Fund therefore concentrated on protecting the finances of voluntary hospitals, and argued that Exchequer grants based on a notional loss of income from the contributory schemes would prove inadequate to post-war needs, that capital funds should not come through the local authorities, as this would lead to their 'domination', and that voluntary hospitals should be allowed to retain their invested funds in order to give them scope for autonomous development.[121] The BHA's representatives did, however, offer one lifeline to the contributory schemes. They made the suggestion that individuals should have the right 'to contract out of purchasing the health portion of the stamp' and choose to support a voluntary scheme instead.[122] However, their memorandum did not elaborate on the mechanics of this idea, such as how a service run on this basis would avoid free-riders or facilitate planning, and the BHA did not pursue it in face-to-face meetings with the Minister.

Thus, the priorities for the representatives of the voluntary hospitals during 1944 were to avoid local authority control and to improve the state grants, not to rescue the contributory schemes. The BHA deputation made only a general appeal for their retention, on the grounds of the 'financial stability' they conferred on hospitals and the civic engagement in management which they encouraged.[123] Willink was unmoved by this and emphasised that they 'must accept as settled Government policy' that the national insurance fund would now cover hospital risks. He then reiterated his challenge: 'Unless the claim of the hospitals that they enjoy widespread public support for the voluntary system was unfounded – which he did not believe – they had a solid ground for appealing for funds to retain their voluntary status'.[124] He also gave assurances that the arrangements for state funding did guarantee stability of finance: the Exchequer grant would increase if voluntary funding fell, and charges would be at fixed rates, not subject to the whim of local authorities.[125]

There were several reasons why the Ministry of Health made no concessions on the dropping of the hotel charge. First, the hospitals had sent contradictory signals. The BHA had initially raised no objection, and had even claimed that it had enunciated the '100 per cent principle' for the service before Beveridge.[126] Second, civil servants had understood from earlier BHA statements that hospitals welcomed the idea of a 'gap' between their total expenditure and the various state payments, precisely because this gave a rationale for ongoing voluntary support.[127] Third, the movement's supporters had sent mixed messages: some argued that a 'free' service would remove the incentive to give, while others asserted that contributors were motivated primarily by belief 'in the voluntary principle'. Civil servants also noted some support for this view in the parliamentary debates, where Storey had claimed that mass subscription could continue, provided the 'workmen' were still allowed to play a part in hospital management.[128] More generally, it seemed clear that as long as the voluntary hospitals received assurances about the adequacy of the state funding, they would not press for the retention of the schemes. They were far more determined to gain concessions on the question of administrative structure and the unwelcome prospect of local authority control.[129] It was on this issue that Willink relented, by allowing voluntary hospital representation on the joint authorities, which now were to have only planning rather than administrative functions – these would remain with hospital governors.[130] In addition, there was also to be a tier of regional councils and hospital planning groups, on which the ratio of voluntary sector to municipal representatives was more favourable.[131]

By the end of the war, then, official policy envisaged a health service which would retain the contributory schemes, albeit in a drastically reduced role. Although their main function would be gone, they would still offer additional benefits, such as convalescence care and ambulance fleets, and they would supplement national and local tax-funding of the voluntary hospitals. In doing so, they would play a crucial role in perpetuating the existence of a voluntary sector in health care.

The NHS Act 1946 and the exclusion of the schemes

Labour's landslide victory in 1945 brought the appointment of Aneurin Bevan as Minister for Health, whose strategy was to move decisively and rapidly to publish a Bill, with a minimum of consultation.[132] Despairing of the intransigence of the various interested parties, Bevan's radical solution was the nationalisation of the voluntary hospitals, which would receive state rather than local authority financing and be administered by unelected hospital management committees (HMCs), subject to centrally appointed regional hospital boards (RHBs).[133] Consultants were partly appeased by gaining payment for their services and the teaching hospitals retained much of their independence; local government objections were disregarded.[134] Historians have generally interpreted this solution as a masterly piece of political pragmatism, motivated partly by the desire to bring forward the legislation alongside the social security reforms.[135] By antagonising and rewarding the interested parties in roughly equal measure, Bevan's uneasy consensus carried the Bill through Parliament. As to who originated the idea of nationalisation, John Hawton, the civil servant who drafted the 1944 White Paper, is one of several likely candidates.[136] Another key influence was the publication in 1945 of the NPHT's hospital surveys, which provided the intellectual justification and geographical basis for regional unification organised around the major teaching hospitals.[137]

Was the nationalisation of the voluntary hospitals, and the consequent demise of the contributory schemes, determined by Bevan's ideological position? In Cabinet he argued that public control should follow public money.[138] Civil servants' estimates suggested that under the Willink proposals between 80 and 90 per cent of the income of voluntary hospitals would come from central funds.[139] Thus it was the logic of democratic politics and Treasury prudence which suggested full ministerial responsibility. The left's preferred course, of local authority control and the gradual disappearance of the voluntaries, was rejected, to the consternation of the SMA's leaders.[140] This is not to say that Bevan did not share the long-standing socialist antipathy towards philanthropy. Introducing the second reading of the NHS Bill he inveighed against voluntary hospitals' fundraising as 'repugnant to a civilised community' and castigated the 'caprice of private charity', which distributed public goods so irrationally.[141] However, he was motivated primarily by a technocratic conviction that a higher standard of medical care would be achieved in a planned system based on large hospital centres, rather than a host of well meaning but inefficient local institutions.[142]

The fate of the contributory schemes seems not to have been pressed on Bevan by his advisers. Their chief advocate at the Ministry, Maude, had now left his post, while key civil servants such as Pater and Hawton were veterans of the earlier debates and hardly likely to reverse the position established in the White Paper. An early briefing paper for the new Minister advised that mass contribution was set to 'largely cease', lending weight to Bevan's belief that public funding must be dominant.[143] The Nuffield surveys made only brief and critical mention of the schemes, in the context of the fragmentation of services and the lack of inter-availability agreements.[144]

In the absence of external policy advice, what was Bevan's personal view of mass contribution? This was undoubtedly coloured by his experience as a young political activist in the valleys of South Wales. Here he had sat on the Committee of the Tredegar Medical Aid Society, an idiosyncratic manifestation of working-class mutualism, in which steel workers, miners and white-collar workers paid into a club which provided full health cover for them and their families.[145] The Society subscribed to the local voluntary, Tredegar Park Cottage Hospital, whose hospital committee was dominated by the young Bevan's adversaries, the Tredegar Iron and Coal Company.[146] He had won a seat on this committee in a deliberate piece of left-wing entryism, and recalled his experience in the Commons in 1946:

> In the mining districts, in the textile districts, in the districts where there are heavy industries it is the industrial population who pay the weekly contributions for the maintenance of the hospitals. When I was a miner I used to find that situation when I was on the hospital committee. We had an annual meeting and a cordial vote of thanks was moved and passed with great enthusiasm to the managing director of the colliery company for his generosity towards the hospital; and when I looked at the balance sheet, I saw that 97 per cent of the revenues were provided by the miners' own contributions; but nobody passed a vote of thanks to the miners.[147]

Thus Bevan's reading of the relationship between contributors and hospital managers was not of harmonious working but rather as a site of class antagonism.

These remarks came in the second reading of the NHS Bill and their context is revealing. Bevan made them in a departure from the text of his speech, when an interruption reminded him that workers' contributions had been an important aspect of hospital funding. He digressed, to argue that it was 'a misuse of language' to call them 'voluntary hospitals', given their reliance on mass contribution from workers who were effectively obliged to pay into the schemes for fear of being charged if they were hospitalised.[148] Here again was the perspective articulated in the PEP report, in Beveridge's writing and in the Pater/McNicholl memorandum, which held that mass contribution was a pragmatic response to a gap in state provision rather than a manifestation of popular voluntarism. Bevan also ignored the schemes in his discussion of popular representation on RHBs and HMCs, when he argued instead that people with existing expertise, and particularly the medical profession, should dominate the new committees, in preference to 'any proposal which made the members delegates'.[149] Nor, when he announced the decision to continue with pay-beds for fee-paying patients, was there any mention of a desirable role for non-profit provident insurance; instead, private medicine within the NHS was justified as a necessary evil designed to ensure top consultants did not opt out of the service.[150] Finally, the Conservative defence of the voluntaries focused not on the schemes' fate but on the need to preserve the hospitals' charitable endowments. Bevan could deal easily with this by pointing to precedent, and he had, anyway, agreed that teaching hospitals in England and Wales would keep their endowments.[151] Otherwise, the opposition stance echoed its performance in 1944, with some hand-wringing for the loss of local pride and the 'spirit of service', but no concrete suggestions on how contributory schemes might be preserved.[152] Thus neither the advice which he received, nor the politics of the Bill's passage, nor his personal convictions, gave Bevan cause to consider the fate of the schemes in this final phase of preparation for the NHS.

Conclusion

At what point did the elimination of the contributory schemes from the structure of the NHS become inevitable? Despite Honigsbaum's verdict, it was only with Bevan's NHS Bill that the 'death-blow' was finally struck, though it is certainly possible that mass contribution would have quickly dried up if the arrangements proposed in the White Paper had gone ahead. Perhaps the precise date at which the schemes were abandoned by policy-makers is unimportant, given a widespread view that voluntary contribution was a transitory phenomenon which would ultimately be incorporated into some system of statutory funding. Even a conservative thinker like Lord Dawson could write that 'although contributory schemes are sound in idea and practice they are likely someday to evolve into a nation-wide scheme of comprehensive social insurance'.[153] In this reading, the schemes were always doomed, and once government and public had accepted Beveridge's plan for a comprehensive social security system the exact moment of their demise became academic.[154]

Or was it? The final shape of the NHS was not the outcome of an unproblematic consensus but a product of negotiation between the interested parties. Even at the final stage Bevan had set aside the Labour Party's blueprint in favour of a structure which accommodated some of the concerns of doctors and voluntary hospital leaders.[155] Thus we are bound to ask why the representatives of the contributory scheme movement proved incapable of asserting themselves in the same manner as other participants. After all, the environment in which they had to operate was by no means hostile. Whatever Beveridge's own view of the schemes, his report was scrupulous in preserving the option of separate, non-profit hospital insurance for the new service. And even if such an option was administratively complicated, it was hardly unthinkable, as the place of Blue Cross in the post-war North American health system demonstrates. Moreover, right up until the end of 1943 the schemes had the support of the Minister of Health and his department's top civil servant, as well as the backing of the BMA and the BHA. Why, then, were the representatives of the schemes, particularly the BHCSA leadership, unable to influence the policy process? To explore this more fully, the next chapter treats the coming of the NHS from the perspective of the schemes themselves.

Notes

1　C. Webster, *The health services since the war, vol. I* (London, 1988), pp. 94–107.
2　C. Webster, *The National Health Service: a political history* (Oxford, 1998, 2nd edn 2002), pp. 1–30.
3　B. Abel-Smith, *The hospitals 1800–1948: a study in social administration in England and Wales* (London, 1964), pp. 478–9.
4　Abel-Smith, *The hospitals*, p. 499.
5　Webster, *Health services since the war*, pp. 31, 36, 46–7.
6　F. Honigsbaum, *Health, happiness and security: the creation of the National Health Service* (London, 1989), pp. 157–60.
7　J. Pater, *The making of the National Health Service* (London, 1981), p. 58.
8　A. Willcocks, *The creation of the National Health Service: a study of pressure groups and a major social policy decision* (London, 1967); H. Eckstein, *The English health service* (Harvard, 1964), pp. 109–63; H. Eckstein, *Pressure group politics: the case of the British Medical Association* (London, 1960).
9　J. Dodd, 'Editor's preface', in G. Palliser *et al.*, *The charitable work of hospital contributory schemes* (Bristol, 1984), p. 9. Dodd was a leading official of one of the Bristol contributory schemes and after 1948 became secretary of the continuing schemes' national association; the quotation is from a retrospective analysis of the schemes' charitable activities, in which Dodd signalled his bitterness at the destruction of the pre-NHS movement.
10　PEP, *Report on the British health services* (London, 1937), p. 234.
11　Webster, *Health services since the war*, pp. 16–22.
12　M. Gorsky, J. Mohan and M. Powell, 'The financial health of voluntary hospitals in interwar Britain', *Economic History Review*, 55 (2002), pp. 533–57; M. Gorsky and J. Mohan, 'London's voluntary hospitals in the inter-war period: growth, transformation or crisis?', *Nonprofit and Voluntary Sector Quarterly*, 30 (2001), pp. 247–75.
13　B. Abel-Smith, *A history of the nursing profession* (London, 1960), ch. 9.
14　Gorsky, Mohan and Powell, 'Financial health', pp. 537–42.
15　Consultative Council on Medical and Allied Services, *Interim report on the future provision of medical and allied services*, Cmd 693 (London, 1920) (Dawson report); this was commissioned by the newly established Ministry of Health to advise on future development of the health services.
16　M. Powell, 'An expanding service: municipal acute medicine in the 1930s', *Twentieth Century British History*, 8 (1997), pp. 334–57.
17　Abel-Smith, *The hospitals*, pp. 380–2; J. Pickstone, *Medicine and industrial society* (Manchester, 1985), pp. 279–93; J. Mohan, *Planning, markets and hospitals* (London, 2002), ch. 3.
18　D. Fox, *Health policies, health politics: the British and American experience, 1911–1965* (Princeton, NJ, 1986), p. 58; Eckstein, *English health service*, pp. 111–12; Abel-Smith, *The hospitals*, pp. 412–15.

19 BHA, *Report of the voluntary hospitals commission* (London, 1937), pp. 22–5, 27–8.
20 *Ibid.*, pp. 33–4.
21 A. T. Page, *Pennies for health: the story of the British Hospitals Contributory Schemes Association* (Birmingham, 1949), pp. 13–14.
22 D. Ritschel, *The politics of planning* (Oxford, 1997), pp. 145, 152; A. Marwick, 'Middle opinion in the thirties: planning, progress and political agreement', *English Historical Review*, 79 (1964), pp. 285–98.
23 J. Pinder (ed.), *Fifty years of Political and Economic Planning: looking forward, 1931–1981* (London, 1981), pp. 27, 45, 148.
24 PEP, *Report on the British health services*, p. 237.
25 *Ibid.*, p. 399.
26 *Ibid.*, pp. 227, 410–11.
27 J. Stewart, *The battle for health: a political history of the Socialist Medical Association, 1930–51* (Aldershot, 1999).
28 J. Stewart, '"For a healthy London": the Socialist Medical Association and the London County Council in the 1930s', *Medical History*, 42 (1997), pp. 417–36.
29 J. Stewart, 'Ideology and process in the creation of the British National Health Service', *Journal of Policy History*, 14 (2002), pp. 113–34.
30 D. Stark Murray, *The future of medicine* (Harmondsworth, 1942), pp. 39–40, 86, 88.
31 A. Bourne, *Health of the future* (Harmondsworth, 1942), pp. 116–17.
32 A. Marwick, 'The Labour Party and the welfare state in Britain, 1900–1948', *American Historical Review*, 73 (1967–68), pp. 380–403, at pp. 389–91; R. Earwicker, 'The labour movement and the creation of the National Health Service 1906–1948', unpublished PhD thesis, University of Birmingham (1982), pp. 11–12, 106–7, 152–5, 176–83.
33 Marwick, 'The Labour Party', p. 396; Labour Party, *Report of the 34th annual conference held in the Garrick Theatre Southport October 1st to 5th, 1934* (London, n.d.), pp. 256–7.
34 *House of Commons Debates*, vol. 374, cols 1116–18, 9 October 1941.
35 TNA: PRO, MH 80/34, Post-war hospital policy, E. Brown, 14 October 1941; Webster, *Health services since the war*, pp. 31–2.
36 *House of Commons Debates*, vol. 374, col. 1119, 9 October 1941.
37 *House of Commons Debates*, vol. 374, cols 1668–9, 1678, 1685–6, 21 October 1941.
38 *House of Commons Debates*, vol. 379, col. 521, 21 April 1942.
39 *House of Commons Debates*, vol. 379, cols 528–30, 21 April 1942.
40 TNA: PRO, MH 77/25, Note for office committee, 24 January 1941; de Montmorency to Maude, 12 February 1941.
41 TNA: PRO, MH 77/25, Brock to Maude, 4 September 1941.
42 Honigsbaum, *Health, happiness and security*, pp. 25–6, 28.
43 TNA: PRO, MH 77/25, Brock to Maude, 4 September 1941.
44 TNA: PRO, MH 80/34, Voluntary hospital contributory and provident schemes, 19 December 1941. Pater played a key supporting role at the Ministry of Health throughout the planning for and subsequent implementation of the NHS, in the posts of principal (1938–43), assistant secretary (1943–45) and principal assistant secretary (1945–60).
45 *Ibid.*, p. 2.
46 TNA: PRO, MH 80/34, Voluntary hospital contributory and provident schemes: discussion of the attached paper, 10 April 1941.
47 TNA: PRO, MH 80/34, Goodenough to Maude, 25 May 1942, Appendix May 1942, Contributory schemes; TNA: PRO, MH 80/34, Notes on methods of obtaining patients' contributions, 28 April 1942, pp. 1–2.
48 *Ibid.*, Notes on methods, pp. 2–3.
49 TNA: PRO, MH 80/34, Memorandum on contributory schemes development, 21 May 1942, p. 3.
50 TNA: PRO, MH 80/34, Memorandum: the contributory schemes, pp. 4, 6.
51 *Ibid.*, pp. 4–5.
52 TNA: PRO, MH 80/34, Maude to Pooley, 2 May 1942, Notes on methods, p. 3.
53 TNA: PRO, MH 80/34, Maude to Goodenough, 9 May 1942; Honigsbaum, *Health,*

happiness and security, pp. 158–9; TNA: PRO, MH 77/26, Maude to Fraser, 21 April 1942.

54 'Hospital services and contributory schemes', *British Medical Journal*, 26 December 1942, p. 764.

55 W. Beveridge, *Social insurance and allied services*, Cmd 6404 (London, 1942), p. 6; R. Lowe, 'A prophet dishonoured in his own country? The rejection of Beveridge in Britain, 1945–1970', in J. Hills, J. Ditch and H. Glennerster (eds), *Beveridge and social security: an international retrospective* (Oxford, 1994), pp. 118–33.

56 Beveridge, *Social insurance and allied services*, p. 158.

57 *Ibid.*, pp. 160–1.

58 *Ibid.*, p. 160; though see also TNA: PRO, MH 80/34, Memorandum on contributory schemes development, 21 May 1942, p. 2.

59 Beveridge, *Social insurance and allied services*, p. 160.

60 *Ibid.*, pp. 143–5.

61 TNA: PRO, MH 80/31, Beveridge to Maude, 2 February 1942.

62 PEP, *Report on the British health services*, p. 410.

63 W. Beveridge, *Voluntary action: a report on methods of social advance* (London, 1948), pp. 115–16.

64 *Ibid.*, pp. 116–17, 292.

65 W. Beveridge, *Social insurance and allied services. Appendix G, Memoranda from organisations*, Cmd 6405 (London, 1942); Beveridge, *Social insurance and allied services*, pp. 247–8.

66 Beveridge, *Social insurance and allied services. Appendix G*, pp. 14, 19.

67 *Ibid.*, pp. 45, 73.

68 TNA: PRO, CAB 87/78, SIC (42), 24 June 1942.

69 'Hospital policy', *The Times*, 16 December 1942.

70 *House of Commons Debates*, vol. 386, Anderson col. 1662, 16 February 1943.

71 *House of Commons Debates*, vol. 386, Morrison col. 2040, 18 February 1943.

72 TNA: PRO, MH 80/34, Pater and McNicholl, Hospital contributory schemes and the Beveridge plan, 31 December 1942.

73 *Ibid.*, pp. 2–4.

74 *Ibid.*, p. 2.

75 TNA: PRO, MH 80/34, NHS 10, National Health Service, pp. 3–4.

76 Beveridge, *Social insurance and allied services*, p. 161.

77 TNA: PRO, MH 77/62, Assistant private secretary to Newstead, 7 August 1943; Memo, 25 August 1943.

78 From November 1943 the Reconstruction Committee: see Honigsbaum, *Health, happiness and security*, p. 67.

79 Honigsbaum, *Health, happiness and security*, pp. 161–4; Pater, *The making of the National Health Service*, pp. 71–3; Webster, *Health services since the war*, pp. 53–4.

80 TNA: PRO, MH 80/34, National Health Service, payment by patients in hospital, 11 December 1943.

81 Department of Health for Scotland, *Report of the committee on post-war hospital problems in Scotland* (Hetherington committee) (London, 1943), pp. 17–19.

82 *Ibid.*, p. 19.

83 National Archives of Scotland, HH 65/69, Finance, April 1943; Beveridge to Hetherington, 16 March 1942; HH 65/66, Stirling and Clackmannan Voluntary Hospital Joint Committee; HH 65/67, Russell Paton, Memorandum.

84 TNA: PRO, MH 80/34, Extract of conclusions of a meeting of the committee held on Friday 15 October 1943.

85 TNA: PRO, CAB 87/13, PR (43) 90, Sources of income of voluntary hospitals; this claimed, misleadingly, that contributory schemes in Scotland raised only 6 per cent of hospital income, though in 1935, the final year for which national figures are available, contribution amounted to 13 per cent.

86 *The Hospital*, November 1943, p. 336.

87 TNA: PRO, CAB 87/7, RC (44) 3, 10 January 1944.

88 TNA: PRO, MH 80/34, Brown to Anderson, 8 November 1943; CAB 87/7, RC (44) 2, Memo.
89 TNA: PRO, CAB 124/442, NHS: position of voluntary hospitals, 18 January 1944.
90 Honigsbaum, *Health, happiness and security*, p. 163.
91 Webster, *Health services since the war*, p. 53; TNA: PRO, MH 80/34, Extract of conclusions of a meeting of the committee held on Friday 15 October 1943, p. i.
92 TNA: PRO, MH 80/34, Johnston to Sir John Anderson, 10 November 1943.
93 Webster, *Health services since the war*, pp. 53–4; Honigsbaum, *Health, happiness and security*, p. 201.
94 Honigsbaum, *Health, happiness and security*, pp. 68, 104, 200.
95 TNA: PRO, MH 80/34, Johnston to Sir John Anderson, 10 November 1943; TNA: PRO, MH 80/34, Contributory schemes, Notes on methods of obtaining patients' contributions, p. 1; *The Hospital*, November 1943, p. 336.
96 Honigsbaum, *Health, happiness and security*, p. 164; the phrase is ascribed to Pater, but see TNA: PRO, MH 80/26, Voluntary hospitals and the cost of maintenance of inpatients, 4 November 1943.
97 Honigsbaum, *Health, happiness and security*, p. 163; Ministry of Health, Department of Health for Scotland, *A National Health Service*, Cmd 6502 (London, 1944), though see Appendix A.
98 TNA: PRO, MH 77/62, Hawton to Haddow, 18 May 1944.
99 Webster, *Health services since the war*, pp. 55–75.
100 Ministry of Health, *A National Health Service*, pp. 23–4.
101 *Ibid.*, p. 23.
102 See also 'Minister's replies to questions', *British Medical Journal*, 13 May 1944, p. 651.
103 *House of Commons Debates*, vol. 398, col. 437, 16 March 1944.
104 *House of Commons Debates*, vol. 398, cols 544–5, 17 March 1944.
105 *House of Commons Debates*, vol. 398, cols 545–7, 17 March 1944.
106 *House of Lords Debates*, vol. 131, cols 76–7, 16 March 1944.
107 *House of Commons Debates*, vol. 398, Howitt col. 490–2, 16 March 1944, Gridley col. 560, 17 March 1944; *House of Lords Debates*, vol. 131, Lord Southwood cols 52–3, 21 March 1944.
108 *House of Commons Debates*, vol. 398, Graham-Little col. 448–9, Colegate col. 517, 16 March 1944.
109 *House of Lords Debates*, vol. 131, Lord Luke, cols 111–13, 16 March 1944; *House of Commons Debates*, vol. 398, Jewson col. 470, 16 March 1944.
110 TNA: PRO, MH 80/27, Notes on points raised in the debate on the NHS.
111 *House of Commons Debates*, vol. 398, Storey cols 506–8, 16 March 1944.
112 *House of Commons Debates*, vol. 398, Watt cols 588–90, 17 March 1944.
113 *Ibid.*, Howitt cols 490–2, 16 March 1944.
114 *Ibid.*, Jewson col. 469–70, 16 March 1944.
115 *Ibid.*, Craik Henderson, cols 462–6, 16 March 1944.
116 *Ibid.*, Johnston col. 629, 17 March 1944.
117 *Ibid.*, Walkden cols 474–6, 16 March 1944.
118 *Ibid.*, Messer cols 563–4, 17 March 1944.
119 TNA: PRO, MH 80/34, Nuffield Provincial Hospitals Trust: National Health Service, July 1944, p. 6.
120 *Ibid.*, p. 1.
121 TNA: PRO, MH 80/34, King Edward's Hospital Fund, Memorandum on National Health Service, July 1944, p. 13; 'Voluntary hospitals and the White Paper', *British Medical Journal*, 16 September 1944, p. 60; TNA: PRO, MH 80/34, Nuffield Provincial Hospitals Trust: National Health Service, July 1944, pp. 6–7; TNA: PRO, MH 80/34, The British Hospitals Association: comments of the voluntary hospitals on the proposals in the White Paper, n.d., pp. 5–6.
122 TNA: PRO, MH 80/34, The British Hospitals Association: comments of the voluntary hospitals on the proposals in the White Paper, n.d., p. 6.

123 TNA: PRO, MH 80/34, NHS (44) 16, National Health Service: meeting with representatives of British Hospitals Association, 18 October 1944, p. 2.
124 *Ibid.*, p. 3.
125 TNA: PRO, MH 80/34, NHS (44) 9, National Health Service: meeting with representatives of the British Hospitals Association, 3 August 1944, p. 3.
126 Honigsbaum, *Health, happiness and security*, p. 163.
127 TNA: PRO, MH 80/34, Voluntary hospital finance White Paper proposals.
128 *Ibid.*; *House of Commons Debates*, vol. 398, Storey, cols 506–8, 16 March 1944.
129 TNA: PRO, MH 80/34, NHS (44) 9, National Health Service: meeting with representatives of the British Hospitals Association, 3 August 1944, pp. 1–3; TNA: PRO, MH 80/34, NHS (44) 16, National Health Service: meeting with representatives of British Hospitals Association, 18 October 1944, pp. 1–2.
130 Pater, *The making of the National Health Service*, pp. 102–3.
131 Honigsbaum, *Health, happiness and security*, pp. 169–70.
132 Abel-Smith, *The hospitals*, pp. 472–87; Stewart, *Battle for health*, p. 233; Honigsbaum, *Health, happiness and security*, pp. 169–71, 216–17; Webster, *The National Health Service*, pp. 14–15; Pater, *The making of the National Health Service*, pp. 116–17.
133 Webster, *The National Health Service*, pp. 16–19; Webster, *Health services since the war*, pp. 89–90; F. Honigsbaum, *The division in British medicine* (London, 1979), p. 290.
134 Honigsbaum, *Health, happiness and security*, pp. 179, 215–16; Abel-Smith, *The hospitals*, pp. 484–6.
135 J. Campbell, *Nye Bevan and the mirage of British socialism* (London, 1987), pp. 166–8, 177–8.
136 Honigsbaum, *Health, happiness and security*, pp. 173–4; Abel-Smith, *The hospitals*, p. 475.
137 Pater, *The making of the National Health Service*, pp. 31–3, 174–5; Webster, *Health services since the war*, pp. 264–8.
138 TNA: PRO, MH 80/34, Draft Cabinet paper, National Health Service, the future of the hospital services.
139 *Ibid.*, p. 2.
140 Stewart, *Battle for health*, pp. 153, 188–98; Stewart, 'Ideology and process'.
141 *House of Commons Debates*, vol. 422, A. Bevan, cols 46–7, 30 April 1946.
142 TNA: PRO, MH 80/34, Draft Cabinet paper, National Health Service, the future of the hospital services, pp. 3–4; 'Health Service Bill', *British Medical Journal*, 15 June 1945, p. 934.
143 TNA: PRO, MH 80/34, Minister's questionnaire, 7 August 1945, p. 2; TNA: PRO, MH 80/34, Sources of income of voluntary hospitals, 31 August 1945, p. 3; TNA: PRO, MH 80/34, Draft Cabinet paper, National Health Service, the future of the hospital services, pp. 2–3.
144 NPHT, *The hospital surveys: the Domesday Book of the hospital services* (Oxford, 1946), pp. 14–15.
145 Campbell, *Nye Bevan*, p. 21.
146 M. Foot, *Aneurin Bevan, a biography. Vol. I: 1897–1945* (London, 1962), pp. 63–4.
147 *House of Commons Debates*, vol. 422, A. Bevan, col. 47, 30 April 1946.
148 *Ibid.*, A. Bevan, cols 47–8.
149 *Ibid.*, A. Bevan, col. 51.
150 *Ibid.*, A. Bevan, col. 57.
151 *Ibid.*, A. Bevan, cols 61–2.
152 *Ibid.*, Richard Law, cols 73–4; Viscountess Davidson, col. 89.
153 Viscount Dawson of Penn, 'Medicine and the public welfare', *British Medical Journal*, 9 May 1942, p. 574.
154 Abel-Smith, *The hospitals*, p. 500.
155 Stewart, 'Ideology and process'.

Chapter 8

The contributory schemes and the coming of the National Health Service

Reflecting on the BHCSA's efforts to influence the NHS policy debates, its first historian concluded that: 'it can certainly never be said that … the Association failed for lack of trying'.[1] This chapter reassesses this verdict, through an exploration of the responses of both the BHCSA and individual schemes to plans for the new health service. Its premise is that the shape of the NHS was the outcome of a process of discussion within a policy community of politicians, civil servants, medical professionals and interest groups from civil society. Although a broad consensus in favour of reform was shared by 1939, it was by no means clear, at least until 1944 (and only definitely by late 1945), that the contributory schemes would have no place in the new dispensation. In this they were not alone: among other voluntary sector institutions which lost ground as Attlee's welfare state was formed were the friendly societies, which had hitherto administered health insurance, and the voluntary hospitals. However, others gained concessions: the BHA achieved its goal of keeping hospital management independent of the local authorities, with considerable autonomy for teaching hospitals, while the BMA averted plans for a full-time salaried service, retained private hospital beds and won improved remuneration.[2] Why did the contributory schemes come away from negotiations empty-handed?

The first section examines the response of the BHCSA to the policy process at two key junctures, the periods between Ernest Brown's parliamentary statement of October 1941 and the 1944 White Paper, and between the White Paper and the NHS Bill of 1946. The picture which emerges for the contributory schemes is one of strategic inconsistency and marginalisation in the policy discussions. Next, the NHS debates are viewed from the perspective of the localities, and it is shown that while some elements supported continuation of the status quo, other sections of the movement embraced the idea of a tax-funded NHS. Finally, the schemes' failure to influence events is analysed in the context of the literature of pressure group politics.

The BHCSA and the policy process

In the wake of Brown's statement and the initiation of policy debate (on which see chapter 7), the BHCSA pursued a strategic alliance with the BHA. The aim was to drive forward plans for regionalisation and greater uniformity between the constituent schemes through a combined BHCSA/BHA Income Limits Sub-committee. As the name suggests, this was convened following the rise in the income limit for NHI, for which eligibility had initially been confined to those earning less than £160 per annum, since NHI was intended only for the working class. It had then had risen successively to £420.[3] For the schemes this raised the questions of whether they should adopt a similar limit and whether they should also cater to the middle class. The sub-committee therefore began by debating the desirability of establishing schemes for the insured and their dependants ('grade A'), alongside provident schemes ('grade B') for higher earners.[4] Following hints of the Beveridge report's likely contents, the sub-committee's brief expanded to a consideration of a standardised national contributory system, to head off the anticipated proposals for a state health service.[5] The first method adopted was a survey of members' attitudes towards standardisation, in which the key proposals were: regional groupings of schemes; a national minimum contribution (4*d* per contributor, 1*d* per employer); full inter-availability and reciprocity of vouchers in voluntary and municipal institutions; standardised hospital and ancillary benefits; adoption of the NHI income limit; and the payment of hospital consultants.[6] This was a tactically astute approach, given civil servants' concerns about the schemes' heterogeneity. Moreover, it aligned the Association closely with the BHA, in a regionalisation project articulated in the Sankey report and by the NPHT (see chapter 7).[7] An air of realism pervaded the leadership's presentation of the sub-committee's endeavours in 1942; plans had to be based not on what 'might have been desirable a few years ago … but on a realisation of the present and completely changed position'.[8]

However, the tactic of promoting change through consensus and encouragement quickly faltered, as the consultation procedure failed to convey sufficient urgency to grassroots members. Only fifty of the BHCSA's 160 affiliates replied to the canvas of proposals for uniformity, of which forty-five gave support in principle, though with various reservations.[9] There followed a conference in London and four regional meetings, which were intended to provide a platform for agreement. However, these were poorly planned and attended. To the delegates' irritation, copies of the sub-committee's interim report were not circulated beforehand and scheme members were far outnumbered by the representatives of the voluntary hospitals (in Glasgow, by sixty-seven to five).[10] The BHCSA then collated responses and moderated the proposals to meet concerns, deciding, for example, that the cost of policing the NHI income limit should be borne by the hospitals.[11] Thus, as the Beveridge report was published, the BHA and BHCSA approved the sub-committee's standardisation plans.[12]

Unfortunately, this joint front soon collapsed, as William Newstead, the BHCSA's secretary, disagreed with his BHA counterpart, Percy Wetenhall, over the next step. The BHA wanted to proceed with the plan for regionalisation, allotting a single scheme to each hospital area. Newstead counselled against, arguing that inviting the smaller schemes to 'commit hari-kari' was impractical, and even if it could be achieved would still exclude those funds in the North East of England which rejected the southern contributory scheme model in favour of the 'open door' policy.[13] Convinced that Beveridge signalled the delivery of hospital cover through NHI, the BHCSA now made a crucial decision to change its strategy. Rather than ratcheting up the pressure on its members to accept greater uniformity, it advanced a different, more ambitious vision of the schemes' place within the NHS.[14] It also broke from the BHA and sought separate access to Whitehall to press its case.[15] Building on the earlier ideas of T. W. Place (his forerunner at the BHCSA), Newstead's plan proposed that the schemes should be the main distribution agency for national insurance payments, linking individual contributors to the hospitals. The plan envisaged a National Hospital Contributory Scheme, which would oversee service delivery, Area Schemes in the regions, and Sub-area Schemes, conforming to local authority boundaries, which would reimburse the hospitals for maintenance costs on the basis of vouchers submitted to them.[16] This went far beyond Sir John Maude's proposals (see chapter 7), which were to persist with the current arrangements, albeit with greater uniformity.[17] It also lacked unanimous internal support. In a scathing attack, Sydney Lamb, doyen of contributory organisation in Sheffield and Liverpool, condemned the departure from the regionalisation policy and the failure to act in concert with the BHA and BMA. Newstead, he argued, was a defeatist who had accepted the 'impending abolition' of the schemes.[18]

Newstead's rhetoric was also poorly chosen. Instead of emphasising the schemes' role in ensuring the democratic input of patients, he argued that voluntary institutions were needed to 'prevent the loss of virile and robust self-reliance and self-dependency' on the part of 'John Citizen', who might otherwise be 'ready to claim the advantages of organised Society, but reluctant to honour the attendant obligations'.[19] Given civil servants' doubts about the extent of popular commitment to the schemes, it is probable that this argumentation played poorly. Lamb caustically dubbed it 'beautiful idealism' and doubted that 'the country would entrust the cultivation of such virtues' to the BHCSA.[20] Also, the Newstead plan was contradictory, for if the BHCSA was now simply to channel the 'Beveridge fund' to hospitals, where was the scope for it to inculcate self-help?

Having cut itself adrift from the existing BHA strategy, the BHCSA became increasingly marginalised in the policy discussions of 1943. The leadership was dismayed that it was not granted an audience with the minister, but instead met with Maude, his finance officer, H. H. George, and civil servants John Pater and John Hawton.[21] Nor was there any interest in the Newstead plan. Instead, the officials set out their proposal – for the schemes to indemnify patients against a 'hotel charge' of £1 per week.[22] Again they stressed the need for full inter-availability and reciprocity between hospitals and gave assurances about their enthusiasm for 'voluntary initiative'.[23] BHCSA delegates Bertram Ford and Newstead did not highlight the contributory schemes' potential for democratic representation. Instead the discussion centred on those services – such as ambulances, district nursing and convalescence – which would now fall within the NHS's remit. Maude suggested such auxiliary benefits could be offered under contract from the government. The schemes might also cover dental and optical appliances and extended benefits for the better-off who preferred treatment 'in more expensive surroundings'.[24] Any hopes that the health service would provide a 'national minimum' beyond which the schemes could still appeal were dashed.[25] The BHCSA's leaders were asked to prepare estimates of the level of charges required to meet hotel expenses, and Newstead swiftly accomplished this, drawing on the experience of the Birmingham scheme.[26] When they finally met with Brown, he was reassuring as to their continuance but offered no concrete information on their future role.[27]

The decision to cooperate over the hotel charge rather than persisting with the BHA's regionalisation plans proved to be a further miscalculation, for once the White Paper abandoned this option the BHCSA was left with no coherent strategy. Ford met Henry Willink (Brown's successor as Minister of Health) in March 1944 to clarify the size of the funding gap which the schemes were now expected to fill, and wondered how the Minister expected 'working class folk' to carry on their voluntary contributions alongside the tax-based system. Again he floated the Newstead plan for a national and regional structure of contributory schemes to distribute the social insurance fund.[28] Willink, however, summarily disabused the BHCSA of the hope that the schemes might act as private agencies for public purposes, making it clear that they could have no official collecting or distributing function. Nor was there room for an alternative model in which the schemes offered cover for those outside the NHS, since the proposed service would not operate an income limit nor offer scope for contracting out.[29] The dropping of the hotel charge was justified (rather disingenuously) because it was based on a false distinction, in that maintenance was 'an indispensable condition' of treatment.[30] More positively, Willink sketched out the scope for the schemes' future work: contracting ambulance fleets and convalescent homes to the NHS, provident insurance for private patients, indemnifying against charges for 'surgical appliances'[31] and, most crucially, filling the shortfall in hospital income by voluntary fundraising.[32] Willink also expressed his conviction that 'custom' and 'individual interest' would sustain working-class voluntarism.[33]

By spring 1944 the BHCSA had adopted a defeatist position. Ford informed BHCSA affiliates that resistance to the White Paper's proposals was 'wishful thinking' and had to be abandoned; the Minister's mind was made up and it was clear that 'the country generally approve' the planned service.[34] The Association now had to address the substantive issues which the transition to the NHS raised, such as maintaining the level of contributions until the new service began, considering whether to offer provident insurance to patients wishing to pay for it and developing 'constructive and practicable ideas' about how to appeal for the maintenance of voluntary contribution under a tax-based system.[35] Even at this stage, some schemes protested over their exclusion from the NHS and Ford was subjected to angry denunciations. However, an attempt by the Manchester district schemes to launch a new campaign against the White Paper rapidly foundered on lack of support from the

BHCSA executive, and from the BHA and BMA, which were invited to join it.[36] Lobbying by individual funds against the Minister's intention to 'destroy the … goodwill' of the schemes 'with the stroke of a pen' was also fruitless.[37] Thus, from mid-1944, BHCSA members were debating their future on Ford's terms, and Willink congratulated him on his 'statesmanlike attitude'.[38]

Before the general election of July 1945, several additional initiatives were suggested for a future role within the White Paper's framework. The HSA proposed that schemes should participate in choosing the governing bodies of voluntary hospitals, which the Ministry approved but noted was a purely internal affair.[39] Ford's internal consultations produced various ideas about continuation, and a BHCSA planning sub-committee drafted a proposal for the 'retention and reconstruction' of the movement.[40] Despite some resistance to calls for a unitary approach, Newstead succeeded in putting a document before the Ministry, co-signed by the BHA's Wetenhall, in May 1945.[41] This codified the changed functions, including fundraising, the insurance for surgical, dental and optical appliances, and coverage for pay-beds.[42] Scheme membership would permit the 'patient-user' to gain representation on hospital management boards, and the movement would support health education and research into industrial diseases. Other ancillary services they could provide included transport to hospital, travel and accommodation allowances for patients' visitors, support for patients needing home help or social services, and convalescent and rest home facilities. Finally, Newstead revived his plan for a unitary regional administrative structure, though now bereft of formal integration with NHS regions, other than geographical contiguity.[43]

Whether Newstead could really have delivered the support of the doggedly localist contributory scheme movement for this new arrangement is uncertain. It arrived on civil servants' desks just as the war in Europe, and with it the coalition government, was nearing its end. To the BHCSA leadership the political auguries of the 1945 election were depressing. Ford gloomily expressed shock that Churchill's removal from office had been effected, 'strangely enough, by the direct action of his own fellow countrymen swayed by some powerful reactions'.[44] With respect to the schemes' future, this pessimism was well founded.

Aneurin Bevan's proposals immediately placed the BHCSA in a difficult position. Having already signalled in 1944 its willingness to submit to the government's wishes, it could hardly object to the new Bill, which went even further in undermining the basis of its appeal. In addition, Newstead's 'retention and reconstruction' proposals were stalled at the BHCSA's annual meeting in 1945, which resolved not to adopt them until the new government's plans were set out.[45] Hamstrung by this 'wait and see' resolution (from a strong supporter of the NHS who doubted the schemes should continue), and excluded from ministerial discussions, the BHCSA now became a bystander.[46] A special committee scrutinised the Bill, attempting to discern from opaque clauses on convalescent homes and appliances whether anything now remained of the role negotiated with Willink.[47] The only ray of hope was the preservation of pay-beds, through which the extended benefit schemes might survive. Here, though, the BHCSA quickly descended into infighting over a proposal to amalgamate the provident arms of existing associations. This provoked angry dissent from some delegates, presumably out of hostility to private wards.[48]

Once the NHS Acts were passed, the movement could do little but focus on immediate questions, such as the fate of the schemes' paid employees under the new service, and the problem of sustaining contributions before the 'appointed day' of the NHS's launch (5 July 1948).[49] Ford's speech to the BHCSA conference of 1947 was a last salute, made while 'the Sword of Damocles is still suspended above':

> we are maintaining a Bridge of Security for the hospitals and for our people, over the stream of change and reorganisation which we hope, at its flood tide will lead to the Land of Fulfilment, where if success should crown our efforts we shall find that we have been of no small assistance in the creation of the most effective and far reaching Health Service that the world has ever seen.[50]

Throughout the period, then, the strategic goals of the BHCSA lacked consistency and tended to follow events rather than pre-empt them. There is evidence neither of any systematic appeal to public opinion, nor of the articulation of a clear and constant position in Parliament through friendly MPs. After initially working closely with the BHA, the united front was ruptured by the first Newstead plan, and subsequent attempts at a coordinated approach were not seriously pursued. There is no reason to suppose that the BHCSA exercised any significant influence on decision-makers.

The view from the localities

How was the establishment of the NHS viewed at the grassroots? This section considers the response to national developments in various individual schemes. It reveals that divisions of opinion within the movement not only damaged the effort to achieve uniformity but also undermined popular support for the voluntary system. However, even among contributors who were strong supporters of the state health service there was anger at the absence of democratic mechanisms in Bevan's new structure.

First, though, how did the war affect the schemes? Despite early fears, the war years saw impressive leaps in their income, as rising wages and female employment sustained membership and allowed executives to impose increases in contribution rates.[51] The exception was the HSA, whose fall in membership was presumably related to London's distinctive experience of labour mobility and evacuation, and whose income exceeded 1939 levels only in 1944. Major urban schemes made a significant commitment to the war effort. Their rural convalescent homes, for example, joined the EHS to house patients referred from areas vulnerable to enemy bombs.[52] Ambulances and drivers were put at the disposal of civil defence planners and rendered vital service during the Blitz. In Liverpool the MHC's war emergency committee channelled significant sums towards charitable initiatives such as refuges for Blitz victims, emergency distributions of clothes, bedding and food, blood donor organisation, canteens and hostels for transient soldiers, and an enquiry bureau to advise on war-related health issues.[53]

Thus, when the NHS policy debates began, the schemes were in robust condition despite the challenges of war and, if anything, had augmented their position as important civic institutions. Public pronouncements at first confidently rehearsed pre-war loyalties: a 'system of State and Municipal ownership', Merseysiders were told in 1939, was inconceivable since it would 'be subject to many of the vagaries of party politics' and would imperil freedom of medical research.[54] Here was the prevailing view of scheme hierarchies, shaped by the philosophy of the BHA and BMA conservatives, for whom a state medical service was anathema.[55] In most English schemes this view prevailed until at least 1943, at which point the leadership began signalling a more fundamental transformation, as the following case studies show.

Multi-hospital schemes: from resistance to acceptance

In large multi-hospital schemes led by BHCSA luminaries, public discussion closely followed the twists in national policy. In Birmingham Brown's statement was met with equanimity and the local press predicted a future for the schemes.[56] Ford emphasised the moral and social benefits of the schemes within the welfare state: 'something of inestimable value will have been lost to the nation if there should grow up a generation of people well-versed in their rights, but totally ignorant of their duties'.[57] The progress of the BHA/BHCSA Income Limits Sub-committee was noted approvingly, and the BHSF's response to Beveridge was lukewarm, with fears voiced about 'bureaucratic control' and neglect of patients' needs.[58] On the eve of the White Paper, Ford confidently outlined the Newstead plan for scheme administration of NHI, and reassured contributors of official awareness of the BHCSA's activities and of the psychological value of voluntary effort.[59] Liverpudlians were similarly well informed of BHCSA policy, since Sydney Lamb was the local advocate of close cooperation with the BHA and the regionalisation plans.[60] After publication of the Beveridge report, hopes were pinned on rapid progress towards full reciprocity and standardisation, and a combative rhetoric was maintained, with dark warnings about sacrificing the 'freedom and elasticity' of the voluntary system and its 'leaven of individual responsibility … an inseparable part of the spiritual and moral fibre of this loved country'.[61]

From 1944, however, the tone of published discussion altered. Ford's address to the BHSF suggested resignation: 'we must be prepared to scrap our regrets and say "If anything we have done in the past can help – then take it and Godspeed"'.[62] Similarly, Newstead argued by early 1945 that the White Paper's proposals were broadly accepted and 'the promise of something better has captured the public imagination'.[63] In Liverpool a less emotive tone prevailed from 1945, by which point Lamb had resigned and the chair of the contributors' association was the staunch Labourite Jack Braddock: indeed, Labour members blocked a late gesture towards uniformity, in the proposal to impose a flat rate rather than the 'penny in the pound'.[64] Here, too, there was acknowledgement that 'all shades of opinion' favoured reform, and hostility towards Bevan's proposals was limited to the issue of employees' rights: voluntary hospital administrators were to be incorporated into the NHS, while officials of independent schemes had no such privilege.[65] The HSA likewise accepted the inevitable and, in a clear reversal of its earlier position (see chapter 5), a *Contributor* editorial acknowledged that there was now no difference between a voluntary and a state hospital.[66]

In their final phases the multi-hospital schemes concentrated on sustaining local hospital funding in the run-up to the 'appointed day', but they did not develop a common strategy for continuation (a reflection of their different local traditions and inheritance). Thus, in Birmingham, the case for continuation rested on the survival of assets (nine convalescent homes) and human capital (in the form of experienced officials).[67] After the war, convalescence benefit therefore became the main focus, along with a charitable trust set up to administer the residual capital of the fund for the provision of patient and staff amenities.[68] On Merseyside a more far-reaching scheme was conceived in an effort to 'augment' the NHS.[69] In addition to convalescence benefits, the MHC proposed cash grants for hospital patients, home-helps, sickroom equipment, health advice bureaux and charitable support for hospital amenities.[70]

Paradoxically, the death throes of the schemes also saw the birth of Britain's private medical insurance funds, as the extended benefit plans inspired future activities. These had witnessed a period of development in the mid-1940s. The HSA, for example, had launched a 'Group B' scheme in 1944, under which those earning over the NHI income limit subscribed at 7*d* per week.[71] The Merseyside Private Patients Scheme was begun in 1947, based on its 'Group B' plan, opened in 1945.[72] More significantly, a new organisation, the British United Provident Association (BUPA), was set up, with the Birmingham extended benefits scheme the largest constituent member. An amalgam of several other bodies, including the British Provident Association and the Oxford and District Provident Association, BUPA offered provident health insurance for private medical care.[73] Thus the provisions in the NHS Acts for the retention of pay-beds and private consultation accelerated a trend towards expansion which had been underway since 1937, when a federation of provident funds had been formed under the presidency of Bertram Ford, later BUPA's vice-president between 1947 and 1951.[74]

Wolverhampton: a divided membership

The perspective articulated by scheme executives is only part of the story, and the case of Wolverhampton provides insight into grassroots attitudes. Here, a cleavage between the leadership and the local labour movement is suggestive of broader divisions of opinion among ordinary contributors. Wolverhampton contributors' association was a generally passive group dominated by Alderman Alan Davies, a one-time member of the Sankey commission and thus closely identified with the preservation of the voluntary hospital system.[75] Indeed, in 1944 it passed a resolution expressing its 'concern' over the White Paper. However, when members debated their willingness to continue making voluntary payments if hospitals became tax funded, it soon became apparent that many would not.[76] Davies and the executive argued that the retention of the voluntary system was the ideal way forward, and in this he was supported by local MPs Robert Bird (Conservative) and Geoffrey Mander (Liberal), who warned that an extension of government grants would inevitably mean the end of voluntarism. Members, however, expressed a 'considerable divergence of opinion' over future voluntary contributions.[77]

The movement's fissure was fully exposed when the association voted on acceptance of the White Paper. Speaking for the shop stewards' committee of a local engineering firm with over 2,000 workers, a Mr Holloway moved that 'the voluntary contributions system be abolished and the Social Security propositions, as embodied in the White Paper should be supported in full. Any gap in existence to cover further expenses should be chargeable to the rates.'[78] Davies and the executive were then attacked for seeking to influence opinion by sending out a BHCSA circular, which they hoped would rebut 'anything the Trades Council Representatives may bring forward'; they denied this had 'showed contempt for the intelligence of the delegates.'[79] Challenging claims that the voluntary lobby represented 'vested interests', Davies asserted that the scheme was democratic and transparent, and defended the board of Wolverhampton's Royal Hospital as 'progressive and extremely generous'. An amendment favouring the preservation of the Royal's voluntary status was then carried by sixty votes to twenty-four. However, this victory for the establishment was tarnished by objections that delegates wielded only a single vote, rather than a bloc vote in accordance with the number of contributors represented: this would presumably have weighted the ballot towards large firms where trade union influence was stronger.[80]

The result of all this was an injection of greater democratic fervour into the hitherto quiescent Association, as the defeated trade unionists retaliated. The local branch of the National Association of Local Government Officers (NALGO) demanded 'larger representation' for contributors on the Royal's board of management and several new nominations to the executive committee were made.[81] At the next AGM, new representatives were formally elected to the committee, including Jarrett, a NALGO man (and water board employee) and Morris and Holloway (engineering firm employees), who were prominent in the row over the White Paper.[82] The tenor of executive committee proceedings then changed, as the new members raised objections about such matters as income limits, the coverage of the ambulance service, the almoner's procedures and the treatment of old age pensioners in arrears.[83] Morris pressed for a sub-committee to consider AGM voting rules, on which the three new men sat, and this granted larger firms proportionately more representation.

In sum, then, after years of passive collaboration, the White Paper debate forced the issues of popular representation and democracy onto the agenda and made the Wolverhampton contributors' association, for a short period at least, a genuine forum for the defence of patients' rights. More crucially, this episode reveals the depth of division at the grassroots over the preservation of voluntary contribution.

The Winchester scheme: an example of loyalism

A contrasting example is the Winchester and District Contributory Scheme, where no evidence of dissent was revealed at contributor meetings. Founded and dominated by officers of the Royal Hampshire County Hospital, this exemplifies a smaller scheme in a non-industrial setting. Here the likelihood of a state health service signalled by the Beveridge report was viewed unfavourably by the chair of the hospital's court of governors, Sir George Cooper, at the contributors' AGM: 'in spite of bureaucrats and highbrows … "people baked on one side," there was much good in the old order'. He then successfully appealed for contributors' endorsement of bringing the scheme into uniformity with others in the BHCSA's Mid-Southern Group.[84] This, however, was a dilatory process, as the group was still deliberating on uniformity of benefits and contributions one year on, and a further mandate for standardisation had to be sought. Nor was there a clear sense, even in mid-1945, that the status quo was threatened: 'They had had … voluntary hospitals for over 100 years and it was a fine thing for a country to say it had got them'.[85] With a traditionalist leadership, this scheme supported the BHCSA/BHA initiative and proceeded willingly, if not urgently, towards regional standardisation.

Once the Act was passed, the fund decided to wind itself up. At its final meeting speakers lamented the impending demise of voluntarism and celebrated its importance to democracy.[86] Despite discussion of establishing a new association to provide patients' amenities, the scheme then fell into abeyance until 1953, when a meeting was convened to dispose of the remaining funds. Under the aegis of Cooper, now chair of Winchester HMC, it decided to devote these to a new hostel and reception department for the hospital, with the residue going to a trust for patients' comforts; a league of friends was also planned.[87]

Scotland and the North East: objection to the loss of democracy

Given their opposition to standard contribution rates and the means test, it is not surprising that the schemes in Scotland and the North East of England viewed the coming of the NHS with more equanimity than their southern counterparts. Here there were fewer public encomia for the voluntary system, and less interest in continuation after 1948, although these schemes also mourned the loss of contributor representation under the new system.

Edinburgh's League of Subscribers illustrates the BHCSA's difficulties in marshalling a united front in 1942–43. Though aware of BHCSA efforts to promote regionalisation and standardisation in order to 'strengthen it in its negotiations with the Government', the League took no action in this direction.[88] Once the White Paper had been published it was acknowledged that resistance was 'impracticable and would be unacceptable'.[89] Indeed, the League regarded the White Paper as an endorsement of its 'open door' policy, which was now 'to become the rule for all Hospitals'.[90] Newstead's 1945 visit to address contributors on the scope for future activity drew only some thirty people.[91] Bevan's plans were received with 'general support ... as a necessary enactment', though an initial proposal to welcome the Bill was set aside on the grounds that the League should avoid 'party political propaganda'.[92] Some vain efforts were made by the executive to start a continuing scheme (see chapter 9), but these foundered and the League was wound up in March 1949.[93] Alongside this support for government, however, rising concern was expressed about the arrangements for representation on the new hospital management boards. The League proposed instead that the hospitals should be empowered to recommend members to the Secretary of State, so as to 'give a more democratic and local flavour' to hospital governance.[94] Discussion of the Bill's text deepened worries that it was 'leading to a separation of Hospital Management from popular control'. The 1946 AGM saw further expression of frustration at the 'surprising distrust of the people and of popular representation'; there was anger that the appointed boards would not be accountable to the public, who 'are to be taxed, rated and insured to provide Hospital finance'.[95]

In Glasgow the publication of the Beveridge report was the point at which contributor sentiment swung against the preservation of the voluntary system. Initially, managers of the Royal Infirmary actively sought to sway worker delegates' opinion against both the White Paper and NHS Bill.[96] Ministerial authority, they argued, would allow 'no form of effective democratic control', would divert charitable monies against donors' wishes, and would squander 'as a social asset the sense of common effort which has played so important a part in the building up of Voluntary Hospitals'.[97] It seems unlikely that rank-and-file members shared these reservations by the mid-1940s. Certainly, pre-war contributors had a keen preference for voluntary hospital treatment, even when the quality of municipal care had improved,[98] but by 1939 they were beginning to discuss the extension of state support more enthusiastically.[99] The Beveridge report was the catalyst for attitudinal change.[100] Worker delegate John Inglis summarised perceptions thus: 'the social conscience of the public had been awakened' and, if peacetime organisation matched the war effort, 'the world would be a better place to live in'.[101] The final demise of the scheme in 1948 also suggests that there was no abiding commitment to voluntary hospitals on the part of the ordinary contributor. The executive offered no proposals for reconstitution, beyond suggesting individual firms might maintain their collecting committees to raise charitable funds for equipment and special purposes.[102] Once again, though, the absence of direct representation on NHS boards troubled labour movement spokespersons. In 1945 William Cross contrasted the present 'great system', in which hospitals were 'the most democratically controlled Institutions in this Country', with a putative future in which governance was no longer transparent and responsive.[103] Cross's final address included a rueful comment about the failure to secure direct representation of employee contributors on the new Regional Hospital Board for the West of Scotland.[104]

Finally, brief mention may be made of Sunderland Royal Infirmary, which also demonstrates a pattern of rejection of BHCSA regionalisation proposals, followed by support for the NHS reforms, and ultimately dismay at the absence of representative procedures. As noted in chapter 6, Sunderland's worker governors had resisted moves in the 1930s towards a formal contributory scheme. The issue appeared again in 1941, during the BHCSA/BHA drive towards regionalisation, with proposals to establish the 'Sunderland Divisional Contributory Scheme'.[105] The main features of this were: a flat-rate contribution from workers earning below the NHI income limit; a HSA-style voucher system for admissions; the assessment of non-contributors as paying patients; equitable allocation among local hospitals according to utilisation rates; and transfer and reciprocal arrangements with other hospitals and schemes.[106] At first the workers' committee seemed amenable, and negotiated concessions such as free membership for pensioners.[107] Ultimately, though, two special meetings culminated in rejection, against the wishes of management.[108] Thus the principles of free access and variable rates were retained: at this point some workplaces contributed at rates as low as 1*d* per week, and clearly the BHCSA-recommended flat rate (4*d*) would have meant higher deductions for many.[109] Given this stance, and the strong trade union presence among the governors, it is unsurprising that no resistance to the NHS proposals was recorded. In 1948 the governors considered continuation but resolved to take no action until they saw how the NHS Act operated; thus the scheme terminated. The governors' final meetings also discussed membership of the Sunderland area HMC, and they nominated several members for this, including five colliery representatives.[110] On discovering later that though their secretary had been appointed to the HMC the worker governors had been rejected, their final act was to pass a resolution 'representing organised labour in Sunderland and district' to 'protest against the undemocratic method of appointment' of the HMC.[111]

Various key points emerge from these diverse local cases. In some contributory schemes a strong lead was given by executives in the early 1940s in favour of the preservation of the voluntary hospital system with their support. However, the fierceness of their rhetoric softened after the Beveridge report, and particularly after the 1944 White Paper. The BHCSA/BHA standardisation drive was well received by the large multi-hospital schemes, though single-hospital funds, which perhaps had less cause to consider issues of uniformity and reciprocity, were either slow to embrace regional groupings or reluctant to concede cherished features like the open door or variable rates. In schemes where trade unionists were prominent there was a clear support for the White Paper's plans for state funding, and later for Bevan's proposals. However, even contributors who were untroubled by the prospect of the schemes' demise resented the system of central appointment to NHS management bodies, which was seen as curtailing existing opportunities for democratic participation.

The BHCSA and pressure group politics

Having considered both national and local responses of the contributory schemes to the coming of the NHS, this section develops an explanation of why the movement was unable to secure its place within the new health system. Its analytical framework is drawn from the political science literature which examines the workings of pressure groups in the policy process. In particular, criteria which are held to determine the likelihood of a group's success are identified, then utilised to assess the BHCSA's performance.

First, though, it is useful to divide the policy-making process into three notional phases at which groups can intercede: an agenda-setting phase, a policy formation phase, and a policy implementation phase.[112] Evidence from post-war pressure groups underlines the importance of entering the debate at the agenda-setting stage, the period of initial discussion in the media, civil society and political parties. Successful groups use this phase to shift public opinion by dramatising their case early on. Once the policy formation phase begins, it is vital that pressure groups work with civil servants to shape the parameters of policy debate.[113] Early action is essential, as once the policy formation process leaves Whitehall there is less room for manoeuvre.[114] As we have shown, the BHCSA was not prominent in the agenda-setting phase and failed to assert a strong line with civil servants in the policy formation phase of 1942 and 1943. What features of the Association and its operating environment determined this?

The BHCSA as a pressure group: internal features

A pressure group's effectiveness hinges partly on features of the group itself. Is it a producer group, such as a trade union, a representational group, serving or representing a particular set of members, or a promotional group, speaking on behalf of others?[115] Of these, the producer group, which has the sanction of the withdrawal of its goods or services, has the greatest advantage in negotiation (as the BMA's success in extracting concessions demonstrates).[116] A group's size and wealth are obviously important, as are its membership density and internal cohesion. In practice, groups which appear to be large and representative can have very loose relations between members and leaders, with low levels of participation and office-holding.[117] These factors bear on the level of activism it can call on and the degree of seriousness with which government must view its cause.[118] A minimum size is also important to the effectiveness of the secretariat and organisational bureaucracy, though large representational groups may be less successful than small, professional promotional groups.[119] Moreover, large representative organisations may suffer from 'stifling breadth', where 'leader–member responsiveness' (ideally a perfect alignment of views) is weakened by too much internal diversity.[120] In this case, effectiveness depends on internal structures and formal democratic arrangements which minimise splits and allow more centrist views to predominate. Groups also need to be able to marshal expertise, and to mobilise members' interests and activism through their decision-making machinery.[121]

Alongside issues of size, structure and mandate, much depends on the quality and strategic ability of the leadership. Tactics might involve sophisticated propaganda techniques to persuade the public, and co-optation of and collaboration with MPs to ensure that arguments are aired in Parliament. The essence of pressure group activity is a clear, consistent message and a professional approach to putting it before both the public and policy-makers.[122]

How did the BHCSA measure up to these various criteria for pressure group success? With respect to membership density and internal structures, it is arguable that it did have both a mandate and an appropriate organisation to act effectively on behalf of its members. It represented a clear majority of contributors, with its affiliated schemes accounting, in 1942, for about 90 per cent of contributory scheme membership and income.[123] It also had operational procedures for representation and decision-making, ranging from the elections to the executive committee and the AGM for delegates to the provision for special general meetings. There was an annual subscription for administration, which funded the activities of the executive, and arrangements for the regular briefing and consultation of affiliated schemes.[124] In theory, then, the BHCSA could genuinely claim to speak for a significant body of people and could draw on organisational resources to mount a campaign.

However, the BHCSA leadership adopted an inconsistent strategy and tended to react to events rather than forcefully set the agenda. It did not seek to shape public opinion until it was arguably too late, for example considering the employment of a public relations officer only in 1944 and rejecting the idea of a press campaign. Nor did it secure representation in the House of Commons, other than through untargeted appeals for members to lobby their MPs.[125] Here it may be compared with the BMA, which, though it also eschewed public relations, was well represented by doctors in Parliament and had good channels of communication with Whitehall.[126] By contrast, the BHCSA was regarded as peripheral. As noted, although it submitted written evidence to the Beveridge committee, its marginality is illustrated by the omission of this from the printed appendix to the report (see chapter 7).[127] Its weak impact is also demonstrated by the persistent incorrect usage by policy-makers of the generic term 'hospital saving associations' (after the metropolitan HSA), rather than 'contributory schemes', until as late as March 1943.[128] Alongside its low profile, there was also a tendency throughout the whole the policy formation process for the BHCSA to incline towards a 'wait and see' approach.[129] This reactive stance was by no means approved by all members, some of whom lambasted BHCSA leaders for their 'dilatory procedure' and publicly urged them to put 'more ginger … into the fight'.[130]

Having failed to establish an independent position that was grasped by the public and by Whitehall, the BHCSA was not well placed when, in 1943, it decided to change strategy. Indeed, the split from the BHA and the adoption of the Newstead plan were, in retrospect, tactical errors. The original advantage of aligning itself with the BHA had been that the regionalisation policy was widely understood and supported by the voluntary hospitals' defenders; moreover, the joint approach alongside hospital elites improved its access to the corridors of power. The accompanying risk was that Whitehall would regard the BHCSA as very much the junior partner, whose interests were subsumed within those of the BHA.[131] This is precisely what happened, because when the BHCSA later sought to assert an independent line it found the Newstead plan quickly dismissed. There was also tactical ineptitude. Newstead's inability to secure the support of his own constituency for his proposals has already been mentioned, but his wrecking of the earlier strategy went further than this. At the crucial meeting between the Ministry and the BHCSA to discuss the 'hotel charges' model, Newstead frankly informed the already sceptical bureaucrats of his own doubts that smaller schemes would accept regional uniformity.[132]

Is it fair to criticise the BHCSA leadership for its strategic vacillation and reactive approach to the policy arena? Essentially it was a representational group, set up initially not to lobby government but to provide a national forum for resolving practical issues of reciprocity, territorial disputes and so on. It is anachronistic to consider the BHCSA a 'pressure' or 'promotional' group, in the post-war sense of a body representing the interests of members as consumers. Nor were its leaders full-time professionals versed in political lobbying. Ford, the BHCSA's president (1930–48), and Newstead, its secretary (1943–47), were respectively chair and manager of the BHCA. Thus they conceived of their role essentially as public servants animated by the voluntary impulse. They explicitly rejected the idea that the BHCSA should be 'fighting for sectional interests' and deliberately 'kept out of the newspapers ... to escape the charge of being moved by self-interest'.[133] Here again it is important to recall the duality that characterised the inter-war movement: on the one hand a traditionalist manifestation of philanthropic voluntarism, and on the other a new-model, non-profit, mutual insurer. The BHCSA leadership clung to the former conception, viewing contribution as essentially voluntary giving, entailing no rights to treatment.[134] Hence they did not see their role as defending the interests of contributors *qua* consumers; rather they believed the Association had a duty to adapt itself to changing notions of the broader public good. This was the context for the 'wait and see' approach. Whatever their personal views, Ford and Newstead acted as patriotic citizens, accepting that the NHS proposals 'genuinely expressed the needs of the time' and that it would be 'undignified and against the interests of the country' to oppose them.[135]

The BHCSA leadership therefore lacked the conviction and fixity of purpose needed to marshal such a heterogeneous movement. Theirs was a large representational group in which diversity of opinion was so great that leader–member responsiveness was bound to be poor. There were two key splits within the affiliated schemes which prevented them acting in unison. First, there was a split between the more parochial single-hospital funds and the independent multi-hospital schemes, which were more receptive to calls for regional coordination. Even among the latter schemes, however, the 1942–43 uniformity drive was thwarted by attachment to local diversity. Indeed, efforts by the BHCSA in the 1930s to promulgate a 'model' scheme constitution

had quickly aroused localist resentment.[136] This went beyond the concerns
of economically depressed areas about proposals for uniform subscription
rates. In Sheffield, for example, contributors were reluctant to adopt income
limits to exclude the middle class, and preferred instead to retain a 'gentleman's
agreement' predicated hitherto on trust; here the extension of the 'penny in
the pound' rate to higher earners was deemed more equitable.[137] Something
more dynamic than the BHCSA's consensus-building approach was therefore
required to herd these diverse associations towards standardisation. The second
split was that between hospital leaders and organised labour, for at the grassroots many members came to regard a state-run NHS as desirable. BHCSA
delegate meetings in the mid-1940s regularly heard from 'Labour men' who felt
that with a state health service in prospect the schemes were now irrelevant.[138]
Conceivably the BHCSA might have appealed to this constituency by more
forcefully emphasising the schemes' role as guardians of democratic involvement. Instead, its rhetoric foregrounded the moral virtues of voluntarism for
'John Citizen', an idiom unlikely to appeal to leftists who disliked charity as a
manifestation of class hierarchies.

The BHCSA as a pressure group: external environment

Analysis of the BHCSA's internal features therefore highlights issues of leadership, strategy and cohesiveness which militated against success. The outcome of
pressure groups' efforts can also be determined by the external political environment in which they operate.[139] Clearly, the chances of success increase when
a group's objectives are in tune with broader currents of opinion, above and
beyond its own agenda-setting endeavours.[140] Also crucial, as an issue becomes
more politicised, are relations with other groups within the policy community,
particularly where more powerful groups have different or opposing goals.
Studies of policy networks illustrate how weaker groups can be excluded or
marginalised, thus restricting policy options and biasing outcomes towards the
interests of dominant producer or professional groups.[141] The party political
environment is also important, as in general politicians tend to favour those
groups whose objectives are closest to their own 'policy dispositions' and perceptions of electoral interest.[142]

   In the case of the BHCSA, its role as the 'poor relation' in the policy debates
was the result not simply of its reactive approach but also of the dominance
of more powerful interests. The key player was the BMA, which, unlike the
BHCSA, already functioned as a self-assured pressure group.[143] Not only did it
have a powerful sanction but it also had a high-profile metropolitan leadership,
confident in its mandate to represent a producer interest. A BHCSA/BMA
alliance was always unlikely. Historically, doctors had been hostile to the contributory schemes, suspecting that they included a stratum of white-collar
workers who should more properly have been paying patients.[144] There was,
for example, no considered discussion of the schemes' place in the NHS in
the BMA's *British Medical Journal*, though the readership was regularly alerted

to the development of provident schemes for the middle class.[145] Hospital consultants were probably less concerned with the sources of hospital finance than with the question of avoiding local authority control, and may have regarded stable government funding and remuneration as more desirable. The correspondence of Charles Hill, the BMA's deputy secretary, suggests he was impatient with the BHCSA, regarding it as poorly led and lacking a clear policy, and by 1944 he was 'somewhat gloomy' about the schemes' future survival.[146]

The BHCSA's actual ally, initially at least, was the BHA, though here too there was a divergence of interests. For the BHA, the foundation of the alliance did not rest on any inherent admiration of worker governors; as we have seen (chapters 5 and 6), their representation was only grudgingly conceded by the voluntary hospital leadership at the outset, while trade unionists could cause difficulties for hospital boards. Rather, it was rooted in financial necessity, for only by resisting state funding could the voluntaries fend off public sector control. Following the 1944 White Paper, and the realisation that the government was settled on a predominantly tax-based funding system, the basis for the alliance was weakened, regardless of Newstead's change of strategy. Henceforth, the BHA's financial goal was to press for direct grants rather than local taxation, on the assumption that this would preserve administrative independence.[147] This confluence of BHA and BMA objectives around resistance to local authority control led to the formation of their own liaison committee. Despite its requests, the BHCSA was accorded no permanent seat on this, and now found itself largely shut out.[148]

The prominence of the BMA and BHA was not the only reason for government's tendency to disregard the schemes in the policy formation process. Abel-Smith's observation about the BHCSA's lack of 'power and influence' is also pertinent: ministers and advisers turned instead to representatives of the NPHT and the King's Fund, whose leaders were of a higher social status than the provincial scheme executives.[149] Nor were the schemes able to counter Whitehall perceptions that their mass membership was testimony to pragmatism rather than to popular voluntarism. Parliamentary debates demonstrated that some MPs were willing to voice support for the contributory schemes in the context of a broader defence of the voluntary hospital. However, in the absence of parliamentary lobbying by the BHCSA, there was no independent caucus presenting a coherent case for their retention; instead, speakers alluded loosely to the 'interest', 'pride' and 'spirit' which they embodied.[150] Thus there was no reason for government to suppose that ignoring the BHCSA would be unpopular with backbenchers or carry an electoral penalty.

Conclusion

Is it possible that if the BHCSA's leaders had possessed greater resolve, guile and charisma they could have succeeded in embedding a non-profit hospital insurance element in the NHS? Two alternatives might be envisaged: one in which a solid BHCSA/BHA alliance, supported by the NPHT and the King's Fund, had forced through the regionalisation model envisaged in the Sankey report; and another in which the Newstead plan of converting the schemes primarily to approved agencies for distributing tax receipts to the hospitals had been accepted. The latter was always unrealistic, though the BHCSA leaders clearly failed to mobilise internal support around a more contemporary appeal to democratic engagement, which might have been married to Newstead's model. Instead, an opportunity was provided by the debate concerning hotel charges, but this could have been seized only if the voluntary sector had been able to achieve standardisation of schemes within hospital regions; by 1942 its own slow progress towards this stood in contrast to the regional organisation of wartime hospital services achieved by the state's EHS. A significant aspect of this collective failure of the voluntary hospital movement was attributable to the contributory schemes but, given the BHCSA's internal divisions, an alternative outcome must be deemed unlikely. And while, judged by contemporary standards of pressure group politics, the leadership proved ineffective, its tendency to place public interest before sectional interest was a reflection both of the nature of the movement and of the philanthropic tradition from which it sprang. Finally, the conviction of other key interest groups that they could achieve concessions without the support of the BHCSA meant that the schemes were indeed (in Abel-Smith's words, quoted at the start of chapter 7) 'swept into the background'.

Notes

1   A. T. Page, *Pennies for health: the story of the British Hospitals Contributory Schemes Association* (Birmingham, 1949), p. 21.

2   C. Webster, *The health services since the war, vol. I* (London, 1988), pp. 107–20.

3   B. Harris, *The origins of the British welfare state: society, state and social welfare in England and Wales 1800–1945* (Basingstoke, 2004), pp. 162–3.

4   BLPES, BHCSA 4/2, Preliminary memorandum by the president, 1 August 1942; BLPES, BHCSA 16/7, Abridged notes of a series of conferences, 2 September 1942, p. 6.

5   BLPES, BHCSA 4/2, BHA, *First interim report of the Hospital and Contributory Scheme Income Limits Sub-committee*, 27 July 1942, pp. 3–5.

6   *Ibid.*, pp. 6–11; BLPES, BHCSA 4/2, Preliminary memorandum by the president, 1 August 1942, pp. 3–4.

7   Webster, *Health services since the war*, pp. 263–5.

8   BLPES, BHCSA 4/2, Preliminary memorandum by the president, 1 August 1942, p. 3.

9   BLPES, BHCSA 4/2, *First interim report of the Hospitals and Contributory Scheme Income Limits Sub-committee*, Summary of replies, 4 October 1942, p. 1.

10 BLPES, BHCSA 16/7, Abridged notes of a series of conferences of voluntary hospitals and contributory schemes, 2 September 1942, p. 4.

11 BLPES, BHCSA 4/2, Memorandum on replies received from associated contributory schemes, n.d., pp. 1–2.

12 BLPES, BHCSA 18/3, Ford to scheme secretaries, 23 December 1942.

13 BLPES, BHCSA 4/2, Newstead to Wetenhall, 19 January 1943.

14 BLPES, BHCSA 18/3, Newstead, 'What is the issue before us?'

15 BLPES, BHCSA 19/2, Newstead to Ministry of Health, 29 March 1943, Ford to Wetenhall, 19 April 1943, Newstead to Ford, 19 April 1943.

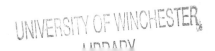

16   TNA: PRO, MH 77/62, W. F. Newstead, Statement of suggestions leading to the develop-
     ment of a national policy for contributory schemes, 10 January 1943 (this document can
     also be found in BLPES, BHCSA 16/7).
17   BLPES, BHCSA 14/2, Report of preliminary and informal conversation held at the
     Ministry of Health, Friday, 2 July 1943.
18   BLPES, BHCSA 18/3/62, Statement by Sydney Lamb, 26 January 1943.
19   TNA: PRO, MH 77/62, Newstead, Statement of suggestions, pp. 10–11.
20   BLPES, BHCSA 18/3/62, Statement by Sydney Lamb, p. 2.
21   TNA: PRO, MH 77/62, Ford to Brown, 19 March 1943; Newstead to Brown, 20 July
     1943; BLPES, BHCSA 14/2, Report of preliminary and informal conversation; J. Pater,
     The making of the National Health Service (London, 1981), p. 178.
22   TNA: PRO, MH 80/34, J. E. Pater, Contributory schemes, 28 June 1943.
23   TNA: PRO, MH 80/34, NHS 27, National Health Service, p. 1; BLPES, BHCSA 14/2,
     Report of preliminary and informal conversation, pp. 3, 4.
24   BLPES, BHCSA 14/2, Report of preliminary and informal conversation, p. 3.
25   TNA: PRO, MH 77/62, Newstead, Statement of suggestions, p. 3.
26   TNA: PRO, MH 77/62, Newstead to Maude, 22 July 1943.
27   TNA: PRO, MH 77/62, Assistant private secretary to Newstead, 7 August 1943; TNA:
     PRO, MH 77/62, Memo, 25 August 1943.
28   BLPES, BHCSA 19/2 197, Notes for interview with the Minister of Health, 10 March
     1944, pp. 1–2.
29   TNA: PRO, BHCSA 19/2 190, Short statement by the president on his interview with
     the Minister of Health, 10 March 1944, p. 1; TNA: PRO, MH 77/62, F. B. Elliot,
     director of HSA, 26 August 1944; TNA: PRO, MH 80/34, Rucker to Anderson, 21
     March 1945.
30   TNA: PRO, BHCSA 1944/4, Confidential circular to affiliated schemes' delegates:
     National Health Service, p. 1; TNA: PRO, BHCSA 1944/4, Short statement, p. 2.
31   The term 'surgical appliances' actually denoted a wide range of support and prosthetic
     items, such as elastic hosiery, wigs, trusses and corsets.
32   TNA: PRO, BHCSA 1944/4, Short statement, pp. 1–2.
33   Ibid., p. 1.
34   TNA: PRO, BHCSA 1944/4, Confidential circular to affiliated schemes' delegates, p. 3;
     BLPES, BHCSA 18/2 52, Précis of proceedings at the special general meeting, 18 April
     1944, p. 4.
35   BLPES, BHCSA 18/2 52, Précis of proceedings at the special general meeting, 18 April
     1944, pp. 4–5, 11; TNA: PRO, BHCSA 1944/4, Confidential circular to affiliated
     schemes' delegates, pp. 2–3.
36   BLPES, BHCSA 16/7 185, Circular to schemes, CSA 1944/45, p. 1; BLPES, BHCSA
     18/7, Newstead correspondence with Charles Hill, passim.
37   TNA: PRO, MH 77/62, Stevenson to Willink, n.d.; Paulton and District Hospital
     League to Willink, 10 May 1944; Dart to Willinck, 31 March 1944.
38   TNA: PRO, MH 77/62, Willink to Ford, April 1944.
39   TNA: PRO, MH 80/34, Rucker to Anderson, 2 December 1944.
40   BLPES, BHCSA 4/5, Minutes of the planning sub-committee, 20 July 1945; Page,
     Pennies for health, p. 23.
41   TNA: PRO, MH 80/34, Proposals to form a basis for the retention and reconstruction
     of the voluntary contributory schemes, May 1945; Page, Pennies for health, p. 24.
42   TNA: PRO, MH 80/34, Proposals to form a basis for the retention and reconstruction
     of the voluntary contributory schemes, May 1945, p. 2.
43   Ibid., pp. 2–4.
44   BLPES, BHCSA 7/4, AGM, 19 September 1945, president's address.
45   TNA: PRO, MH 80/34, British Hospitals Contributory Schemes Association: Debate
     on future policy.
46   BLPES, BHCSA 7/4, AGM, 19 September 1945; Page, Pennies for health, pp. 24–5.
47   BLPES, BHCSA 6/8, Memo accompanying minutes of AGM, 19 September 1946;

BLPES, BHCSA 6/8, NHS Bill 1946 statement by ad-hoc committee to examine Bill; TNA: PRO, MH 80/34, British Hospitals Contributory Schemes Association, National Health Service Bill, 20 May 1946.

48 BLPES, BHCSA 6/8, Memo accompanying minutes of AGM, 19 September 1946.
49 TNA: PRO, MH 80/34, Notes of meeting, 13 March 1946.
50 BLPES, BHCSA 6/8, AGM, 18 September 1947.
51 MRO, M610 MED 4/1, MHC, annual report, 1939.
52 For Birmingham: *The Samaritan*, 9 (2) (summer 1942).
53 MRO, M610 MED 4/1, MHC, annual reports, 1939, 1970, p. 16; MRO, M610 MED 2/3/1/1, MAHC MB, 12 March 1940.
54 MRO, M610 MED 4/1, MHC, annual report, 1939.
55 *The Samaritan*, 6 (1) (spring 1939).
56 *House of Commons Debates*, vol. 374, cols 1116–18, 9 October 1941; *Birmingham Post*, 17 September 1943.
57 BLSL, BHCA, annual report, 1942.
58 *The Samaritan*, 10 (1) (spring 1943), 10 (2) (summer 1943).
59 *The Samaritan*, 10 (4) (winter 1943).
60 MRO, M610 MED 4/1, MHC, annual reports, 1940, 1941.
61 MRO, M610 MED 4/1, MHC, annual reports, 1942, 1943.
62 *The Samaritan*, 11 (1) (spring 1944).
63 *The Samaritan*, 12 (1) (spring 1945).
64 MRO, M610 MED 4/1, MHC, annual report, 1945; MRO, M610 MED 2/3/1/1, Merseyside Association of Hospital Contributors: minutes of contributors meetings and the executive committee, 4 September 1945.
65 MRO, M610 MED 4/1, MHC, annual report, 1945; and see BLSL, BHCA, annual report, 1946.
66 *The Contributor*, August/September 1945.
67 BHSF Archive, BHSF, annual report, 1948.
68 BHSF Archive, BHSF, annual report, 1949.
69 MRO, M610 MED 4/1, MHC, annual report, 1947.
70 MRO, M610 MED 2/3/1/1, Merseyside Association of Hospital Contributors, Minutes of contributors meetings and the executive committee, 25 May 1948; MRO, M610 MED 4/1, MHC, annual report, 1947.
71 TNA: PRO, MEPO 2/7318, *The Hospital Saving Association: contributory scheme for class B contributors*, May 1944.
72 MRO, M610 MED 2/3/1/1, Merseyside Association of Hospital Contributors, Minutes of contributors meetings and the executive committee, 29 May 1945, 28 October 1947; MHC, News Bulletin No. 8, July 1945.
73 A. Bryant, *BUPA 1947–1968: a history of the British United Provident Association* (London, 1968), pp. 17, 21.
74 *Ibid.*, pp. 7, 9–18.
75 PAAA, Wolverhampton and Staffordshire Hospital, Hospital Saturday Committee minute book, 4 December 1935; British Hospitals Association, *Report of the voluntary hospitals commission* (London, 1937), pp. 4–5.
76 PAAA, Royal Hospital Wolverhampton Contributory Association, Minute book, 3 May 1944, 16 September 1944.
77 *Express and Star*, 15 May 1944, 18 September 1944; PAAA, Royal Hospital Wolverhampton Contributory Association, Minute book, 13 May 1944, 16 September 1944.
78 PAAA, Royal Hospital Wolverhampton Contributory Association, Minute book, 16 December 1944.
79 *Ibid.*, 5 November 1944, 3 December 1944.
80 *Express and Star*, 18 December 1944; PAAA, Royal Hospital Wolverhampton Contributory Association, Minute book, 16 December 1944.
81 PAAA, Royal Hospital Wolverhampton Contributory Association, Minute book, 14 January 1945.

82 HRO, 5M63/150, Royal Hampshire County Hospital at Winchester minute book, 17 February 1945.
83 *Ibid.*, 4 March 1945, 2 May 1945, 5 September 1945, 3 October 1945, 7 November 1945, 5 December 1945, 9 January 1946, 8 May 1946.
84 HRO, 5M63/150, Royal Hampshire County Hospital at Winchester, Minute book, *Hampshire Chronicle and General Advertiser*, 4 September 1943.
85 *Ibid.*, *Hampshire Observer*, 28 July 1945.
86 *Ibid.*, 17 August 1946, 26 July 1947; *Hampshire Chronicle*, 26 June 1948.
87 HRO, 5M63/150, Royal Hampshire County Hospital at Winchester, Minute book, 20 June 1953.
88 LHSA, LHB 1/18/3, Minutes of meetings of the League of Subscribers to the Royal Infirmary of Edinburgh, 14 July 1943, 20 January 1943.
89 *Ibid.*, 19 April 1944, 27 February 1944; LHSA, LHG 1/18/3, League of Subscribers to the Royal Infirmary of Edinburgh, annual report, 1947, typescript appendix.
90 LHSA, LHB 1/18/3, Minutes of meetings of the League of Subscribers to the Royal Infirmary of Edinburgh, 19 April 1944, 19 November 1944.
91 *Ibid.*, 21 January 1945, 1 March 1945.
92 LHSA, LHB 1/18/3, Minutes of meetings of the League of Subscribers to the Royal Infirmary of Edinburgh, 31 March 1946.
93 LHSA, LHB 1/18/4, Minutes of meetings of the League of Subscribers to the Royal Infirmary of Edinburgh, 27 March 1949.
94 LHSA, LHB1/18/3, Minutes of meetings of the League of Subscribers to the Royal Infirmary of Edinburgh, 31 March 1946, 17 April 1946, 16 October 1946.
95 *Ibid.*, 12 and 17 November 1946.
96 ML, HB 14/1/97, Minute book, Joint consultative committee of the Royal, Western and Victoria Infirmaries and the Royal Hospital for Sick Children Glasgow, 13 April 1944, 14 December 1944.
97 ML, HB 14/1/53, Glasgow Royal Infirmary minutes, 2 April 1946.
98 ML, HB 14/1/45, Glasgow Royal Infirmary minutes, 8 January 1938.
99 *Ibid.*, 14 February 1938; ML, HB 14/1/46, Glasgow Royal Infirmary minutes, 14 January 1939.
100 ML, HB14/1/50, Glasgow Royal Infirmary minutes, 9 January 1943, 23 November 1943.
101 ML, HB14/1/51, Glasgow Royal Infirmary minutes, 8 January 1944.
102 ML, HB14/1/54, Glasgow Royal Infirmary minutes, 10 January 1948.
103 ML, HB14/1/52, Glasgow Royal Infirmary minutes, 13 January 1945; J. Jenkinson, M. Moss and I. Russell, *The Royal: the history of Glasgow Royal Infirmary 1794–1994* (Glasgow, 1994), p. 192.
104 ML, HB14/1/54, Glasgow Royal Infirmary minutes, 10 January 1948.
105 TWAS, HO/SRI/3/6, Sunderland Royal Infirmary, Workmen's governors minute book, 24 May 1941, 11 October 1941.
106 TWAS, HO/SRI/3/7, Sunderland Royal Infirmary, Workmen's governors minute book, inset 1942.
107 *Ibid.*, 4 October 1942, 16 January 1943.
108 TWAS, HO/SRI/3/6, Sunderland Royal Infirmary, Workmen's governors minute book, 6 February 1943, 13 March 1943.
109 *Ibid.*, 22 January 1944.
110 TWAS, HO/SRI/3/7, Sunderland Royal Infirmary, Workmen's governors minute book, 10 April 1948, 26 June 1948.
111 *Ibid.*, 26 June 1948.
112 B. Coxall, *Pressure groups in British politics* (Harlow, 2001), p. 36; W. Grant, *Pressure groups, politics and democracy in Britain* (Hemel Hempstead, 1989), p. 117.
113 Grant, *Pressure groups*, pp. 48–50.
114 I. Budge, *The new British politics* (Harlow, 1998), pp. 277, 283; Grant, *Pressure groups*, pp. 55–6.

115   Budge, *The new British politics*, pp. 282–3; H. Eckstein, *Pressure group politics: the case of the British Medical Association* (London, 1960), pp. 33–5; P. Whiteley and S. Winyard, *Pressure for the poor* (London, 1987), pp. 3–5, 27.

116   Coxall, *Pressure groups*, p. 21; Eckstein, *Pressure group politics*, pp. 98–103.

117   S. E. Finer, 'Groups and political participation', in R. Kimber and J. Richardson (eds), *Pressure groups in Britain: a reader* (London, 1974), pp. 255–75, at pp. 261–3.

118   Coxall, *Pressure groups*, pp. 141–2, 146–7.

119   Grant, *Pressure groups*, pp. 118, 122; Whiteley and Winyard, *Pressure for the poor*, pp. 132–3.

120   Grant, *Pressure groups*, pp. 120–1; Finer, 'Groups and political participation', pp. 259–63.

121   Coxall, *Pressure groups*, pp. 121, 142–3.

122   A. Potter, *Organized groups in British national politics* (London, 1961), pp. 257–8, 271–80, 285–7, 315–6; R. Baggot, *Pressure groups today* (Manchester, 1995), pp. 134–51.

123   BLPES, BHCSA 4/2, Preliminary memorandum by president, 1 August 1942.

124   BLPES, BHCSA 7/1, AGM, 24 September 1932.

125   BLPES, BHCSA 16/7, Special general meeting, 18 April 1944; BLPES, BHCSA 16/7, Circular to schemes, 7 June 1944, pp. 2–3; BLPES, BHCSA 16/7, Minutes of special meeting of the executive committee, 13 July 1944, p. 2.

126   Eckstein, *Pressure group politics*, pp. 73–9.

127   W. Beveridge, *Social insurance and allied services. Appendix G, Memoranda from organisations*, Cmd 6405 (London, 1942); W. Beveridge, *Social insurance and allied services*, Cmd 6404 (London, 1942), pp. 247–8.

128   Beveridge, *Social insurance*, Cmd 6404, p. 160; TNA: PRO, MH 80/34, NHS 10, p. 3.

129   BLPES, BHCSA 7/4, Report of the executive committee, 30 June 1943.

130   BLPES, BHCSA 7/4, AGM, 23 July 1942; BLPES, BHCSA 7/4, AGM, 16 September 1943; BLPES, BHCSA 18/2, Précis of proceedings special general meeting, 18 April 1944, speeches by Steen, Lesser and Brown (quotation p. 13); BLPES, BHCSA 14/2, Newstead to Ford, 29 April 1944; BLPES, BHCSA 19/2, Chance Brothers Ltd to Newstead, 3 May 1943.

131   TNA: PRO, MH 80/34, NHS 14.

132   BLPES, BHCSA 14/2, Preliminary and informal conversation, p. 7.

133   BLPES, BHCSA 18/2, Confidential circular to affiliated schemes' delegates, 30 March 1944; BLPES, BHCSA 19/2, Newstead to Wetenhall; see also BLPES, BHCSA 7/4, Confidential circular to affiliated schemes, 1944/45.

134   Page, *Pennies for health*, pp. 12–13.

135   *Ibid.*, pp. 23, 25–6; BLPES, BHCSA 7/4, Special general meeting, 18 April 1944.

136   BLPES, BHCSA 22/1, Norwich Hospitals contributors' association to Place, 20 May 1936.

137   BLPES, BHCSA 4/2, BHA, *First interim report*; BHCSA, Minutes of the meeting of the Sheffield Regional Group, 15 October 1941; WHSA, Sheffield and District Association of Hospital Contributors delegates meetings, p. 2.

138   BLPES, BHCSA 7/4, AGM, 19 September 1945 (Ross); BLPES, BHCSA 6/8, AGM, 19 September 1946 (Boyland); TNA: PRO, MH 80/34, Ross to Hawton, 26 April 1946.

139   Budge, *The new British politics*, pp. 282–3.

140   Coxall, *Pressure groups*, pp. 156–7; R. Rose, *Politics in England: persistence and change* (London, 1965, 4th edn 1985), pp. 254–6; Grant, *Pressure groups*, pp. 126–7.

141   Coxall, *Pressure groups*, p. 68; R. Alford, *Health care politics: ideological and interest-group barriers to reform* (New York, 1975).

142   J. Dearlove, 'Councillors and interest groups in Kensington and Chelsea', in R. Kimber and J. Richardson (eds), *Pressure groups in Britain: a reader* (London, 1974), pp. 210–41, at pp. 225–6.

143   Eckstein, *Pressure group politics*, pp. 40–72, 96–115.

144   Sheffield City Archives, SCA 640 (48), City of Sheffield Town Clerk's Department, Local Government Act 1929, Correspondence, Sheffield Royal Infirmary memo relating

to finance, 24 May 1929; *British Medical Journal*, 3 December 1938, p. 1171; BLPES, BHCSA 18/7, Notes on interview with Dr Hill, p. 3.

145 *British Medical Journal*, 25 October 1941, p. 258; *British Medical Journal*, 26 December 1942, pp. 758–9; *British Medical Journal*, 20 February 1943, p. 1995; *British Medical Journal*, 5 June 1943, pp. 705–6.

146 BLPES, BHCSA 18/7, Newstead/Hill correspondence, April 1944, quotation, Hill to Newstead, 25 April 1944.

147 BLPES, BHCSA 14/6, BHA (Scottish Branch), Memorandum by executive committee, 16 March 1945.

148 BLPES, BHCSA 18/7, Newstead–Wetenhall correspondence, 5 and 8 May 1944; Newstead to Steward, 25 May 1944, Wetenhall to Newstead 8 May 1944.

149 Abel-Smith, *The hospitals*, p. 499.

150 *House of Commons Debates*, vol. 398, Graham-Little, cols 448–9, Colegate, col. 517, 16 March 1944.

Chapter 9

'Where the shoe pinches': reorientation under the National Health Service

In an address to the schemes at their 1948 conference, a few months after the creation of the NHS, Aneurin Bevan advised the schemes that, in the changed circumstances, they should 'Watch to see where the shoe pinches first because it is where the shoe pinches, and if the nation cannot do it, there your voluntary services will be required'.[1] This quote has entered the folklore of the contributory scheme movement. This chapter considers the response of the schemes to the establishment of the NHS. First, the debates that took place in 1946–48 are outlined, when the schemes had to decide whether or not to continue in existence and, if they were to continue, what their role ought to be. Both the attitudes of the schemes and the response by government are considered: despite Bevan's rhetoric, how supportive was government of proposals for continuation? Second, the success of efforts by the surviving schemes to develop a market niche is traced and developments are related to socioeconomic changes in post-war Britain and to the evolution of policy towards the NHS. Further, the evolution of the schemes – or health cash plans (HCPs), as they were known by the end of the century – is set against the emergence of private health insurance and the degree of complementarity (or otherwise) between these two markets is examined.

Finding a new role, 1946–48: scheme proposals and official reactions

The attitude of the BHCSA leadership in the spring of 1946 remained cautious and reactive.[2] The Association continued to channel its campaigns and suggestions for amendments through the BHA. It therefore failed to have a distinctive voice, as it operated through an organisation that was now marginalised, since the BHA's purpose was to represent the interests of voluntary hospitals, whose demise was now certain.[3]

There were, nevertheless, efforts to carve out a distinctive niche for future activities. In July 1947 the BHCSA's secretary, William Newstead, produced a set of proposals, though they differed little from those originally produced in 1945 (see chapter 8).[4] The document's purpose was to consider whether continuation was a 'good and necessary thing for the community', rather than a self-interested 'means of keeping Contributory Scheme office doors open'. This implied developing ancillary services for which the need could 'most appropriately be met' by the contributory scheme movement. Newstead suggested reconstruction on the basis of regional units, the boundaries of which would be co-terminous with NHS regions. There was a recognition of the 'intense local patriotism' in the movement and consequently Newstead envisaged a 'number of schemes in some regions working together under a common policy', rather glossing over the historic difficulties that had been experienced in this regard (see chapter 4).[5] Possible activities included convalescence and grants for spa treatment, prevention of illness, loan of sick room equipment, and grants for surgical and optical appliances, dental treatment and domestic help. The plan also recommended cash benefits for in-patients and their extension to include not only episodes of acute illness but also tuberculosis, other infectious diseases and mental illness, on the grounds that 'the economic need [for cash benefits] will be much the same' for those suffering from these conditions.[6] Other possibilities included grants for hospital amenities and for medical research. There was a hint, however, that the new schemes might be less inclusive than previously, with a suggestion that costs could be kept down by excluding men over sixty-five and women over sixty.

These proposals would appear to have demarcated a sphere of activity for the schemes which was distinctive, consistent with their pre-war ethos and activities, and which differentiated them from the nascent provident associations (which sought to develop insurance against the cost of private hospital treatment). Local evidence also suggests that there was a determination to continue, for at least three reasons. First, some schemes had substantial assets, such as convalescent homes, which were disclaimed by the government on nationalisation of the hospitals, and schemes therefore retained them. This provided a physical and symbolic asset base on which to draw. Second, at the ideological level there was a commitment to 'perpetuating the great tradition of voluntary service' under the welfare state.[7] 'It is democracy at work', argued the MHC, appealing to 'the sense of real sportsmanship, to the desire for self help and to the sound moral outlook of the average British citizen'.[8] Third, many schemes were ingrained features both of workplace culture, with most members subscribing through their firm's payroll,[9] and of civic life, in the form of public events such as carnivals and rallies (see chapter 5); their sterling contribution to the war effort has also been noted (in chapter 8).

Support for continuation was not universal, however. The attitude of some left-wing groups and trades councils ranged from outright hostility to continuation, to grudging acceptance subject to guarantees about representation for members. For example, when the BHSF announced that it would be continuing outside the NHS to provide convalescent homes for its members, the president of the Birmingham trades council threatened to arrange a boycott on payments to the Fund by union members in 1947 unless the trades council was given adequate representation on its committee.[10] In Liverpool in 1949 the MHC won a libel case against a shop stewards' newspaper, the *Mersey Clarion*, which had claimed that the continuation of the Merseyside scheme would be contrary to the interests of the Labour government and that the scheme organisers simply wished to maintain their positions of employment, salaries and pensions.[11] However, some prominent socialist figures supported continuation; John Braddock (MHC chair 1947–63) considered the 'penny in the pound fund' to be 'a proven money-spinner which ought not to be allowed to die' and the fund duly reconstituted itself.[12] Proposals to maintain the benefits of the provident schemes also aroused union opposition, as in Wolverhampton (where a grant towards costs of pay-beds was one example). Here the trades council attacked the proposed scheme on what appears to have been two counts: employees felt it meant a needless deduction from wages, and the support of private medicine threatened the principles of the NHS.[13]

Despite such opposition there were demands for continuation. Discussions in the Edinburgh League of Subscribers indicate some of the options considered, but the eventual termination of this fund helps illustrate why the survival of the contributory scheme movement was patchy. The early hope of the League's leaders, such as Russell Paton, was that the fundraising and representative roles would be combined and approved by the Scottish Department of Health, but this was not to be. By mid-1947 two options were under discussion: either developing into a provident fund for the middle class, or continuing principally as a small-scale charity providing amenities for patients.[14] The former option was not pursued, but by the start of 1948 proposals were developed for continuation through the provision of a cash sickness benefit, domiciliary aid and charitable gifts to patients of the Edinburgh Royal Infirmary.[15] Weighing against this was uncertainty about the attitude of the new Infirmary board; its support would be vital as hitherto the hospital had provided the League's accommodation, staffing and accounting services. Also, word came that Co-operative Society members thought 'that there was now no need of the League' and members observed that the new local authority social services department was providing much of the domiciliary welfare service which the League had planned to offer.[16] None the less, shortly after the NHS came into existence in July 1948 a special meeting of 170 subscribers and members of the executive resolved to continue on a regional basis as the South-East of Scotland League of Hospital Subscribers. This was to be a charity for 'our less fortunate brethren', on the basis of a penny per week subscription, which would principally provide 'additional comforts and amenities', though it was hoped that the League would also offer 'collective representation' in the 'interests of the patients'.[17]

This was arguably a limited role, but since care had been taken to formulate proposals for activities which were complementary to the NHS, one might have expected the government at least to endorse and welcome such initiatives. The attitude of the Ministry of Health can be gauged from records of discussions between officials and representatives of surviving schemes in early 1948. The Ministry agreed that there was scope for the schemes in the provision of convalescence facilities; it was also aware of plans to offer cash benefits for the sick, and for the replacement and repair of appliances supplied to individuals. However, officials admitted that they had 'been rather discouraging – we clearly do not want the idea to arise that appliances provided by the Service are inferior'. The position they adopted was a somewhat hands-off one: the activities of the surviving schemes were 'entirely their own affair'. The main concern was that the schemes organised directly by voluntary hospitals should close; as regards the independent schemes, 'that is a matter for themselves'.[18]

Officials may have felt obliged to adopt this rather circumspect tone but both in public and in private Bevan was rather more effusive. He insisted that the hospitals would still need public service and enthusiasm, both in governance and in 'voluntary work of many kinds'.[19] Most famously, in the speech to the BHCSA with which this chapter began, he argued that the government was putting the 'coping stone' on work begun by the schemes, wished them 'Godspeed to whatever you may do in supplementing what we have already done', and advised that they should not determine their future orientation too quickly; they should wait to see precisely where the 'shoe pinches'.

Not unreasonably, the schemes interpreted this as an endorsement of their work and an encouragement to find new avenues to explore. However, this apparently supportive statement was not backed by action. Hospitals were instructed to cease their charitable fundraising activities and to wind up 'contributory schemes run by the hospitals themselves',[20] while fears of conflicts of interest led to the disbarment of committee members of continuing schemes from serving on RHBs and HMCs.[21] The Ministry of Health also declined to guarantee employment for scheme officials, even though their continued efforts had kept hospitals afloat financially between the end of payments to voluntary hospitals via the wartime EMS and the inception of the NHS in July 1948. This problem particularly affected employees of multi-hospital schemes. Clause 64 of the 1946 NHS Bill guaranteed to find NHS employment for (or pay compensation to) staff of those schemes that were attached to individual hospitals, but there was no such protection for employees of independent contributory schemes.

The Edinburgh League's experience is instructive. The Infirmary's new board of management refused to offer financial help or permanent office space, while the majority of firms canvassed said they intended to cease contributions.[22] Support was not forthcoming from the Scottish Department of Health, which might have permitted the Infirmary to use the residue of the League's last payment to support its continuation, nor from the RHB, which favoured smaller leagues of friends, affiliated to individual hospitals.[23] Russell Paton (secretary of both the Infirmary and the League) continued to press the RHB in late 1948, arguing that since the Infirmary's catchment was so large a regional league was justified; he also developed a lengthy list of 'comforts and amenities' which might be provided, and suggested the League might be a vehicle for representation of patients' interests and welfare on a 'broad democratic basis'.[24] By early 1949, however, the League's executive was forced to admit defeat. The RHB argued that, given the establishment of various local leagues of hospital friends in south-east Scotland, the proposed regional league was unnecessary, while works' representatives now reported lack of interest on the part of their members. The League then dissolved.[25] At its final AGM the Edinburgh Royal

Infirmary expressed gratitude and promised a plaque in its memory, though the occasion was marred by a dissenting member from the Leith branch of the National Union of Railwaymen, who complained: 'This league has become an institution, but you fellows are murdering it'.[26]

The failure of the Edinburgh League's continuation plans also provide insight into why a *national* network of contributory schemes did not emerge after 1948. In areas without means tested hospital charging, subscription rates had been low and no additional benefits were offered, other than the 'open door' of local hospitals. There was therefore no tradition of extra-hospital benefits which could have been developed into an attractive new package. The proposal for a fund which would be solely charitable had little appeal. The League also illustrates the fate of a single-hospital scheme, which in contrast to the city-wide funds of Sheffield, Birmingham, Leeds and Merseyside had no staff, premises or other assets. Freed from its dependence on League income, the hospital now had no incentive to commit precious resources to such a marginal association, while the attitude of the RHB and the state appears to have been benign indifference.

Such restrictions on the schemes and indifference to their fate were criticised (by John Dodd, joint secretary of the BHCSA) as an 'attack on liberty',[27] while the BHCSA deplored the small number of RHB members who had experience of the contributory schemes.[28] In reality, the schemes' fate had been sealed on the passage of the 1946 Act, and the final AGMs of the BCHSA were occasions for eulogies, tributes to key individuals, assertions as to the quintessentially British and Christian virtues of the movement, and dire warnings to governments if they diminished the scope for voluntary action.[29] The organisation was wound up in October 1948. It was clear that a number of schemes intended to continue in existence, and a new representative organisation was formed. Dodd proposed that it should be titled the British Hospitals Voluntary Service Association, to mark a break from the old organisation while 'perpetuating the great tradition of voluntary service'.[30] In fact, efforts to re-establish the schemes along these lines, as Hospital Leagues of Friends, proposed by Percy Wetenhall (of the BHA) came to nothing at the time.[31] It was finally agreed that the new association would be called the 'BHCSA (1948)' to 'maintain goodwill and draw attention to the fact that something fundamental happened in 1948', though for simplicity it is still referred to hereafter simply as the BHCSA.[32]

Continuation under the NHS

> The employees were of the opinion that as the government have now taken over they must provide a full service, and owing to increased insurance deductions they do not feel prepared to pay further to a nationalised hospital.[33]

So wrote James Winyard, timber merchant, in response to an enquiry in 1948 from the Wolverhampton Royal Hospital contributors' association as to whether the firm favoured the scheme's continuation. It might have been expected that this negative sentiment would have been well nigh universal among the movement's members since, by financing hospitals from direct taxation, nationalisation would appear to have removed the *raison d'être* of the contributory schemes. The great majority of schemes folded after 1948, but thirty-five of them thought it worth continuing. These were mostly those which had been independent of the local voluntary hospital, and had their own board of trustees or were registered under the Companies Act.[34] They included the London-based HSA and numerous large schemes in major cities such as Birmingham, Leeds, Liverpool, Manchester and Sheffield (all of these had had a membership of at least 250,000 contributors immediately before the establishment of the NHS) and several smaller funds. When the national picture of continuing membership became clear in 1950, the schemes could claim some 3.4 million contributors, a figure which may be compared against the 56,000 who subscribed to the early provident health insurance plans.[35] Given that the majority of pre-1948 members had been workers in the lower income brackets, this apparently surprising level of support illustrates the extent to which the major multi-hospital schemes were an ingrained feature of civic and workplace life. No survey data have been located which illuminate the attitudes of those who continued as members (or who joined the remaining schemes). However, scheme reports and accounts reveal the market niches which they colonised and their patterns of recruitment and membership over time.

Benefits offered by the surviving schemes

There is no continuous record of the pattern of benefits offered – the BHCSA began to collate and publish this annually only from 1970 – but a summary for 1952 indicated that 59 per cent of scheme expenditure went on cash grants to hospital in-patients, followed by convalescence (12 per cent), optical and dental grants (8 per cent each) and various smaller items.[36] This provides a useful baseline but for more detail it is necessary to examine the records of individual schemes. A full sequence detailing the proportion of expenditure allocated to the various benefits survives for the Leeds Hospital Fund (figure 9.1), which, with between 160,000 and 220,000 members for much of this period, is typical of a large urban scheme.[37] Initially, claims were mainly for accommodation in the scheme's convalescent homes, along with limited grants towards consultations with specialists, and two benefits which were soon dropped: grants for chiropody and for 'surgical appliances'. Here such items are grouped in the 'miscellaneous' category, which also included provision of home-helps. However, by the early 1950s three key benefits had emerged: a cash payment while members were hospitalised, and grants towards the costs of spectacles and dental care. Then, from the 1960s, a cash payment for members sick at home was introduced. The principal long-run trends in expenditure were: the consistent importance of the hospital cash benefit for the first two decades, until a decline set in from the 1970s; the marginal significance of convalescence; and the growth in expenditure on the dental and optical grants. Trends in the

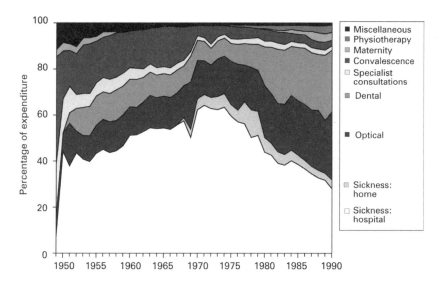

Figure 9.1. Composition of the expenditure of Leeds and District Workpeople's Hospital Fund, 1949–90.

numbers of claims, as opposed to spending on particular benefits, would show a different pattern, because of the relatively small size of many claims; there were far more claims for optical and dental benefits than for hospital cash benefits. For example, in Leeds, around 60 per cent of claims were for optical and dental benefits from the early 1950s but, as can be seen from figure 9.1, hospital cash benefits at that time accounted for a much higher proportion of benefits paid (around 50 per cent, rising to 60 per cent by the early 1970s).

Other scheme records present variations on this theme, depending on the timing of the introduction of new benefits. For example, the Merseyside scheme did not introduce optical and dental benefits until several years after the institution of NHS charges, while the Birmingham and Sheffield schemes initially offered only convalescent home accommodation. By the late 1960s, however, the reports of these schemes show that the hospital in-patient grant was the most popular benefit in cash terms, and that optical and dental expenditures grew steadily from the late 1970s, a trend which is consistent with increases in charges for NHS prescriptions. Other schemes also conformed to this general pattern, and regional variation gave way towards greater uniformity by the 1980s.[38]

In interpreting the relationship between the schemes and the NHS, Mossialos and Thomson's classification of voluntary health insurance is helpful. They distinguish between insurance according to whether it substitutes for the statutory health care system, provides complementary cover for services which the state provides partially or not at all, or offers supplementary cover, thereby enabling faster access and increased consumer choice.[39] Of these, substitutive voluntary health insurance (whereby individuals opt out of statutory coverage) is unknown in the UK. In this classification, the contributory scheme/cash plan market has been complementary to the NHS, in that it provides a range of benefits which fall outside the state scheme. Only the grants towards specialist consultations can genuinely be deemed supplementary, and similar to private medical insurance (PMI), in that they allow claimants to purchase a service they might otherwise have received free from the NHS. These grants, however, were not a very large component of expenditure, since they typically covered only a proportion of the consultation fee and were subject to restrictions on the frequency of claims. They were also frowned upon by the BHCSA leadership, which believed they were 'aiding and abetting queue jumping'.[40]

Beyond this, the schemes colonised areas which were excluded from the ambit of the NHS. Convalescent homes had multiplied during the early twentieth century. They were either affiliated to voluntary hospitals, which used them to prevent bed-blocking, or operated by associations such as trade unions, friendly societies and contributory schemes, which offered accommodation as a welfare benefit. In 1948 the government decided to 'disclaim' some 230 institutions which were deemed surplus to the requirements of the NHS, including many convalescent homes.[41] In some cases these homes were disclaimed because of strenuous opposition by the schemes which had established them, such as the BHSF.[42] Resource constraints prevented the NHS from developing such services and this created a market for the schemes, which offered this additional benefit either in their own institutions or through contractual arrangements with independent homes. Popular locations for convalescent institutions were in rural areas or coastal resorts, which were thought to be conducive to recuperation. A medical recommendation was necessary to claim the benefit, which might also include travel expenses and pocket money.

By contrast, the hospital cash grants were essentially a new product, developed on the premise that, despite the universal NHI ushered in by the welfare state, an episode of sickness was still likely to entail a loss of earnings. The BHCSA considered that the idea had originated with the Bristol Medical Institutions Contributory Scheme, which in 1930 had set up a 'Section II' extended benefits scheme, which for an additional 1d contribution paid a guinea per week cash grant on hospitalisation.[43] In 1936 this section was reconstituted as the Bristol Contributory Welfare Association, which claimed to be 'the pioneers of the scheme in England'.[44] Intriguingly, the cash payment idea also echoed earlier traditions of friendly societies' sickness pay, since its instigator, J. S. Tudor, secretary of the Bristol scheme, was a friendly-society activist.[45] BHCSA discussion documents in the late 1940s had promoted the cash grant idea and by 1952 twenty-two out of twenty-seven affiliated schemes operated it.[46]

The dental and optical grants responded more clearly to consumer demand in an area where, from the outset, government had allowed some scope for patient charges. These were initially intended to be for repairs and replacements, though in 1951 charges were imposed of about half the cost of dentures, and for spectacles the full price of frames and 10s per lens.[47] Having promoted a repairs benefit since 1948, the BHCSA was well placed to advise its affiliates on grants towards these new costs.[48] In 1951 one of the most prominent figures in the pre-war contributory scheme movement, Sir Alan Anderson of the HSA, foresaw the opportunities which the imposition of charges would bring: 'new needs would arise which were not contemplated when the health service was formed'.[49] Soon after NHS charges were introduced, patterns of take-up in Leeds showed that claims for optical benefits increased dramatically, and those for dental treatment climbed from the 1970s onwards. This experience was repeated elsewhere, though, as shown below, there was no obvious association between the introduction of charges and changes in scheme membership. The introduction of these charges led the chairman of the Hull Voluntary Health Contributory Scheme to comment publicly that Bevan's shoe 'now pinches in the wrong place'.[50] The schemes had not been prepared for the sharp increase in claims following the introduction of charges, and the upsurge in demand for spectacles had compelled one scheme to 'knock off the whole of our ophthalmic benefits'.[51] This prompted consideration of the scope and limits of the activities of the surviving schemes. One suggestion was that effort should be concentrated on cash benefits in time of sickness, the incidence of which could not be predicted, and convalescence, rather than dental or optical benefits where potential subscribers could anticipate a high probability of needing assistance. The matter was left to individual schemes, but it is clear that dental and optical benefits constituted a major proportion of their activity from the 1950s onwards. From the late 1970s optical and dental benefits grew to around 35–40 per cent of the total benefits paid in Sheffield and Merseyside, while in Leeds, by the late 1980s, as NHS dentistry declined, dental expenses accounted for some 40 per cent of all claims. A survey of the attitudes of present-day contributors to the Bolton and District Hospital Saturday Fund revealed that optical and dental grants are still those deemed most important by members.[52]

The growing popularity of these two benefits helps explain why the incidence of claims steadily increased throughout the post-war period. In the Leeds fund there were typically between twenty and thirty claims per hundred members in the 1950s, but by the late 1980s the incidence was nearer ninety claims per hundred members, and recent data indicate that the total number of claims made exceeds the number of subscribers. This reflects the small size of the claims and does not signal a threat to actuarial viability. Another long-run trend discernible in all the schemes surveyed was the decline of convalescent home benefits. This is best understood in the light of changing norms of non-acute care, as doctors became less inclined to recommend institutional convalescence to patients who did not require active nursing or treatment.[53] A Ministry of Health enquiry in 1959 questioned the therapeutic value of what officials described as 'recuperative holidays'.[54] The BHCSA preferred the epithet 'traditional convalescence', though it was frankly acknowledged that this meant 'a recuperative stay in pleasant surroundings ... the sort of rest that the more well to do are able to provide for themselves in a suitable hotel'.[55]

There is evidence that the 'seaside holiday' element of convalescence, rather than its medicinal aspects, was central to its appeal. Thus the Leeds fund reported that take-up of its inland homes on the Yorkshire Moors had fallen off in favour of the coastal institutions, particularly in the winter months.[56] Consumer preferences were also shifting away from the old-fashioned, institutional atmosphere of the homes.[57] In 1966 the Merseyside scheme summarised matters thus: 'Changes in social conditions, the advent of the Welfare State, increases in wage rates, and improved standards of medical diagnosis and treatment have … created different outlooks on convalescence'.[58] BHCSA appeals to the Ministry of Health to open up spare capacity to local authority contracting for after-care (and thus to public monies) therefore met with a negative response.[59] The Ministry did not believe that there was evidence of unmet demand for the convalescence facilities which the schemes provided and it seems the BHCSA's protestations were a rather ineffectual effort to garner state support. This was not forthcoming; the NHS was operating within tight revenue constraints and there is evidence elsewhere (e.g. from the provision of geriatric services) of efforts to limit the growth in expenditure at that time.[60] Thus, without statutory backing for a reorientation of these recuperative facilities, decline in their utilisation continued apace; convalescence benefit fell as a percentage of the total distribution of schemes affiliated to the BHCSA, from 15 per cent in 1969, to 10 per cent in 1973, to 5 per cent in 1982.[61] With it went a vital part of the identity of the movement, which to BHCSA leaders had represented a 'shop window of our schemes', and in the long term several schemes divested themselves of their convalescent homes.[62] The Birmingham fund, which had attached great importance to and invested substantial sums in its convalescence facilities, closed its last home in 2004, disposing of the property shortly after.[63]

Recent data on benefit claims show that, of some 6.1 million claims made in 2002, 3.6 million were for dental and optical benefits, which averaged £24 and £55 per claim, respectively. This is consistent with data from individual schemes; grants for dental and ophthalmic services accounted for around 60 per cent of the total number of claims on the Leeds fund from the early 1950s.[64] In cash terms the largest category of benefits was still payments associated with in-patient stays (26 per cent), with dental (21 per cent) and optical (24 per cent) claims close behind. The declining significance of cash benefits is partly an artefact of reductions in lengths of stay in hospital since the 1950s, when such payments accounted for over 40 per cent of scheme expenditure. In terms of the total number of claims made, the largest recent increases have been in claims for dental and optical benefits, which increased by 75 per cent between 1999 and 2002. Also notable has been the growth in claims for physiotherapy and chiropody, which together now represent some 12.5 per cent of benefits paid, and at least some schemes also now cover the costs of treatments such as acupuncture and osteopathy, reflecting a growing consumer interest in such therapies.[65] These trends indicate, in part, the extent to which dental and optical services are now a private responsibility, in part the growing cultural acceptance of alternative therapies, and in part the difficulties of obtaining services such as physiotherapy on the NHS.

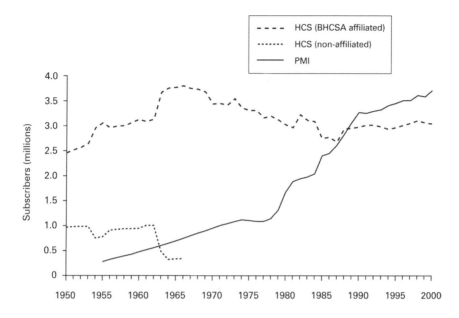

Figure 9.2. Numbers of subscribers to hospital contributory schemes (HCS) and to private medical insurance (PMI), 1950–2000.

Membership

Figure 9.2 shows the membership numbers of the hospital contributory schemes/HCPs from 1950 to 2000, set against the trend in numbers of PMI subscribers. Estimation of membership data is subject to a margin of error. Since the majority of contributions continued to come through workplace payroll deductions, rather than individual payments, schemes typically kept no record of the exact numbers of subscribers. Instead they estimated their membership based on potentially obsolete records of the size of constituent firms and few published totals in their annual reports. The main source for these figures is therefore the collated statistics of the BHCSA – renamed the British Health Care Association (BrHCA) in 1989 – which is an aggregation of these imprecise estimates.[66] Even these do not give the full picture, as some schemes were not affiliated to the national association, while others suspended their affiliation from time to time. However, the numbers in non-affiliated schemes declined quite markedly, particularly after the early 1960s, when the BHSF joined the BHCSA. From then on it seems that less than one in ten members was in an unaffiliated fund, and it is reasonable to presume that these national figures fairly reflect actual trends,[67] though the withdrawal of the HSA for part of this period means that the data underestimate the true membership totals.

Two further difficulties with the data should be noted. First, it would be interesting to distinguish between individual members and those whose membership was by dint of joining a participating firm, but there is no national record of this. Individual scheme records show that firm membership predominated at first: in Wolverhampton and Sheffield it was estimated that only 9.5 and 11.5 per cent of subscribers were individual members in 1959, while on Merseyside individual subscription income was 9 per cent of the total.[68] A BHCSA examination in 1970 broadly confirmed this pattern but noted that individual membership was unusually high in areas such as Bristol, Exeter, Hull and Reading.[69] In the 1980s the balance began to change, with the Merseyside fund, for example, drawing about one-third of its income from individuals by 1990. This is likely to reflect the impact of recession on firm membership as well as a shift in the marketing of schemes towards the individual member. The second aspect which these data obscure is the varied geography of contribution. The essentially urban basis of the movement persisted, with rural areas considered to be 'difficult and expensive in which to campaign'.[70] Nor did the funds have a genuinely national constituency: the large 'uncovered' areas (where schemes had not continued in existence) included Scotland, Northern Ireland, the North East of England and the far North West. Notwithstanding this, some schemes recorded increased recruitment and take-up within their defined catchment areas.[71]

With all these caveats in mind, figure 9.2 shows that if non-affiliated schemes are included, scheme membership rose from about 3.5 million at the start of the NHS to reach about 4 million in the 1960s. There is some indication of growth in the mid-1950s and this might suggest an association with the introduction of NHS charges. However, the monthly membership totals calculated for one scheme – the Patients' Aid Association in Wolverhampton – show steady growth in the 1950s, with no discernible 'break of slope' around 1951, which suggests that recruitment decisions reflected the overall benefit package rather than specific changes in NHS policy.[72] Given the industrial base of many major schemes, the high level of membership in the late 1950s and early 1960s is not surprising, as it coincided with an era in which British manufacturing employment peaked. Membership then shrank slowly during the 1970s and 1980s, reflecting the decline in manufacturing, before it stabilised and then recovered slightly in the 1990s.

This pattern contrasts vividly with the trend in subscriptions to PMI, which, after slow growth in the post-war period, entered a period of rapid expansion in the last two decades of the century. The forces driving the growth of PMI are well known and include aggressive advertising strategies which capitalised on disenchantment with the NHS, the advent of US commercial insurers, the growth of employer-paid insurance (offered as a perk, either to circumvent incomes policies in the 1970s or to attract scarce staff in competitive labour markets) and the rising real incomes of social groups most likely to purchase it.[73] Thus there was a strong social gradient in the distribution of PMI, with coverage reaching 28 per cent in the professional and managerial socioeconomic groups. There were also strong regional contrasts.[74]

Quite different factors determined trends in membership of the contributory schemes, for PMI products were not direct substitutes for HCPs. Three issues underpinned the rise in scheme take-up in the 1950s: first, the re-establishment of cordial relations with local trades councils, which overcame opposition to payroll deductions and encouraged the voluntary work of collectors, both inside and outside the workplace; second, the success of the schemes in tailoring benefits packages and subscription levels (on average 3½d per week in 1956) to their market; and third, the imposition of NHS optical and dental charges, which boosted demand.[75] Yet concerns were expressed in the early 1960s that the schemes were not developing a new constituency. Premiums remained low in an era of prosperity; in 1963 the question was posed whether there could be 'any serious virtue in these coppers while there can scarcely be anyone unable to afford at least 6d per week?' Failure to develop new markets was attributed to the 'unenterprising' nature of recruitment efforts, as well as to complacency and indifference.[76] The implication was that the schemes ought to develop a greater range of benefits and extend their clientele beyond their traditional working-class base.

This does not appear to have happened and the beginnings of decline in the late 1960s were initially explained in terms of profile and publicity: 'are we hiding our light under a bushel?' wondered the BHCSA president in 1967.[77] By the mid-1970s, though, real problems were developing. It became harder to replace the ageing, long-serving volunteer collectors;[78] at the same time, strikes, inflation and unemployment meant that for the BHCSA 'signals are firmly set at danger', with 'factory closures, and redundancies' undermining membership in the movement's heartlands.[79] Matters became 'gloomier still' at the end of the 1970s: membership was static and recruitment efforts were at best only matching losses through deaths, redundancy or job change. In Manchester, for example, scheme membership had been 'decimated' by the closure of large engineering firms. Such was the reduction in the manufacturing base in the North West that, by the late 1980s, the public sector, led by the NHS, had become the largest source of membership, while annual reports even in more recent years have continued to cite the steady decline in British manufacturing, especially in the Midlands and North West, as a cause of reductions in membership in individual schemes (though total membership was recovering by the end of the century).[80] A further consequence of economic restructuring was that many members who had lost their jobs continued their subscriptions but now either through their new employers (which were typically smaller firms than those for which they had previously worked) or as individual members.[81] Either way, the result was increased overhead costs for the schemes and BHCSA reports for the 1970s and 1980s make reference to reductions in the proportion of income paid out in benefits.[82]

The BHCSA's leaders ruefully contrasted this situation with the acceleration of PMI membership, with one comment being that 'what we have to sell is less attractive and our marketing methods are less efficient'.[83] Unfavourable comparisons with PMI may be somewhat harsh. Much of the growth in the latter was through company-paid schemes in the booming sectors of the economy in the south of England; many of the losses in contributory scheme membership were through factory closures in the industrial heartlands. The two were not substitutes, nor were they really targeting the same markets.

What is undeniable is that the schemes clearly now needed to reach out to constituencies which they had not previously tapped.

There was a push to raise the schemes' profile in the late 1980s and early 1990s, with the engagement of two parliamentary representatives, the employment of a public relations firm and the renaming of the national body as the BrHCA, with a full-time secretary.[84] The rebranding of the schemes as 'health cash plans' and a concerted effort to update their image also aided recovery, as did the restructuring of benefits to include grants for complementary medical care, though these account only for a small proportion of benefits paid. Finally, there is some suggestion that the rising tide of PMI in the 1990s may also have lifted the HCPs. The Family Resources Survey for 2000–1 estimated that 18 per cent of the population had some form of health insurance, whether through HCPs or PMI, and that since an estimated 10 per cent of the population was covered by HCPs and 12.3 per cent had PMI, it was probable that some 5 per cent subscribed to both products.[85] The suggestion, then, is that the greater visibility of cash plan products promoted by provident and commercial insurers may now be boosting scheme membership too. Even so, only some 15 per cent of HCP policies are company paid; this contrasts sharply with PMI, where only approximately one-third of policies are individually paid.[86]

Consideration of the whole post-war period points to two further aspects of the schemes' constituency which have influenced membership trends: first, they have retained strong local and urban identities; and second, they have attempted to retain the support of their traditional social base. On the first point, local loyalties were vital to their post-war recovery and recent research into the relationship between a scheme's town of origin and its brand recognition has suggested that these remain an important motivator for purchase of an HCP.[87] Indeed, one scheme estimates that nearly half its members live in the town in which it is based and that some 20 per cent of the town's working-age population are covered.[88] At the same time, such localism could inhibit expansion into parts of Britain where coverage was low. For example, some schemes were restricted by their articles of association to a defined territory; in the case of Birmingham, this meant organising within twenty-five miles of the city centre.[89] Scheme executives were well aware of those areas in which expansion was desirable. The failure of schemes in the North East to continue after 1948 meant that this was one area in which expansion would now be possible, Teesside being noted in particular. Other areas identified included the North West (north of Manchester) and Shropshire.[90] However, schemes were reluctant to commit 'limited resources for development in new areas for uncertain returns'; they still relied heavily on voluntary labour by group secretaries, who could not reasonably be expected to travel long distances on speculative recruitment drives.[91] A somewhat different perspective on this was given by John Dodd, who commented that the effect of these early attempts to delimit territory was simply to 'prevent schemes fighting over small areas where there are great open spaces for future development'.[92] He clearly felt that such attempts at cooperation were a distraction.

Efforts to establish regional groups to promote the movement over the whole country got underway in the 1960s and initially made some headway in the Midlands, the South West, East Anglia, Yorkshire and the North West (the latter group continuing to meet into the 1990s).[93] However, just as in the 1930s, an element of parochialism and local patriotism militated against such initiatives. A representative of the Bolton fund informed the 1965 AGM of the BHCSA that his committee attached great importance to the fact that they were 'a local body'; they would not support any regionalisation initiatives if this implied standardisation of contributions and benefits.[94] The president of the Association poured oil on these troubled waters, by arguing that the aim of regionalisation was simply to 'identify untilled ground'; if a scheme was operating in, or near to, an area and was not 'developing' it, then it could not adopt a 'dog in the manger' attitude and prevent another scheme from doing so. However, as in the 1930s, the BHCSA had no sanctions at its disposal; it could not enforce national resolutions, and individual schemes or regional groups could simply choose to ignore them.[95]

On the second point – the social background of subscribers – their post-1948 development suggests that the HCPs have attempted, while introducing a range of higher-cost products, to retain the support of their traditional social base. Although concerns have occasionally been expressed that schemes whose contribution rates were 'unduly influenced by the needs of the elderly, the retired or unemployed cannot give the required service to the mass of the working population,'[96] the movement has been reminded from time to time that its 'historical strength – and great advantage over provident and commercial insurance schemes – has been provision for those not able to help themselves…. There must be provision for these groups.'[97] Hence, while schemes have generally moved upmarket over the past two decades, to offer an extended range of benefits, they have not always phased out their cheapest benefit packages, though they have been closed to new subscribers, and some have indicated their determination to adhere to this ideal.[98] The problem this posed for schemes adhering to their traditional role was evident in the following quote, from a small, rural scheme in the 1980s. The scheme reported that: 'to go too far [raise subscriptions too much] would take us too close to private hospital schemes, but not to go far enough will soon make us totally unnecessary.'[99] Such schemes faced a difficult balancing act: their subscription rates were low but were still not attracting much new custom, but raising them excessively would have meant catering for a quite different market. As a result, it is clear that social gradients in take-up of HCPs are much less than for PMI: coverage varies between 8 per cent and 13 per cent across socio-economic groups for the cash plans, while PMI has a coverage of over 25 per cent of the professional and managerial groups and some 3 per cent in the unskilled manual groups. For the HCPs, the highest rates of coverage are in the intermediate socioeconomic groups (skilled manual workers), at 13 per cent. According to one scheme, those who are self-payers are broadly representative of the community as a whole, in contrast to company or group schemes, where there is still something of a preponderance of the traditional working class.[100] However, the evidence from another HCP on the age distribution of membership suggests that approximately 10 per cent of its self-paying policies have been taken out by the under-thirty-fives, whereas as many as 30 per cent of members of its various company-paid or group plans are aged thirty-five or under. Care should be taken in generalising from this evidence but if this were the experience of other HCPs it might imply that they were not persuading those in younger age groups to take out policies, other than through their workplace.[101]

Labour movement ties also remained important. For example, when the Leeds fund attempted in 1965 to recruit members at a shipbuilding firm in Sunderland, it found that the employees were more receptive to approaches made 'through the trade union side' than through management.[102] During the coal dispute of 1984–85 many miners fell into arrears with their subscriptions, but by agreement reached between the National Union of Mineworkers and the respective schemes, the miners paid off the arrears through double contributions once they returned to work, the additional administrative costs of this being borne by the National Coal Board.[103] Trade union support has featured more recently; for example, in 2001 Medicash was operating a 'Unison endorsed' HCP.[104]

Has such an orientation been a help or a hindrance? Some felt that just as the movement's localism constrained geographical expansion, so its rootedness in the culture of workplace association circumscribed its social appeal. The dilemma was nicely captured in a letter of 1989 from a scheme member to the secretary of the BHCSA; he noted that membership of the main private health insurance schemes:

> can be boasted of in the clubhouse after 18 holes. [However] Flashing your contributory scheme membership card would probably get you drummed out of the club. Sadly our image just hasn't been updated; we are still a cloth cap and muffler set up. We are working class and there is nothing wrong with that but unlike years ago there is no longer any pride in being working class.[105]

In this reading, then, the fate and image of the movement were tied into its local and industrial heritage. The schemes therefore appeared worthy but old-fashioned, while their reliance on workplace subscription exposed them to losses in membership and income during economic recession. These factors provide a plausible account of the difficulties experienced by HCPs in reinvigorating their membership in the late twentieth century; they needed to find new markets and attract the support of a younger, upwardly mobile constituency.

Conclusion

The schemes had to carve out a new niche after 1948 but they also had to steer a careful course. First, they could not colonise territory now occupied by the NHS and, in contrast with other European health care systems, where co-payments of various kinds are common,[106] the scope for developing new products to complement NHS services was limited. Second, they could not move into provident insurance without compromising their ideals, though there was a determination to resist encroachment from commercial insurance providers. In rebuilding the movement, activists could draw on a reservoir of strong community support, certainly in several large cities where pre-war expansion into non-hospital benefits had established products that could still be offered after 1948. However, this was not the case everywhere and the fate of the Edinburgh League of Subscribers exemplifies the problems confronting a scheme whose socially progressive policy of concentrating solely on open access to hospital treatment meant that it was completely redundant under the NHS, while its proposed alternative – charitable fundraising to support the hospitals – generated little enthusiasm.

The benefits offered by the surviving schemes were influenced broadly by NHS decisions which delimited their scope for developing new products. An obvious example is official policy towards convalescence, which made it clear that the NHS was not likely to develop new capacity in this area. Connections between other NHS policies – such as charging for services – and changes in scheme benefits and membership are, however, harder to separate from the effects of changing social conditions and attitudes. For example, despite the impact of recession in the 1970s and 1980s, some (though not all) schemes experienced growth in membership, but we cannot determine whether this was a response to increased NHS charges or a reaction to the broader product mix offered by the schemes. It is therefore not possible to assess the effect on recruitment of the regular increases in NHS charges from 1979. Any positive effect is masked by the negative impacts of economic decline. It is also possible that recruitment of new members was not a response to NHS charges but instead reflected a response to the more up-market packages offered by schemes in a bid to attract a new clientele (see also chapter 10).

The latter point signalled a wider concern for the movement. Growing affluence posed a challenge for recruitment and product development. The schemes attached great importance to catering for their traditional low-income membership base, which was the 'historical strength' of the movement, but a corollary was an outmoded image. Even in the 1950s and early 1960s one can detect signs of concern that the schemes were not attracting younger age groups and that they were failing to tap rising the discretionary expenditure associated with increased prosperity.

Thus, while the major surviving schemes had a strong membership base in many of the principal cities, efforts to expand into areas where coverage was low met with limited success. The schemes went through a period of stagnation in the 1970s and early 1980s, reflecting recessionary effects on their core membership. By the early 1980s there were around a million fewer contributors than in the mid-1960s. Economic growth, the rising tide of PMI and greater diversification of the product mix subsequently led to a modest upward turn in membership trends, and coverage is presently slowly returning to levels experienced in the 1960s. However, while in terms of membership numbers and benefit packages a case could be made that little has changed, there have been developments both in the ethos of the schemes and in the products they offer, and it is to these issues that the final substantive chapter turns.

Notes

1   BLPES, BHCSA 3/12, Aneurin Bevan, address to the conference of the BHCSA, Folkestone, 1 October 1948.
2   BLPES, BHCSA 2/6, Minutes of the executive committee, 14 February 1946.
3   *Ibid.*, 28 March 1946. The BHCSA bound its interests to those of the voluntary hospitals, resolving 'to support the BHA in its endeavours to secure modification of the Bill in the interests of voluntary hospitals and patients'.
4   BLPES, BHCSA 3/12, Proposals by the planning sub-committee for possible future activities for contributory schemes, July 1947.
5   *Ibid.*
6   *Ibid.*
7   BLPES, BHCSA 3/10, John Dodd to Henry Lesser, 9 September 1948.
8   MRO, M610 MED 2/3/2/2, MHC, The future of the Merseyside Hospitals Council, Memorandum by the secretary, revision sub-committee, 6 May 1947.
9   S. Cherry, 'Hospital Saturday, workplace collections and issues in late nineteenth century hospital funding', *Medical History*, 44 (2000), pp. 461–88.
10 'Saturday fund faces trades union boycott', *Birmingham Evening Despatch*, 3 September 1947.
11 BLPES, BHCSA 18/7, BHCSA circular CSA 49/1, 1949. The issue of staff salaries and pensions in Liverpool was a long-standing bone of contention – see chapter 6.
12 MRO, M610 MED 4/1, MHC, annual report, 1966; J. Braddock and E. Braddock, *The Braddocks* (London, 1963), p. 142.
13 PAAA, Executive council minutes of meetings, 9 May 1948, 23 June 1948, 4 January 1949, 3 May 1949, 29 October 1949, 16 November 1949, 28 January 1950; *Express and Star*, 10 November 1949, 'Firms not willing 1948', letters from Sketchley Dye works, 4 May 1948, James Smith Lock Manufacturers, 30 April 1948; Patients' Aid Association, *For whom we serve* (Wolverhampton, 1984), p. 13.
14 LHSA, LHB 1/18/3, Minutes of meetings of the League of Subscribers to the Royal Infirmary of Edinburgh, April 1947, 15 October 1947.
15 LHSA, LHB 1/18/4, The Royal Infirmary of Edinburgh, League of Subscribers 1947–1948, minute book, 21 January 1948, 12 February 1948.
16 *Ibid.*, 23 April 1948, 5 May 1948, 16 May 1948, 23 May 1948.
17 *Ibid.*, 13 June 1948; LHSA, LHB 1/18/4, Royal Infirmary of Edinburgh League of Subscribers, annual report, 1948.
18 TNA: PRO, MH 99/18, Pater to W. Bain Grey, 4 May 1948.
19 MRO, M610 MED 2/3/2/2, Aneurin Bevan to Bessie Braddock, 27 January 1948.
20 TNA: PRO, MH 99/37, NHS appeals for funds, etc.; Ministry of Health circular RHB (48) 41A, 1948.
21 *Daily Telegraph*, 12 January 1949; Ministry of Health circular RHB (48) 25A, Appendix 1; BLPES, BHCSA 18/7, BHCSA circular CSA, 1949.
22 LHSA, LHB 1/18/4, The Royal Infirmary of Edinburgh, League of Subscribers, Minute book, 13 July 1948, 31 August 1948, 2 September 1948.
23 *Ibid.*, 2 September 1948, 14 September 1948, 26 October 1948, 7 November 1948.
24 *Ibid.*, 19 November 1948, 28 November 1948.
25 *Ibid.*, 21 February 1949.
26 *Ibid.*, 27 March 1949; *Daily Express*, 28 March 1949.
27 *Daily Telegraph*, 12 January 1949.
28 BLPES, BHCSA 7/4, AGM, September 1947.

29 *Ibid.*
30 BLPES, BHCSA 3/10, John Dodd to Henry Lesser, 9 September 1948.
31 BLPES, BHCSA 18/10, Circular CSA 2/67.
32 BLPES, BHCSA 3/12, Report of a meeting of continuing contributory schemes, Folkestone, 2 October 1948.
33 PAAA, 'Firms not willing 1948', 30 April 1948.
34 BLPES, BHCSA 15/6, Summary of questionnaire having regard to the forthcoming implementation of the National Health Service Act 1946, February 1948; A. T. Page, *Pennies for health: the story of the British Hospitals Contributory Schemes Association* (Birmingham, 1949).
35 BrHCA Archive, BHCSA (1948), annual report, 1950; J. Higgins, *The business of medicine* (London, 1988), p. 47.
36 BLPES, BHCSA 3/12, J. Dodd, Thoughts engendered by a study of contributory scheme statistics, 1951–2.
37 Calculated from Leeds and District Workpeople's Hospital Fund, annual reports, by dividing income from contributors by average contributions. Copies of the Fund's annual reports are held in Leeds Central Library.
38 This discussion is based on our analysis of annual reports of several surviving schemes; fuller details are available from the authors.
39 E. Mossialos and S. Thomson, 'Voluntary health insurance in the European Union: a critical assessment', *International Journal of Health Services*, 32 (2002), pp. 18–88, at p. 24.
40 TNA: PRO, BS 6756, BHCSA (1948), Ninth annual general meeting, Manchester, Appendix 2, pp. 4–5.
41 Higgins, *The business of medicine*, p. 32.
42 P. Maskell, *The best of health: 130 years of BHSF 1873–2003* (Birmingham, 2003), p. 34 (available online at www.bhsf.co.uk, last accessed February 2006).
43 Bristol Medical Institutions Contributory Scheme, annual report, 1931, p. 9; the surplus on the Section II fund went to the hospitals, so it remained integral to the parent scheme.
44 Bristol Contributory Scheme Welfare Association, annual report, 1937, p. 8.
45 M. Wren, *BCWA: Half a century of service* (Bristol, 1985), pp. 5, 13.
46 BLPES, BHCSA 3/12, Study of hospital contributory scheme statistics, 1951/52.
47 C. Webster, *The health services since the war, vol. I* (London, 1988), pp. 179–80.
48 TNA: PRO, MH 99/94, BHCSA, Background notes for minister: history of the contributory schemes movement and the Association, n.d. but 1962, p. 2.
49 Letter to *The Times*, 5 May 1951.
50 BLPES, BHCSA 3/12, How far should the contributory scheme movement attempt to fill gaps in the NHS?, Report of discussion at the 1952 (Cardiff) conference of the BHCSA.
51 *Ibid.*
52 P. Green, 'What's in a name? A study of Bolton and District Hospital Saturday Fund', unpublished MBA dissertation, Bolton Institute (2001), p. 146.
53 TNA: PRO, MH 99/94, BHCSA, Background notes, pp. 3–4.
54 TNA: PRO, MH 99/94, Note on convalescence for the minister's address to the conference of the BHCSA, 19 October 1962, pp. 1–2; *The Hospital*, 55 (11) (1959).
55 TNA: PRO, MH 99/94, Note on convalescence, pp. 2–3; MRO, M610 MED 2/3/2/2, The future of the Merseyside Hospitals Council, May 1947.
56 Leeds Central Library, Leeds and District Workpeople's Hospital Fund, annual reports, 1955, 1974.
57 BLPES, BHCSA 18/9, Convalescence and after care sub-committee report, appendix 3 to circular CSA 61/1, 1961.
58 MRO, M610 MED 4/1, MHC, annual report, 1966.
59 TNA: PRO, MH 99/94, Note on convalescence, pp. 3–5.
60 P. Bridgen, 'Hospitals, geriatric medicine and the long-term care of elderly people, 1946–76', *Social History of Medicine*, 14 (2001), pp. 507–23, at pp. 516–17; J. Mohan, *Planning, markets and hospitals* (London, 2002), pp. 119–20, 139–40.

61 BrHCA Archive, BHCSA (1948), annual reports, 1969/70, 1973/74, 1982/83.
62 WHSA, Minutes of the 19th BHCSA (1948) AGM, 1967.
63 *Weston Mercury*, 4 March 2005, 'Members angry over Kewstoke sale' (see www.thewestonmercury.co.uk/archived_material/2005/week_09/news/asp/05-03-04Sale.asp, last accessed February 2006)
64 Leeds Central Library, Leeds and District Workpeople's Hospital Fund, annual reports.
65 Laing and Buisson, *Health cash plans: UK market sector report 2000* (London, 2003).
66 Scheme statistics are compiled from: BLPES, BHCSA 18/7, Thoughts engendered by a study of hospital contributory scheme statistics 1951/52; BLPES, BHCSA 3/12, AGM 1955, Hospital contributory scheme statistics 1953/54; BLPES, BHCSA 18/8, The state of the movement: hospital contributory scheme statistics 1954/56, appendix to CSA 57/3, p. 33; WHSA, Reports of BHCSA AGM, 1956, 1982, 1988; BLPES, BHCSA 18/9, J. Dodd, Summary of the state of the movement 1962: popularity of benefits; BHCSA, annual reports, 1950–81, 1987/88; Laing and Buisson, *Health cash plans*; PMI: Office of Health Economics, *Compendium of health statistics* (London, 2001).
67 BrHCA Archive, BHCSA (1948), annual report, 1963/64.
68 MRO, M610 MED 4/1 MHC, annual report, 1960; PAAA, annual report, 1960; WHSA, SHC, annual report, 1960.
69 BrHCA Archive, BHCSA (1948), annual report, 1970/71
70 WHSA, BHCSA (1948), Minutes of the AGM, Southport, 1965
71 BLPES, BEV VII 4, BHCSA (1948), State of the movement, 1962.
72 PAAA, annual reports.
73 Higgins, *The business of medicine*, ch. 3; M. Calnan, S. Cant and J. Gabe, *Going private: why people pay for their health care* (Buckingham, 1993), pp. 2–18; C. Propper and A. Eastwood, *The reasons for non-corporate private health insurance purchase in the UK* (York, 1989), pp. 12–15.
74 Office of National Statistics, *General household survey* (London, various dates).
75 PAAA, Executive council minutes of meetings, January 1950; Leeds Central Library, Leeds and District Workpeople's Hospital Fund, annual reports, 1957, 1958; BLPES, BHCSA 18/8, AGM, 1956/57, p. 10.
76 BrHCA Archive, BHCSA (1948), annual report, 1963/64, p. 12.
77 BrHCA Archive, BHCSA (1948), annual report, 1967/68; BLPES, BCHSA 18/10, BHCSA circular CSA 2/67, October 1967.
78 BrHCA Archive, BHCSA (1948), annual report, 1971/72.
79 BrHCA Archive, BHCSA (1948), annual reports, 1970/71, 1974/75.
80 BrHCA Archive, BHCSA (1948), annual report, 1987/88, Reports from affiliated schemes, p. 14; British Health Care Association, annual reports, 2000, 2003.
81 BrHCA Archive, BHCSA (1948), annual reports, 1983/84, 1984/85.
82 BrHCA Archive, BHCSA (1948), annual report, 1975/76.
83 BrHCA Archive, BHCSA (1948), annual reports, 1979/80, 1980/81.
84 BrHCA Archive, Executive committee minutes, 14 December 1989.
85 *Family Resources Survey 2000–1* (London, 2002), cited in G. Orros, *The NHS Plan – Health cash plans for older people* (Canterbury, 2002) (available online at http://66.249.93.104/search?q=cache:U_u6aJOPoa0J:www.futurestudies.co.uk/communications/infocus/200.pdf+%22george+orros%22&hl=en, last accessed February 2006).
86 Laing and Buisson, *Health cash plans*.
87 Green, 'What's in a name?', p. 194.
88 Personal communication.
89 BLPES, BEV VIII 4, State of the movement, 1962.
90 BLPES, BHCSA 18/8, Report of the expansion subcommittee, 1956.
91 BLPES, BHCSA 18/8, BHCSA (1948) AGM, 1956.
92 *Ibid.*
93 BrHCA Archive, BHCSA (1948), annual report, 1968; MRO, M610, MED7/1/4.
94 WHSA, BHCSA (1948), Report of AGM 1965, J. N. Briscoe.
95 *Ibid.*

96 BrHCA Archive, BHCSA (1948), annual report, 1976/77.
97 BrHCA Archive, BHCSA (1948), annual report, 1983/84.
98 BrHCA Archive, BrHCA, annual report, 1993/94.
99 BrHCA Archive, BHCSA (1948), annual report, 1986/87.
100 These estimates are based on a national survey provided by one of the cash plans.
101 Personal communication.
102 WHSA, BHCSA (1948), Minutes of the 17th AGM, Southport, 1965.
103 BrHCA Archive, BHCSA (1948), annual report, 1984/85.
104 Medicash (formerly Merseyside Health Benefits Council), annual report, 2001.
105 BrHCA Archive, letter to G. Waite, 15 June 1989.
106 M. Moran, 'The health-care state in Europe', *Environment and Planning C*, 10 (1992), pp. 77–90.

Chapter 10

The health cash plans and the new mutualism in health care

This chapter turns from an empirical examination of the schemes' post-1948 development to some broader considerations regarding their character and ethos, and to a discussion of both their present role and their potential role in the British welfare state. These questions are approached through an investigation of three issues. First, the extent to which the schemes have retained their distinctive orientation and social purpose since 1948 is considered. It is perhaps no surprise that they have lacked a conventional commercial instinct, given their idiosyncratic origins, structure and ethos, and the survivors have retained many features of their predecessors. They are non-profit organisations and, unlike private insurers, they have neither challenged the principle of a collective risk pool embodied in the NHS nor attempted to offer a superior alternative. The surviving schemes are distinguished by: their commitment to charitable activity and their support for the NHS; their reliance on voluntary participation in fundraising and governance; and their commitment to an ethos of mutualism. Second, the impact of social and economic change on the schemes is explored through consideration of the evolving product mix, the strategies used to promote the schemes' products, the importance of the schemes as aspects of occupational welfare, and the changing market structure. Third, the potential future of the schemes is discussed in relation to proposals for reform of the institutions and practices of the welfare state.

The ethos of the surviving schemes: charity, voluntarism and mutualism

Charitable status and fundraising for charitable purposes

The charitable *origins* of HCPs are indisputable, as they lie in the collection of funds for voluntary hospitals. Although pre-NHS subscribers almost certainly viewed scheme membership as a form of insurance, the schemes persisted in presenting themselves as charities, not least because if contributions were treated as 'gifts' to the hospital they were not liable for taxation. In the 1920s there were challenges from the Inland Revenue to the schemes, which wished to view them as insurance. However, it was established that the schemes should be regarded as charities for three principal reasons: their object was to raise money which would be used to support hospital activities; the alleviation of poor health, or the improvement of health, has been regarded as a legitimate charitable purpose for many years; and the mere fact of contribution did not entitle members to any benefits – funds raised were used solely to finance the hospitals.[1]

On the establishment of the NHS the BHCSA leadership was quick to argue for retention of charitable status and in fact the Association's constitution includes several charitable objectives as being defining characteristics of contributory schemes. It was acknowledged that the schemes were now operating in a different environment; John Dodd, joint secretary of the BHCSA, observed that the pre-NHS schemes had been a 'carefree movement' so far as solvency was concerned. Their task had simply been to maximise income and transfer it to hospitals. In contrast, the new movement was 'obliged to conduct its affairs on insurance principles'.[2]

After 1948 the Inland Revenue regarded some surviving schemes as having begun trading as insurers and they therefore faced taxation on their surpluses. In challenging this decision, the general arguments used by the schemes were essentially those on which they had relied in the 1920s. In addition, they were not trading to make a profit but instead were seeking to pool benefits arising as a result of the members' contribution income. The Inland Revenue argued that income spent in providing benefits for members could not be regarded as having been applied for charitable purposes only; a hospital contributory fund which offered mutual insurance without a 'requirement of poverty as a condition for receiving benefit' could not be charitable. An exemption was granted in relation to investment income, as long as that income was free to be applied to the provision of hospital and similar amenities. Concerns were also expressed that an expansion of the range of benefits provided (something which the schemes were contemplating in the 1950s in order to attract new custom) would undermine the 'dominant charitable purposes of the schemes'; people would be joining in expectation of private benefit. On these grounds, claims for charitable status were rejected.[3] Under the 1960 Charities Act the schemes' status as charities was formally removed, which prompted several to establish separate charitable trusts through which their giving was channelled and which were still liable for tax relief.[4] Some were also permitted to finance their convalescent homes through charitable trusts and thus retained some tax benefits for members.

What did the schemes' charitable work mean in practice? The NHS Act had restricted charitable effort in the NHS to the provision of amenities and comforts for hospital staff and patients, and to the furtherance of medical education.[5] Examples of amenities provided by the SHC in the early phase included radios, pianos and twenty-four televisions in time for the Coronation in 1953.[6] It also attracted the support of volunteers for its hospital cinema service and for the wrapping of Christmas presents donated by the scheme (14,000 such gifts were made in 1966).[7] In time, though, the amenities aspect of charity work gave way to systematic donation of grants to health and social service organisations and the provision of equipment to hospitals.

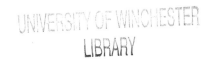

The evolution of such charitable activity over time is hard to gauge at a national level. One estimate was that from 1948 to 1983 the movement gave £7.4 million in charitable gifts.[8] However, there have been variations in the relative amounts committed by the different schemes and not all of them have operated charitable arms: in 1968, for example, only eighteen of the thirty funds affiliated to the BHCSA made charitable gifts out of contributory or invest-ment income.[9] Trends in charitable effort can be reconstructed by measuring the amounts given annually against overall income from contributions. In the early post-war years, charitable spending often represented at least 10 per cent of total income, but subsequent reductions reflect legal redefinitions (e.g. the declaration that providing convalescent homes was no longer a charitable activity). From the 1970s onwards the amounts committed were typically around 3 per cent or less of income, albeit with some variation around this general pattern.[10] The annual reports of the BrHCA for the mid-1990s show that an average of 1.6 per cent of income was committed to charitable causes.[11] This might be seen as a decline and therefore an indication of the distance which the HCPs have travelled from their voluntary roots. Alternatively, the sums involved are typically much larger, proportionately, than those committed by for-profit companies to charitable causes, where many large companies do not donate even 1 per cent of profits, let alone turnover.[12]

Some schemes extended their charitable activities by developing links with hospital leagues of friends (as originally envisaged by the BHA), acting as a 'rallying point' for such leagues and organising them into area associations. Thus the Merseyside Health Benefits Council had run an area association since the mid-1950s, while in Cardiff a scheme had 'sponsored the growth of leagues in Wales'. The picture was uneven, however; in some areas there was very close association between schemes and the leagues of friends, while elsewhere there was virtually no connection.[13] For some, charity was an impor-tant signifier of the schemes' identity; without it, warned Dodd, they were 'in danger of becoming cash mutual insurance societies, rather than voluntary social service organisations'.[14] Dodd wanted the schemes to emphasise their distinctive charitable role and suggested they form a national equivalent of London's King's Fund, with a large endowment for distribution to support the work of the NHS; he wished to call it the Queen's Fund, though this proposal never got beyond the speculative stage.[15]

One final point to note, in respect of corporate social responsibility, relates to the support received from employers in the form of donations. The role of matching contributions from employers in the pre-NHS era was noted in chapter 3; such contributions continued in the 1950s but dwindled thereafter. On Merseyside, many companies initially continued their pre-war practice of matching donations equivalent to one-third of the contributions made by their workers and this accounted for 8 per cent of the scheme's income in the early 1950s. By the late 1960s the equivalent was under 3 per cent, in 1982 approximately 1 per cent and by 1999 it equated to under 0.1 per cent of income.[16] The available data do not allow us to determine whether this decline represents an erosion of corporate social responsibility or whether it simply reflects the growth of company-paid schemes. If this is the case, the nature of the employer contribution is subtly different: a donation to a charitable cause on the one hand, purchase of insurance for its employees on the other.

Voluntarism and participatory structures

The schemes also retained their reliance on voluntary effort in raising their own funds, but this has been a victim of social and technological change. The HSA, for example, still had some 10,700 local groups in the mid-1960s, and Birmingham had several hundred, served by volunteer collectors, but this is no longer the case. Although some schemes retain voluntary workplace representatives, their role is now simply as a point of contact rather than as a collector of funds.[17] Contemporary methods of recruitment and payment (direct mail shots, direct debits and the Internet) have largely eliminated the traditional role of group secretaries. Changing urban form is another reason – the declining population of large cities combined with lower-density residential developments made the job of local group secretaries much more demanding. Aspects of this are regretted by those with decades of involvement, who recall the role played by group secretaries in their communities.[18] Moreover, reliance on voluntary effort had restrained costs, which was helpful in terms of convincing potential supporters of their value *vis-à-vis* commercial insurance companies.[19] However, as it became harder to replace volunteer collectors, costs rose relative to income. In 1973, for example, it was pointed out that the average ratio of benefits to income had dropped from 81 per cent to 75 per cent and that this would make it 'difficult to show convincingly that we provide better value for money than our commercial competitors.'[20]

Another distinctive aspect of the early continuing schemes was their claim to be patients' organisations. On the one hand, this involved the retention of pre-war structures of member participation, whereby branch associations of contributors elected representatives to scheme management committees, so that grassroots opinion influenced policy. On the other, it meant the service of scheme officials on NHS bodies. In relation to the first point, social change and a declining appetite for participation have reduced direct involvement in the governance of the schemes; as was frankly acknowledged at the 1973 AGM of the BHCSA: 'we live in a materialistic world and the first question a potential contributor asks is "what do I get out of it?"'[21] In short, new recruits were not aware of the movement's history and were largely joining for pragmatic reasons, and this situation is not without parallels from the pre-NHS era (see the evidence for this in chapters 5 and 6). As a consequence, annual meetings, which had at one time attracted several hundred contributors, were by the new millennium being attended by only a small number of committed individuals. In relation to the second point, the role of the schemes as a democratic forum for patients was undermined by NHS structures, which had removed agreements for scheme representation on hospital boards (see chapter 8). Despite such setbacks, the BHCSA consistently urged the schemes to develop relationships with hospitals and health authorities, and warned that if they were seen as being concerned only with the interests of their member-ship they could not expect to be given a voice in NHS governance. There were occasional signs of government encouragement – for example, Iain Macleod (Conservative Minister of Health, 1952–55) suggested a role for the schemes as patients' associations that would help patients negotiate pathways through the health and social care system.[22] It was noted that sixty members of con-tributory schemes were on NHS authorities in 1970, which suggested that efforts had been made to take on this role.[23]

Declining participation has prompted organisational restructuring but governance structures have also been streamlined in response to perceptions of inefficiency. For example, the Sheffield scheme introduced a reform of its committee structures in 1974 and renamed itself the Westfield Contributory Health Scheme. Its contributors' association, which had existed since 1921, was wound up, as were the regional committees in Barnsley, Rotherham and Chesterfield. This was prompted by the unwieldy and bureaucratic nature of the organisation; the scheme's central council had over 100 members, a relic of its elaborate and highly democratic pre-war structure of governance. In recent years a further motivation for such reorganisations has been regulatory demands for appropriate corporate governance structures, and the BrHCA annual reports record several instances of organisational reform.[24] This suggests that the role of the contributor in formal governance structures has been reduced. This does not mean that efforts are not made to involve subscribers; in some HCPs there are efforts to consult a sample of the membership through panel surveys, while others retain a small number of voting members and permit other contributors to attend (but not vote at) AGMs. In contrast with, say, building societies, however, large-scale exercises in democracy such as voting at AGMs are not practised because of the cost in relation to the overall income of the schemes.

Mutualism

A third example of the shifting boundary between mutualism and competition is provided by the fate of the so-called 'gentleman's agreement' under which schemes agreed not to canvass or advertise in the territory of another BHCSA-affiliated scheme. Territorial disputes were still in evidence among surviving schemes after the establishment of the NHS, such as complaints about the HSA using its links with the railways to recruit in Yorkshire.[25] The gentleman's agreement was the response; it appears to have dated from 1955, when the BHCSA's executive committee expressed 'strong disapproval of competition between schemes and of disturbance by any other scheme "in possession" in any one contributing establishment'.[26] The schemes saw themselves as a move-ment which had 'eschewed cut-throat competition' and 'had tried to operate on a territorial basis unlike the provident movement'.[27] While private medical insurers and schemes which were not affiliated to the post-1948 BHCSA (such as the Hospital Saturday Fund) competed for business nationally, the agreement was intended to maintain a fraternal spirit by delimiting spheres of operation and by the development of regional groupings. There were certainly echoes here of pre-war efforts at voluntary cooperation. Some suggested that this informal agreement had been beneficial: a 1962 survey argued that 'the advantages and disadvantages of monopoly versus competition' had been 'happily resolved' by the general principle of 'not actively canvassing business in each other's territories, but leaving the consumers with free choice'.[28] Arguably, though, the problems of competition could not really be dealt with by informal agreements of this nature. In the West Midlands, for example, the proximity of several small schemes meant that contributors could easily switch between them in response to changes in benefit offerings. As Dodd acknowledged in 1967, 'the public must be free to choose' and they 'must be allowed to continue in the scheme chosen without regard to residence'.[29]

The agreement came under pressure when, with evidence of declining membership, the need to boost recruitment made the maintenance of restrictive practices problematic. Indeed, one view was that the area boundaries of the agreement were 'perpetuating the inefficient at the expense of the public', since the latter were not being offered the option of HCP benefits.[30] At its 1969 AGM the BHCSA's president deplored restrictions imposed 'by imaginary geographical considerations'.[31] The meeting then terminated the agreement with a resolution that 'the more progressive schemes may develop wherever practicable or desirable without regard to geographical location after giving due notice to and consultation with any local scheme'.[32] This rather half-hearted acceptance of competition led only to further tensions, as in 1979, when the Worcester scheme complained that the Wolverhampton association was advertising in its area and canvassing local firms. The BHCSA's president explained that the terms of the gentleman's agreement (which had in fact been formally terminated a decade earlier) were such that no scheme 'deliberately poached upon another scheme's preserve'.[33] Thus, the spirit of the agreement still acted as a brake on full-blooded competition. As late as 1988 a row developed over the plans of one of the largest schemes to hold countrywide 'road shows'. Its assertion that European competition rules made the gentleman's agreement illegal was met with the protest that 'there was more than legality to consider within the movement', though in the event such objections did not carry the day. It was felt that the movement would be better served if its message and products were pushed effectively everywhere, not merely within 'arbitrary geographical limits'.[34] The idea of the gentleman's agreement fits very well with Halsey's definition of mutualism as a 'sense of common citizenship which leads people not to press their claims for liberty too far and to agree on a certain amount of basic equality of condition', albeit transposed to an organisational level.[35] The schemes thereby agreed to restrain competitive tendencies for the greater good, but in the long term this agreement could not withstand external pressures.

The ideals of mutualism clearly remain important to the public face of the HCPs, as is evident on their websites and in advertising and promotional literature, in the form of references to their history, mutual status and social purpose.[36] However, consideration of charitable giving, democratic structures and the gentleman's agreement suggests that these features are rather less in evidence than was formerly the case. Charitable giving is important to the public face of the schemes but is in quantitative terms less significant than in the past, though the amounts given compare favourably with corporate donations elsewhere in the economy. Large-scale participation and voluntary involvement, such as collection of subscriptions by volunteers, have fallen victim to social and techno-logical change. In addition, developments such as direct debit have superseded this way of gathering subscriptions. Structures to facilitate mass participation have largely disappeared and it is not clear how the surviving schemes might act as patients' associations (as was once envisaged by the BHCSA during the 1950s). Finally, while the schemes' roots in providing low-cost health insurance remain important (as shown in chapter 9), other aspects of mutualism, such as restrictions on competition, have gone. This raises the question of how schemes are responding to contemporary social change and competitive pressures, and of how such developments are affecting the structure of the market.

Social change, competition, diversification and consolidation

There have been a number of external influences on the development of the HCPs. Aside from government NHS policy, which has affected the niche they occupy and the demand for their products, the schemes have long been aware of the threat posed by for-profit insurers. Indeed, as early as 1948 William Newstead had warned that, unless the schemes presented a united front, com-mercial insurers would enter the marketplace.[37] They have also had to respond to recruitment difficulties and membership losses from the 1970s, and to rising prosperity and demand for new services. There has been diversification into new product areas, market segmentation, and careful attention to marketing themselves in an era in which traditional appeals have less purchase.

The appeal of their products is that they offer a way of obtaining assistance with NHS charges, or a means of accessing services which are provided by the NHS but for which there is a lengthy waiting list (physiotherapy and so on). Free NHS optical and dental treatment is now available only for those exempt from charges (on account of their age or unemployment, for example) and this, combined with the growth in demand for services such as physiotherapy and complementary therapies, may explain why some providers have dropped the title 'cash plans' in favour of terms such as 'everyday health plans', 'health care essentials' or 'low-cost health plan'.[38] This rhetoric signals the widespread acceptance that some services are available on the NHS only via a lengthy waiting list, and/or that some health care expenditures are a very frequent occurrence. Marketing is also predicated on a widespread public perception that the NHS is in permanent difficulty. Thus, despite steady growth in NHS expenditure, one can still find references to the 'reducing availability of free immediate treatment on the NHS'.[39] The 'everyday health care essentials' covered by HCPs include the traditional 'teeth and spectacles' benefits, various complementary therapies and now an expanding set of benefits concerned with health screening, private consultations and a range of help-lines. Some schemes have even taken the lead in establishing one-stop providers of the various services covered by the HCPs, as in the One Stop Medical Centre provided by Mercia (formerly the Coventry scheme), and Wakefield's complementary therapy centre, thereby renewing a direct link between funding and provision which had disappeared after 1948.[40]

The schemes have also moved up-market, progressively eliminating their cheapest rates of cover (while allowing long-time contributors to continue at rates of contribution now barred to new entrants) so that a greater range of benefits can be offered in return for larger premiums. The boundary between HCPs and PMI has therefore become blurred; for example, some HCPs offer cover for private consultations, which historically was deplored as likely to lead to queue jumping, although the total number of private consultations funded by the HCPs, at around 200,000 per annum, is small relative to the total numbers receiving private hospital treatment.[41] There is now some overlap in price between the more expensive monthly family plans offered by the HCPs and the cheaper PMI products,[42] and a related overlap in services covered, such as various forms of diagnostic and screening services.[43] The future may see a move in both directions, with private medical insurers seeking to extend their social base through the cash plan market while the HCPs target those who they feel are able to purchase PMI. Symbolising this, there has recently been a merger between HSA, the largest HCP, and the Bristol Contributory Welfare Association, a provider of private health insurance.[44]

Consistent with wider social trends there is evidence of market segmentation in the products offered by the HCPs. There are products targeted at particular groups in the population (singles, over-fifties and amateur sports players), 'stand-alone' plans offering one specific benefit (e.g. physiotherapy, dental or optical treatment, or in-patient benefits) and customised plans for individual companies. Such segmentation is designed to respond to perceptions of particular risks, but this might be contrasted with the generalised notion of social responsibility, if not civic duty, which was used to motivate individuals to contribute to the pre-war schemes. A recent commentary on marketing efforts suggested that subscribers are no longer attracted by messages which stress the apparent complementarity between HCPs and the NHS. Instead, 'most people are more preoccupied with obtaining value-for-money in the pursuit of self-preservation than they are with ethical considerations'.[45]

In addition to direct marketing targeted at individuals, advertising and promotional activities addressed to companies are of growing significance. There is an emphasis on the complementarity between the plans and PMI, with firms offering PMI to senior staff and making HCP coverage available to a broader spectrum of their workforce. The additional cost of adding HCP coverage to company-paid PMI is not large. HCP products are advertised as an element of occupational welfare which are an attractive recruitment perk and which can be used by employers to minimise their exposure to risk (advocates suggest that, in the face of 'increasing pressures of stress and health-related absence on businesses', if employees can go direct to a health care professional without the need for a referral from a general practitioner, this will minimise their time off work).[46] The HCP products cover those hazards of the modern workplace up to a defined limit, which is related to the premium paid, so part of the cost of such treatment may be borne by the employee. Marketing literature also implies that such policies can be an 'affordable and focussed risk management tool' which helps respond to demands from employers' liability insurers for programmes designed to cope with stress in the workplace.[47]

Farnsworth's analysis of occupational social provision has pointed to the ambivalent place occupied by such benefits: they contribute to the maximisation of profits by enhancing loyalty and reducing staff turnover, but they are also of direct benefit to workers by meeting basic physical needs for treatment.[48] As a result of these developments, there is evidence that the balance between individual and company-paid schemes appears to be shifting again in favour of the latter. For example, over 50 per cent of new entrants to the Westfield scheme in 2001–2 had their premiums paid for by their employers,[49] and a recent estimate suggests that although the employer-paid group market accounts for only 15 per cent of HCP contributors, it has recently experienced annual growth rates of 8–10 per cent.[50] This is a reversal of the situation in the 1970s and 1980s, when industrial decline led to a rapid loss of group subscriptions and there was alarm at the difficulty of recovering losses in membership by recruiting individuals.[51]

Socioeconomic changes have also weakened the historic connections between schemes and their localities of origin. This has been viewed as inevitable: 'firm mergers, migration, and nationalised industries' have made 'a nonsense of artificial boundaries'.[52] The decline of territorial restrictions on recruitment has already been noted. In addition, by 1971, five schemes had eliminated references to their place of origin; for example, the Wolverhampton scheme was renamed the Patients' Aid Association (and subsequently PayCare), while that in Bedford became the Provincial Hospital Services Fund. Such manoeuvres were designed to give the impression of a 'wider sphere of operation'.[53] Subsequent similar changes include the renaming of the Sheffield as the Westfield scheme, Coventry and Warwickshire Hospitals Fund as Mercia Health Benefits, and the Bradford scheme, which became known as Sovereign HealthCare from 1986.

Such geographical connections have been further loosened in recent years by several strategic mergers or absorptions of small schemes by larger ones; examples from the past decade include, but were not confined to, those between the HSA and the Leeds scheme; schemes based in Manchester and in Northampton; the Birmingham and Hull schemes; and Westfield (Sheffield) and schemes in Nottingham and Cornwall. Are such developments consistent with an ideal of mutuality? One inference may be that the aim was to extend the sphere of influence of the larger partner, even though the schemes may continue to operate under their own names. An alternative view is that the larger schemes have stepped in to ensure that the contributory scheme movement retains its distinctive character rather than having schemes swallowed up by commercial organisations. As some of the schemes absorbed in this way had as few as 2,000 contributors, it is implausible that they were taken over purely for reasons of market share. On several occasions large schemes have been approached by small ones to try to ensure their survival.[54] This is not interpretable as aggressive, predatory behaviour by the larger partner. Overall, it is fair to say that HCPs are no longer so closely identified with particular communities in the way that was undoubtedly the case with their ancestors. An illustration of this is provided by HSA's sponsorship (until 2005) of Blackburn Rovers Football Club, a club some 250 miles from HSA's headquarters in Andover, Hampshire, or its pre-NHS base in London. There are exceptions to the rule, such as the Bolton scheme, which retains a largely local base.

Regardless of the origin of such mergers and takeovers, recent changes in the HCP sector lend weight to the view, expressed by the trade journal *Health Care Market News* in 2002, that 'the time for the smaller funds looks now to have run out' as a result of competition.[55] The sector is now attracting interest from for-profit commercial cash plan providers, established in most cases by large general insurance companies but with some direct involvement by high street retailers, whose established customer bases provide them with a platform from which to make what the BrHCA described as 'aggressive inroads' into the HCP market.[56] Examples include major general insurers such as Norwich Union, Royal and Sun Alliance, and Standard Life, followed more recently by AXA PPP, and Legal and General. Retail chains are also developing and marketing cash plan products. However, traffic is not all one way, as some of the HCPs are diversifying into products like travel and personal accident insurance.[57]

Where do all these developments in the marketplace leave the remaining non-profit HCPs? For now, the surviving contributory schemes still retain over 80 per cent of the HCP market, with HSA and Westfield accounting between them for 55 per cent of market share.[58] However, the entry of commercial organisations may erode the market position of mutuals, much as was the case when commercial hospital providers moved into private hospital provision in Britain in the 1980s, largely at the expense of the undercapitalised charitable hospital sector. In terms of products, the schemes seem to engage in the processes of differentiation and segmentation that are common in the rest of the insurance sector, while in terms of marketing strategies the HCPs state that they enable individuals or companies to take prudential steps to minimise their exposure to certain kinds of risk. In contrast to the schemes' origins, this does not involve paying into a common fund for the collective good, though it could be argued that a degree of prudential self-interest (the desire to restore workers to employability) also informed company support for the schemes in the pre-NHS era.

The status of the schemes: the new mutualism and the reconstruction of welfare institutions

For government and regulatory bodies, there has always been some confusion about the status and identity of the schemes: are they primarily insurance companies or are they community-based voluntary organisations with strong charitable features? This question has a long history, but it is highly relevant today because there have been renewed questions about the charitable status of HCPs and because of debates about the role of mutuals in a reconstructed welfare state. The HCPs are regarded as examples of voluntary health insurance[59] and a pertinent question here is whether the scope for such insurance in Britain is likely to expand, which in turn will depend on changes in NHS policy.

Following the 1997 election, the Labour government sought to regulate the selling of financial services via the Financial Services Authority, which brought in new and, from the perspective of the surviving contributory schemes, necessary but potentially onerous compliance requirements designed to protect consumers against the mis-selling of financial products. The recent closure or merger of some schemes may in part reflect the cost of compliance with these new regulations, and pro-mutualists such as Birchall have questioned what is seen as the somewhat heavy-handed approach of the government.[60] Perhaps more germane here, however, is the present government's determination to level the financial services playing field. Ironically, this may threaten the HCPs if allowance is not made for their particular character. A paradoxical consequence is that while the government is seeking to expand the scope for what are claimed to be community-based and mutual forms of ownership in one area (e.g. via NHS Foundation Trusts), it may be restricting it in another.

A good example of the difficulties which have arisen relates to a decision by the Inland Revenue in 2000 that some HCPs could no longer be exempt from tax on surpluses from contributions, on the grounds that they could no longer be regarded as mutuals. To qualify for this exemption, their members had to have voting control and to be entitled to a share of any surpluses should the scheme be wound up. Some HCPs could not comply with these regulations because their constitutions required that, if the fund was wound up, its assets would be transferred to another institution with the same objects or charitable purposes; they further stipulated that contributors were specifically not entitled to voting rights at AGMs. These rules had been designed, in the pre-NHS era, to ensure that local hospitals continued to exist for the benefit of the many (those living in the area served) rather than the few (those who happened to be members of a contributory scheme at any point in time). There is an interesting parallel here with the NHS Foundation Trusts, whose members do not have complete voting control (though they elect some of the board), nor do they have an entitlement to a share of surplus assets. Yet these Trusts have been presented as examples of a new mutualism in public policy, even though they do not appear to pass the tests of mutuality applied by the Inland Revenue to other organisations.

Arguments deployed against the Inland Revenue were therefore that while schemes might not strictly be characterised as mutual organisations, their objectives had remained consistent and they were still pursuing their historic social goals. The option of converting to a legal status that the Inland Revenue would recognise as mutual was available, but this would be costly and run the risk that, at some future date, there might be proposals for demutualisation. Conversion was therefore thought likely to inhibit the ability of some HCPs to offer services to people on low incomes. Those aspects of their constitution that were consistent with the broader social purpose of the schemes were now the ones posing difficulties for the Inland Revenue. Correspondence from the government revealed that the review of mutual status had apparently been prompted by 'recent market developments', which the Inland Revenue could not wilfully ignore, as to do so would have been unfair to non-mutual organisations. The irony was clear: it could be argued that the effect of a technical adjustment in tax policy was to place mutual HCPs on the same footing as shareholder-owned companies, at a time when support for mutuals might have been thought to be more in tune with government thinking. What was also ironic was the timing: these discussions about tax status were proceeding while the government was launching its much-vaunted 'new mutualism' in health care through the creation of NHS Foundation Trusts. The Inland Revenue's proposals drew some limited parliamentary condemnation, in the form of an Early Day Motion, signed by some sixty MPs from all parties, which argued that such decisions would undermine the valuable work of HCPs, reduce charitable giving and contradict the government's policy of supporting self-help and voluntarism, while raising premiums. These representations failed to have any effect.[61]

It could be suggested, however, that the government actually had little alternative. European competition law prevents preferential treatment of one type of insurer over another. Furthermore, the Blair government has generally not demonstrated strong objections to the pro-competition legislation from the European Union which was designed to liberalise the service sector, so its apparent indifference in this context is unsurprising.[62] Thus, while the government was extolling the virtues of mutualisation in the NHS it was taking no particular steps to protect the position of established forms of community-based, not-for-profit providers of low-cost health insurance products.

Turning to future developments, the scope for the HCPs will to a degree be set, as it has been since 1948, by the parameters of NHS policy. The present government has substantially increased spending on the NHS, in the belief that the centralised, tax-funded model offers the most equitable way of paying for a national service. One would expect some growth in the HCPs, resulting from rising prosperity and from the difficulties of accessing some NHS services (e.g. dentistry), though as and when increased NHS capacity comes on stream it might be expected to dampen down demand for some of the HCPs' products. Furthermore, some of the government's own policies may provide scope for an extension of voluntary health insurance in ways which have parallels with other health care systems. For example, there is a strong emphasis on choice and consumerism, with the government arguing that this is not incompatible with the aims of the NHS. Ministers are sanguine about the effects of patient choice on the fate of hospitals, and their emphasis on extending choice to all could be read as a response to the challenge of the private sector's marketing devices, which routinely refer to the 'personal' – as opposed to 'national' – health service. The assumption so far is that such extensions of choice would be within the framework of a NHS free at the point of use, with relatively little scope for co-payments for health services. This contrasts with various continental states where the proportion of funds generated by such charges is significantly greater.

However, critics argue that the government's preferred scenario for a patient-led and market-driven NHS is a 'policy roadmap that can only lead to user charges', [63] and if this prediction proves correct, the result would undoubtedly be to open up greater scope for the HCPs to develop products which would insure patients against such charges. The reasoning underpinning such arguments is that the government has let the genie of patient choice out of the bottle, without any way of reining in the consequent increased demands for services, and that these pressures (combined with others, such as rising drugs bills) will render additional sources of finance inevitable. Several think-tanks, such as Civitas and the Adam Smith Institute, use such arguments in support of their view that the only way to save the NHS is to diversify it; they advocate charging for non-core services and they propose that such charges could be covered by self-payment or through supplementary insurance.[64] Discussion of co-payment for services has also featured in the work of think-tanks such as the New Economics Foundation.[65] There is a sense of *déjà vu* about some of this discussion. The contributory schemes were originally designed to cover the costs of maintenance in hospital – the assumption being that the medical care received was provided *gratis*. There have periodically been debates about the possibility of 'hotel charges' for in-patients, for example in discussions of wartime proposals (chapter 7), though these were rejected then and subsequently – even by hawkish Conservative Cabinets in the 1950s.[66] There have always been problems defining the boundary between NHS-funded (and free) health care, on the one hand, and social care funded (and means tested) by local authorities or national social security.[67] The issue is how and where to draw the line. As well as a distinction between core and non-core services, the possibility has also been canvassed of moving towards a social insurance model, in which individuals could opt for several different levels of cover, permitting them to obtain treatment in a range of settings.[68] All such proposals would open up much greater scope for supplementary charges than is currently permitted under the NHS, and this would lead to a much more differentiated NHS than currently exists.[69] In such a scenario, the surviving contributory schemes could develop products which insured individuals against fees for supplementary services, going beyond their present product offerings (cash benefits) but stopping short of fully fledged private insurance. Arguably this would not be without parallels with the role played by the schemes in the pre-NHS era, when treatment was free and the schemes paid for maintenance. Such proposals might well open up new markets for health care products and thereby lead to considerable expansion by the HCPs, but it is not clear that they would revive mutuality, since the attraction to individuals would not extend beyond the rather instrumentalist concerns of obtaining supplementary services.

Conclusion

The surviving contributory schemes initially conceived of themselves as carrying forward a tradition of voluntary sector activity, and a residue of goodwill and habit enabled them to retain and rebuild membership, helped by the rapid development of an attractive benefit package. This was founded on the hospital patient cash grant and optical and dental benefits, and these eventually came to form the core business of the schemes. The HCPs sought to retain a distinctive ethos through their philanthropic work, their representative procedures and their sense that they belonged to a movement characterised by mutualist rather than competitive values. The evidence that they sought to maintain faith with their low-income clientele is also relevant here. By the 1970s, however, the ethos of the schemes was under threat. Doubts were voiced about their public profile and social appeal, more business-like decision-making arrangements were adopted, the relative importance of charitable activity declined, and territorial restrictions on recruitment were gradually loosened. These changes halted the decline in membership, so that by the end of the century, with some 3 million contributors, the movement enjoyed a similar level of support to that which it received in the early 1950s. However, the schemes had not succeeded in sharing in the boom which PMI had experienced in the 1970s and 1980s (see figure 9.2), and they are still searching for a way of tapping significant new markets for their products. At the same time competitive pressures have been exacerbated by the entry of for-profit insurers into the HCP market.

Given these trends, what is the position of HCPs in relation to contemporary debates about and developments in the welfare state? Social changes such as rising prosperity, a more consumerist attitude to public services, and the rolling-back of the state have led commentators to suggest that more of a 'pick and mix' approach to welfare may figure in the future. Diversity and consumer choice will be promoted through provision from the public, private and non-profit sectors.[70] There might be several reasons why HCPs would be attractive in this scenario. One reason relates to trends in the labour market towards self-employment and greater flexibility, which mean that more social risks are met individually; for companies, likewise, HCPs are marketed as ways of minimising or externalising risks, such as those associated with short-term absences from work. Such perks may also aid recruitment in tight labour markets. However, it is difficult to see the schemes as the basis of a revival of mutualism, since HCP policies are marketed as ways in which individuals or companies can insure against individual or corporate risk, rather than to contribute to a common fund. This is particularly so given that some schemes contain many thousands of members spread over large areas; this poses the challenge of restoring the 'sense of involvement which mutuals used to provide when they were small and based in real geographical communities.'[71]

It is somewhat ironic, then, that the government's 'new mutualism' policy discourse has emerged when some elements of mutualism in health care are rather less in evidence than was historically the case; consumerism in the public services does not extend much beyond a desire to maximise individual or family advantage.[72] Evidence on social attitudes to the surviving schemes is lacking and it is therefore difficult to comment on whether mutuality is important to their individual subscribers. While it is possible to demonstrate the social benefits of mutual organisations,[73] it is not clear from marketing rhetoric that the ideal of mutualism per se is important to those taking out subscriptions to HCPs.

At the same time as the government is opening up opportunities, regulation will affect the development of the schemes. A tighter regulatory environment exists than was the case for much of the post-war era. The advent of the Financial Services Authority, the Financial Ombudsman and the General Insurance Standards Council has ushered in customer protection programmes. An emphasis on compliance with regulations is likely to increase the overheads of these mutual insurance companies and to result in more mergers and ultimately fewer and larger HCPs, competing on a national basis for new subscribers in a market which is attracting interest from for-profit providers. Individual mutual schemes will therefore continue in existence, but it remains to be seen whether the notion of mutuality will survive in this environment.

Notes

1 TNA: PRO, BT 298/490, Church to de Keyser, 11 April 1949, summarises the history of these discussions in the 1920s.
2 BLPES, BHCSA 18/7, J. Dodd, Thoughts engendered by a study of hospital contributory schemes' statistics, 1951–52.
3 TNA: PRO, BT 298/490, contains several papers summarising these post-war discussions.
4 G. Palliser et al., *The charitable work of hospital contributory schemes* (Bristol, 1984), pp. 20–3.
5 J. Mohan and M. Gorsky, *Don't look back? Voluntary and charitable finance of health care in Britain, past and present* (London, 2001), pp. 91–5.
6 *Sheffield Forward*, July 1953.
7 WHSA, Sheffield and District Convalescent and Hospital Services Council, annual reports, 1950–68.
8 Palliser et al., *Charitable work*, p. 10.
9 BrHCA Archive, BHCSA (1948), annual report, 1968/69.
10 Our source for this is the annual reports of various schemes (anonymised).
11 BrHCA Archive, BrHCA, annual reports, *passim*.
12 According to research carried out by *The Guardian*, only thirty-four firms in the FTSE 100 gave more than 1 per cent of their profits to charitable causes (see http://business.guardian.co.uk/story/0,,1652384,00.html, last accessed February 2006). For a similar comparison, see J. Michie and J. Blay, *Mutuals and their communities* (London, 2004), p. 22.
13 BrHCA Archive, BHCSA (1948), annual report, 1969/70.
14 BrHCA Archive, Minutes of the 19th BHCSA AGM, 1967.
15 John Dodd, quoted in *British Hospital Journal and Social Service Review*, 25 November 1966.
16 Merseyside HBC/Medicash, annual reports.
17 BrHCA Archive, BHCSA, annual reports (HSA); BHSF, annual reports; personal communication from scheme officials.
18 Personal communication from two chief executives of surviving schemes.
19 BLPES, BHCSA 18/7, State of the movement, 1962.

20   BrHCA Archive, BHCSA, annual report, 1972/73.
21   BrHCA Archive, BHCSA (1948) AGM, Norwich, 1973.
22   *Hospital and Social Services Journal*, 7 October 1955.
23   BrHCA Archive, BHCSA (1948), annual report, 1970/71.
24   BrHCA Archive, BrHCA, annual reports, 1999, 2001.
25   TNA: PRO, MH 99/93, Dodd–Pater, 29 December 1953, 28 June 1954.
26   BLPES, BHCSA 18/8, Report of executive committee, 1955.
27   BLPES, BHCSA 18/10, BHCSA (1948) circular CSA 2/67, October 1967.
28   BLPES, BEV VII 4, BHCSA (1948), Survey of the state of the movement, 1962.
29   BLPES, BHCSA 18/10, BHCSA (1948) circular CSA 2/67, October 1967.
30   *Bradford Telegraph and Argus*, 22 March 1968.
31   BrHCA Archive, BHCSA (1948), annual report, 1969/70, President of BHCSA Sir
     Archibald MacDonald Gordon.
32   BrHCA Archive, BHCSA (1948), annual report, 1969/70, resolution at 1969 BHCSA
     conference.
33   BrHCA Archive, BHCSA (1948), Executive committee, 28 February 1979.
34   BrHCA Archive, BRHCA executive committee minutes, 14 April 1988.
35   A. H. Halsey, quoted in J. Birchall, *The new mutualism in public policy* (London, 2001),
     p. 8.
36   See, for example, P. Maskell, *The best of health: 130 years of BHSF 1873–2003* (Birmingham,
     2003) (available online at www.bhsf.co.uk, last accessed February 2006).
37   BLPES, BHCSA 6/8, Newstead, Memorandum accompanying minutes.
38   See the websites of various individual schemes, which can be found via the BrHCA web-
     site (www.bhca.org.uk, last accessed February 2006).
39   Health Insurance, *The guide to selling cash plans 2004* (available online at http://www.
     hi-mag.com/content/ipi/healthinsurance/images/supps/supp_cashplans.pdf, last accessed
     February 2006).
40   BrHCA Archive, BrHCA, annual reports (e.g. 1992/93, 1994/95).
41   Laing and Buisson, *Health cash plans: UK market sector report 2003* (London, 2003),
     table 3.1.
42   See the CareHealth website (www.carehealth.co.uk, last accessed February 2006) for
     illustrative figures.
43   Laing and Buisson, *Health cash plans*, table 3.1; G. Orros, *The NHS Plan – Health cash
     plans for older people* (2002) (available online at http://66.249.93.104/search?q=cache:
     U_u6aJOPoa0J:www.futurestudies.co.uk/communications/infocus/200.pdf+%22george
     +orros%22&hl=en, last accessed February 2006). Following a merger which was ongoing
     as this book was being finalised, HSA will be known as Simplyhealth.
44   See the HSA website (http://corporate.hsa.co.uk/news/newsitem.asp?articleID=1091,
     last accessed February 2006).
45   Health Insurance, *The guide to selling cash plans 2004*.
46   *Ibid.*
47   *Ibid.*
48   K. Farnsworth, 'Welfare through work: an audit of occupational social provision at the
     turn of the new century', *Social Policy and Administration*, 38 (2004), pp. 437–55, table 1.
49   'Keeping a healthy team', *Sheffield Star*, 3 July 2002.
50   Laing and Buisson, *Health cash plans*.
51   BrHCA Archive, BHCSA (1948), annual reports (e.g. 1975/76, 1984/85) (the latter
     refers to the 'unwelcome prospect of parity between individual and group members').
52   BrHCA Archive, BHCSA (1948), annual report, 1970/71.
53   BrHCA Archive, BHCSA, AGM, 1971.
54   BrHCA Archive, BHCSA (1948), annual reports, 1984/85, 1991/92.
55   *Health Care Market News*, 6 (10) (August–September 2002), p. 35.
56   BrHCA Archive, BrHCA, annual report, 1995/96.
57   Laing and Buisson, *Health cash plans*; Orros, *The NHS Plan*.
58   Laing and Buisson, *Health cash plans*.

59   E. Mossialos and S. Thomson, 'Voluntary health insurance in the European Union: a critical assessment', *International Journal of Health Services*, 32 (2002), pp. 19–88.
60   Laing and Buisson, *Health cash plans*; Birchall, 'New mutualism', pp. 1–3.
61   This discussion is based on information supplied by a scheme involved in these negotiations.
62   Mossialos and Thomson, 'Voluntary health insurance', p. 59; A. Pollock, *NHS plc: the privatisation of our health care* (London, 2004), pp. 60–2.
63   C. Donaldson and D. Ruta, 'Should the NHS follow the American way?', *British Medical Journal*, 331 (2005), pp. 1328–30.
64   Civitas Health Policy Consensus Group, *A new consensus for NHS reform* (London, 2003) (available online at www.civitas.org.uk/nhs/nhsMain.php, last accessed February 2006); N. Bosanquet, *A sustainable health service: from aspiration to delivery* (London, 1999); Mossialos and Thomson, 'Voluntary health insurance'.
65   E. Mayo and H. Moore, *The mutual state: how local communities can run public services* (London, 2002) (available online at www.neweconomics.org/gen/uploads/The%20Mutual%20State.pdf, last accessed February 2006).
66   C. Webster, 'Conservatives and consensus: the politics of the NHS, 1951–64', in A. Oakley and S. Williams (eds), *The politics of the welfare state* (London, 1994), pp. 54–74, at p. 62.
67   P. Bridgen and J. Lewis, *Elderly people and the boundary between health and social care, 1946–91: whose responsibility?* (London, 1999).
68   Civitas Health Policy Consensus Group, *A new consensus for NHS reform*.
69   Mossialos and Thomson, 'Voluntary health insurance', p. 81.
70   R. Klein and J. Millar, 'Do-it-yourself social policy', *Social Policy and Administration*, 29 (1995), pp. 303–16.
71   Birchall, *The new mutualism in public policy*, p. 244.
72   C. Needham, *Citizen-consumers: New Labour's marketplace democracy* (London, 2003).
73   J. Michie and J. Blay, *Mutuals and their communities* (London, 2004).

Chapter 11

Concluding comments

In the course of this project we had a range of reactions to the contributory schemes. One was admiration for the effort and commitment of the schemes and of key individuals within them. A second reaction, arising from the sheer heterogeneity of the schemes, was sympathy with the task facing those officials charged with reorganising the British health services in wartime: they faced the formidable challenge of trying to incorporate over 400 highly diverse schemes into a national structure and it is clear that they could find no practical way of doing this. A third reaction is frustration at the failure of the contributory schemes to act collectively and articulate a plausible alternative in the NHS debates, which meant that the option of preserving some of the attractive features of the movement in the post-war NHS was largely ruled off the agenda. In this brief final chapter we recapitulate the key findings of our work, discuss some pertinent parallels and precedents, and speculate on the prospects for the cash plans.

Key findings

This work shows the attractions and limitations of a form of funding premised on mass contribution by the potential users of the hospital service. The belief that workers' contributions represented a potential 'El Dorado' for hospitals proved to be overoptimistic, but the fact that, at their peak, some 11 million people were members of contributory schemes suggests the need for a reconsideration of their impact. First, the evidence of scheme foundations (chapter 2) suggested that the movement was not entirely a spontaneous manifestation of working-class support, since many initiatives were the product of local elites who recognised the limitations of other sources of funding and the need for diversification. Local circumstances also played their part, both in the formation of schemes and in their subsequent fortunes.

The impact of mass contribution on hospital finances was the subject of chapter 3. This endorsed the findings of Cherry's work, but significantly enhanced them by analysing the finances of a larger sample of hospitals at constant prices and by demonstrating some unintended consequences of mass contribution. It is very clear that the schemes increased demand for hospital services, reflected in rising hospital utilisation; as a result they were something of a mixed blessing. In addition, in some locations at least, this source of income could be unstable, though in truth many communities had little alternative, owing to the absence of a local philanthropic middle class. The schemes also changed the incentive structures facing hospitals and initial efforts were made to respond to this problem through reimbursement mechanisms. The judgement that the schemes had substantial beneficial effects on hospital finances is therefore tempered by an acknowledgement of these unintended consequences.

While significant progress was made in the inter-war period, there remained very substantial variations in scheme membership, and chapter 4 showed how rates of contribution and membership interacted to generate a highly uneven outcome. Had the NHS been based on workplace contributions, it is clear that the large regional disparities in economic performance in recent decades would have generated great variations in hospital funding, requiring substantial inter-regional transfers of resources.

Moreover, localism presented difficulties for cooperation and for the development of regional structures in which problems of competition for members might have been resolved. Such difficulties were sometimes overcome by voluntary cooperation, but acrimonious disputes also developed, and the schemes' national association was unable to resolve these, though (albeit late in the day) some regional committees did develop to address these challenges. Civil servants were therefore entirely correct to identify the variability in the movement, and its local patriotisms, as a major obstacle to reform.

These weaknesses are inherent in voluntarism, but its defenders might argue that they are outweighed by the value of voluntary organisations in providing vehicles for community participation. The schemes certainly recruited in great numbers, engaged in vigorous recruitment activities and developed links with a range of other religious, political and labour organisations to spread their message. On the face of it, therefore, they would appear to have assisted in the process of social capital formation (chapter 5). On closer examination, however, a different picture emerges. There was a disjuncture between the small coterie of committed activists and the mass membership, because social attitude surveys imply that pragmatic considerations were uppermost in the minds of most contributors; they subscribed because it was easy to do so (via workplaces) and because there was little alternative. Further, the schemes recruited from a particular – albeit large – section of the population (those in defined income bands) and they did not generally provide vehicles for the face-to-face associational activity which is held to play a key role in the formation of social capital, although some of the larger funds developed various sporting and social activities. And, crucially, the uneasy relationship between the schemes and the labour movement meant that they were unable to marshal trade union or Labour Party support once discussions began about the organisation of the post-war health services.

A further argument for voluntary provision relates to the participation of the consumer in shaping the delivery of services (chapter 6). There is some evidence that the schemes provided a voice for local concerns, but where such demands were at odds with the wishes of hospital elites they were typically ignored or bypassed. Contributors gained some concessions, for example in relation to the development of extra-hospital benefits, and perhaps the strongest evidence for consumerism was in defence of principles of open, free access to hospital treatment in some areas. This was, of course, the defining characteristic of the post-war NHS.

As the wartime negotiations on the shape of the NHS began, the schemes were playing an important role in hospital finance, but some key problems had not been resolved relating to their comprehensiveness; it was not obvious, therefore, that they could provide a firm basis for a national health service. These difficulties were compounded by their structural position in negotiations (chapters 7 and 8). Once the voluntary hospitals were guaranteed funding, they could afford to neglect the schemes, and it seems that the rhetoric connecting rights and duties had little purchase on decision-makers. Moreover, the schemes proved to be relatively ineffectual as a pressure group. They failed to make common cause with other interest groups and they adopted a relatively deferential approach in negotiations, perhaps reflecting a reluctance to rock the boat at a time of national crisis (not a characteristic shared by the BHA or BMA). They failed to articulate an alternative vision, for example about the need for consumer participation in the new service, and in this respect their policies lacked substance. And from an official perspective, the simplicity of a tax-funded system stood in stark contrast to the sheer heterogeneity of the several hundred contributory schemes.

Once the NHS was established, the scope for voluntary effort and voluntary insurance was unclear, despite supportive speeches from ministers. It is testament to the prominent position of some schemes in civic life, and the attachment of communities to them, that they retained a large membership in the 1950s. However, most of their strongholds in large northern industrial centres were also places vulnerable to post-war economic restructuring, and the consequent decline in membership forced organisational change, the abandonment of some aspects of mutualism and the development of a new product mix (chapters 9 and 10). Today, the democratic and participatory structures of the pre-NHS era are much less in evidence than was formerly the case; a sense of participation in a collective endeavour is also absent from contemporary promotional literature. Finally, competition in the market for low-cost health insurance is leading to a process of concentration, which represents a challenge to the smaller non-profit organisations that remain in the sector. It seems that there are also ambiguities in government's own attitude to the schemes, despite its willingness to explore new forms of service organisation.

Parallels and precedents

Do the schemes offer lessons for contemporary policy-makers in their search for institutional innovation in the welfare state? There are several reasons why it is worthwhile revisiting them.

The first relates to the purchaser–provider split introduced into the NHS in 1991: the establishment of the large, multi-hospital funds, disbursing resources to a range of hospitals, invites consideration of whether the schemes were 'purchasers' of health care. Did they play a role in securing a more efficient service or a more rational distribution of resources? And did they empower consumers, giving them genuine choice of hospital? Though superficially appealing, this parallel with the present day is inappropriate. The schemes did not purchase services on behalf of a defined population. Rather, they raised funds which were then handed over to hospitals. The distinction is important because it relates to the status of the schemes: they were not insurers in a conventional sense, charged with securing value for money on behalf of their insured population. In fact, this placed members of schemes associated with individual hospitals at a disadvantage, because they raised money for hospitals yet had little influence on how it was spent. In the multi-hospital schemes, by contrast, there was greater awareness of potential perverse incentives arising from existing methods of reimbursement and efforts were made to develop appropriate procedures. But consumers did not have choice, in the sense now proposed by the Labour government, nor did they have powers of exit – until reciprocal arrangements developed, they were largely tied to a particular hospital and in practice most could exert only limited influence on hospital policy.

A second possible parallel with present-day concerns relates to the theme of partnership, which is such a pervasive feature of contemporary social policy. The schemes were involved in partnership activities in two senses: they helped foster integration of health care provision through inter-organisational partnerships, and they sought to foster links between workers and employers to facilitate recruitment and fundraising, so that they were said to cut across social divisions. How extensive and successful were such partnerships? There is certainly evidence of the role of the schemes in integrating service provision, in terms of pragmatic efforts to develop links with municipal institutions and reciprocal arrangements with other schemes, but these were certainly not ubiquitous and in some circumstances there was open hostility between schemes. However, there is more variable evidence of partnerships with employers: extensive community and workplace support was not always matched by employer commitment. Thus, in the pre-war era, the success of partnership arrangements depended (as it does today) on the availability and willingness of partners. Importantly, where such arrangements did not exist, nothing could be done to ensure that they were brought into being; employers could continue to lag behind their progressive competitors and schemes could continue to ignore calls for cooperation and reciprocity.

Finally, do the ethos and social purpose of the contributory schemes have lessons for contemporary policy-makers? When advocates of the voluntary sector speak of 'taking the risk of under-government' they mean that the beneficial features of voluntarism outweigh deficiencies such as lack of com-prehensiveness.[1] Though some schemes retain structures to facilitate input into governance (chapter 10), extensive voluntary participation is much less in evidence than in the pre-war period. It is therefore difficult to see that the surviving HCPs could provide a basis for the preservation of a sense of social solidarity as suggested by Green.[2] Some thirty years ago the BHCSA acknowledged that individuals approached the schemes from the perspective of self-interest rather than being motivated by a desire to help their fellow citizens. There is little reason to suppose, from contemporary marketing material, that this situation has changed. Moreover, when a dominant feature of public policy is the use of individual consumerism and choice as a means of incentivising inefficient providers of health care, there is little reason to expect that it will.

Nevertheless, government ministers still evoke the pre-NHS era as one in which there was genuine community control of hospital governance (see chapter 1). Three reflections are apposite here. First, while many people joined hospital contributory schemes this did not necessarily signal a desire to become involved in hospital governance; rather, it was a pragmatic decision to secure some measure of coverage against the costs of hospital treatment. Genuine participation was limited to small numbers of scheme activists, who are unlikely to have been totally representative of the communities served by hospitals. Commitment to wider ideals may also have been short-lived, as is illustrated by the transformation of the HSA's magazine, *The Contributor*, into a family and lifestyle publication (in response to subscribers who wished for more entertaining fare than the staple diet of reports of organisational development) (see chapter 5). The low levels of turnout in the first wave of elections for the new NHS Foundation Trusts, and the possibility that involvement will be subject to the same social imbalances as other forms of participation, indicate that achieving greater public participation is not straightforward and that policy-makers need to think hard about how to engage citizens in hospital governance.[3] Second, the schemes' experience was that representation did not necessarily lead to influence in decision-making, and it is unclear whether the Foundation Trust membership constituencies will actually be able to shape policy. If this form of participation proves to be purely tokenistic, the result may be still greater disillusionment and apathy. Finally, if Labour politicians had the contributory schemes in mind when they advocated Foundation Trusts, they should be aware that the schemes were not an exemplar of Labour's traditions and roots. The schemes were not aligned with any one party and they sought to preserve a studied neutrality. If there was a dominant tradition in Labour thinking in the 1930s, it was in favour of a local government health service. The presentation of Foundation Trusts as the revival of an old Labour tradition is therefore somewhat disingenuous.

Advantages relating to participation and ethos must be set against dimensions such as comprehensiveness and equity, and here the pre-1948 schemes must be found wanting. It might be argued that this is to judge the schemes by post-war collectivist standards, but perceptions of inequalities in access to health services also featured increasingly strongly in public discourse during the 1930s. Once proposals for a genuinely national health service began to develop, the diversity and variability in the coverage of the schemes was a problem for officials concerned with ensuring universal availability of services. Compulsory membership would destroy the voluntary character of the schemes but without compulsion they could not be comprehensive. Only if the health service were underwritten by comprehensive tax funding could the problems of maldistribution be avoided and it is to proposals for a reconstruction of the funding of health care that the final section turns.

Prospects

How might the schemes develop in the future? One scenario is that steady growth in NHS resources is accompanied by parallel growth in the purchasing of cash plans, by individuals and companies, on the back of rising prosperity and tight labour markets. An alternative is that a reconstruction of the NHS along social insurance lines gives a major boost to the surviving HCPs since it would require everyone to purchase an insurance policy of some kind and there would be considerable scope for product differentiation. At the moment, however, this is being canvassed only by the more fervid free-market think-tanks, though the Liberal Democrats have flirted with the idea.[4] Somewhere in between these scenarios are proposals for a substantial expansion of charging for NHS services, possibly through the introduction of an NHS 'core' package of free services and a fee-for-service or insurance-based package of supplementary services.[5] Depending on the nature of the proposals there would be more or less scope for greater inequality in access (the precise effect would depend on the technical features of specific reform proposals).

All of these scenarios would achieve greater take-up of the products offered by the HCPs. The bigger question is whether the resultant increase in take-up would also achieve the promotion of social solidarity, as is often claimed by those advocating organisational reform in the welfare state. For example, Hirst suggested that the welfare state could be pluralised and democratised by a system in which – in the case of health care – the equivalent of vouchers for the purchasing of services (based on weighted per capita spending) would in effect be handed over to individuals rather than being allocated centrally. He hoped that the public would govern how those funds were spent, through active participation in local health purchasing agencies.[6] Similar proposals have emanated from think-tanks such as Civitas.[7] People would join insurers of their choice and the power of exit would, it is argued, guarantee responsiveness. Hirst also argued that such a system would promote participation, since individuals could band together, using their funds to create services responsive to particular needs. Individuals who wished for more than the basic minimum provided through public funds would have the option of purchasing services privately. Likewise, Saunders suggested that privatised welfare offered scope for 'new and active forms of citizenship based on individual competence and the development of genuinely collective forms of association and sociability springing up from below'.[8] Is this true of the cash plans and might it be true in the future? The pre-war schemes did, for a while, offer significant scope for engagement in the governance and financing of health care, though direct effects on hospital policy are hard to identify (chapter 6) and the majority of scheme members were largely passive. And it is not clear that the voluntary effort in support of a collective goal which sustained the schemes in the 1930s can be rekindled easily, given the present-day stress on individual choice. The appeal of the cash plans rests largely on individual self-interest (in terms of assistance with the costs of accessing treatments not otherwise easily available) and so, to paraphrase Hirst, it is not clear how 'associationalist' they are.

For all the rhetoric about participation, the dominant direction of most proposals for reform of the NHS is towards greater use of choice and markets to promote the restructuring of services. A clue to the underlying economic motivation is provided by Civitas, which argues that consumers in the health sector will be truly empowered only if they are able to inflict real economic pain on providers of services (an argument to which the present government appears to subscribe with its emphasis on competition).[9] This is underpinned by a rational choice model of individual behaviour, in which deliberative self-interest is the key motivation, rather than any notion of the public good.[10] According to Taylor-Gooby, this may weaken altruism, stifle intrinsic motivation and exhaust citizenship, with the result that public services will decline in efficiency and support for them will be eroded.[11] Proposals for an extension of choice in the NHS, and the suggestions from conservative think-tanks for an expansion of co-payments, all operate within an individualistic frame of reference. This is an unpromising context in which to make the case for a revived mutualism in health care. In fact, the notion of mutualism is itself threatened by these broader social changes and by recent changes in the regulatory environment in which the HCPs operate (chapter 10). There have already been indications that the entry of for-profit providers is causing problems for the remaining not-for-profit HCPs. It would be ironic if the fate of smaller not-for-profits was put at risk not by nationalisation in 1948, but by a Labour government that has funded the NHS at unprecedented levels and proclaimed its commitment to new forms of ownership and control in the welfare state, while simultaneously pursuing pro-market policies with some vigour.

The history recounted here has testified to our predecessors' search for a form of health services funding which simultaneously succeeded in raising substantial resources, satisfying individual needs and extending community involvement in welfare. Ultimately, the reach of the contributory scheme movement exceeded its grasp, but the conundrum of reconciling efficiency, fairness and democracy remains a core dilemma for health policy. If anything, this challenge is made more difficult in an age of affluence, individualism and economic liberalisation, which limits the ability of not-for-profit organisations to adhere to their traditional role in the face of pressures from commercial competitors. The challenge for the future is to devise a health policy which successfully combines the strengths of public funding with the democratic and participatory ideals which characterised the British hospital contributory scheme movement.

Notes

1   D. Green, *Rediscovering civil society: the rediscovery of welfare without politics* (London, 1993), p. 20.

2   D. Green, 'From national health monopoly to national health guarantee', in D. Gladstone (ed.), *How to pay for health care: public and private alternatives* (London, 1997), p. 30–56, at p. 56.

3   R. Klein, 'Editorial: the first wave of NHS Foundation Trusts', *British Medical Journal*, 328 (2004), p. 1332; P. Day and R. Klein *Governance of Foundation Trusts: dilemmas of diversity* (London, 2005)

4   For example, the think-tank Reform established a Commission on the Reform of Public Services that produced a report entitled *A better way* (London, 2003) (available online at www.reform.co.uk/website/publications/commissiononthereformofpublicservices.aspx, last accessed February 2006); on the Liberal Democrats' proposals, see the *Guardian* website (http://politics.guardian.co.uk/libdems/story/0,9061,1275582,00.html, last accessed February 2006).

5   M. Goldsmith and D. Gladstone, *Road map to reform: health* (London, 2005).

6   P. Hirst, *Associative democracy* (Cambridge, 1994).

7   Civitas, *A new consensus for NHS reform: summary* (available online at www.civitas.org.uk/pdf/hpcgFinalFactsheet.pdf, last accessed February 2006).

8   P. Saunders, 'Citizenship in a liberal society', in B. Turner (ed.), *Citizenship and social theory* (London, 1993), quoted in I. Culpitt, *Social policy and risk* (London, 1999), p. 80.

9   Civitas, 'New consensus'.

10 C. Needham, *Citizen-consumers: New Labour's marketplace democracy* (London, 2003); S. Ruane, 'The future of health care in the UK: think tanks and their policy prescriptions', in M. Powell, K. Clarke and L. Bauld (eds), *Social policy review 17* (London, 2005), pp. 147–66.

11 P. Taylor-Gooby, 'Introduction', in P. Taylor-Gooby (ed.), *Risk, trust and welfare* (London, 2000), p. 13.

Index